Motivational
Interviewing

MOTIVATIONAL INTERVIEWING
A GUIDE FOR MEDICAL TRAINEES

Edited by
Antoine Douaihy, Thomas M. Kelly,
and Melanie A. Gold

Associate Editor
Joshua T. Morra

Foreword by
William R. Miller and Stephen Rollnick

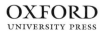

OXFORD
UNIVERSITY PRESS

OXFORD
UNIVERSITY PRESS

Oxford University Press is a department of the University of Oxford.
It furthers the University's objective of excellence in research, scholarship,
and education by publishing worldwide.

Oxford   New York

Auckland   Cape Town   Dar es Salaam   Hong Kong   Karachi
Kuala Lumpur   Madrid   Melbourne   Mexico City   Nairobi
New Delhi   Shanghai   Taipei   Toronto

With offices in

Argentina   Austria   Brazil   Chile   Czech Republic   France   Greece
Guatemala   Hungary   Italy   Japan   Poland   Portugal   Singapore
South Korea   Switzerland   Thailand   Turkey   Ukraine   Vietnam

Oxford is a registered trademark of Oxford University Press
in the UK and certain other countries.

Published in the United States of America by
Oxford University Press
198 Madison Avenue, New York, NY 10016

Library of Congress Cataloging-in-Publication Data

Motivational interviewing : a guide for medical trainees / edited by
Antoine Douaihy, Thomas M. Kelly, and Melanie A. Gold.
    p. ; cm.
Includes bibliographical references and index.
ISBN 978–0–19–995818–4 (alk. paper)
I. Douaihy, Antoine B., 1965– editor.   II. Kelly, Thomas M., 1951–
editor.   III. Gold, Melanie A. (Melanie Ariane), editor.
[DNLM: 1. Motivational Interviewing. WM 55]
R690
610.69—dc23
2014004069

9 8 7 6 5 4 3 2 1
Printed in the United States of America
on acid-free paper

To my patients and trainees, who are my inspiration

—AD

To my parents, brother, sisters, and Jeanine, my life past and present

—TMK

To my patients and trainees, who never cease to amaze me by their resilience and resourcefulness

—MAG

If you talk to a man in a language he understands, that goes to his head. If you talk to him in his language, that goes to his heart.

Nelson Mandela

Contents

Foreword

Medical training involves the assimilation of enormous amounts of information and a strong expectation to always know the right answer. Perhaps it should not be surprising, then, that after medical training it is common practice, when talking to patients, to continue this pattern by dispensing information and providing answers. In acute care medicine this can work: Ask the relevant questions and go down a decision tree to find the right remedy.

This professional expertise model tends to fail, however, when what is needed is a change in patients' behavior and lifestyle. The truth is that we are not experts on our patients' lives—they are—and a lack of knowledge is seldom the most important obstacle to health behavior change. What smoker these days does not already know the health risks of smoking?

We developed motivational interviewing (MI) as an alternative to simply dispensing unwanted information and advice. The evidence base for the efficacy of MI is large and growing rapidly, spanning a broad range of health problems that practitioners encounter regularly. A cutting-edge question now is how best to incorporate MI into medical training and practice. As with patients, dispensing information to health care professionals *about* MI is unlikely to change practice. A single unit on MI early in medical training is quickly overshadowed by what follows.

In this volume, participants in the process of medical training reflect on how they learn, practice, and continue to develop their skills in MI. It speaks specifically to those in training for the practice of medicine. In the spirit of MI it is a truly collaborative effort, reflecting the experience of trainees as well as trainers. For aspiring physicians it offers guidance on how MI can help to lift the burden of chronic disease for both patients and practitioners. It speaks to the heart of medical care: the doctor–patient relationship. May it speak to you as your journey into heath care unfolds.

William R. Miller, PhD
The University of New Mexico

Stephen Rollnick, PhD
Cardiff University

Preface

We, the Editors, wanted to compile a different kind of book about motivational interviewing (MI)—one designed specifically for aspiring physicians. Thus, our intended reader is among the growing number of medical trainees who wish to integrate MI into their medical practice. That said, we believe the content is relevant for psychotherapists, counselors, and practitioners in other health-related fields, and we hope that they too find this book helpful. Our primary objective is to demonstrate how MI can improve the doctor–patient relationship. Our second objective is to provide evidence of the tremendous potential MI has for helping patients change unhealthy behaviors, a task that is central to reducing the epidemic of chronic disease unfolding in our society today.

We applaud our trainees, first, for having recognized that something was missing from their encounters with their patients, and second, for their courage and determination in acquiring and using MI spirit, skills, and strategies to fill that gap. We wish you, the reader, every success as you begin your journey toward helping your patients achieve and sustain meaningful behavior change.

We, the Medical Trainees, have rigorous schedules, an overwhelming amount of information to learn, and very little time in which to accomplish a seemingly endless list of tasks. The Editors of this book believe that trainees who are able to acquire MI skills while in the midst of medical training have a unique perspective based on long-standing experience in learning, practicing, and above all, integrating MI into their medical education. The Editors recruited us—their former and current trainees—to share our experiences and to demonstrate the myriad ways in which MI enriches our encounters with patients. Recognizing the broad applicability of MI across many fields in medicine, our Editors invited a diverse group of specialist trainees from emergency medicine, family medicine, internal medicine, neurology, pediatrics, and psychiatry to contribute to this project.

In a truly collaborative effort, we have been involved in every step of creating this book: from brainstorming the concept and format, to writing the chapters, producing the videos clips, and reviewing the final galley proofs. Throughout this process, our aim has been to produce a practical guide to learning and incorporating the MI approach in patient care. We firmly believe that having good supervision, in-vivo coaching, and modeling are fundamental to learning and practicing MI, and our book facilitates this process. Our guide does not require you to have read William R. Miller and Stephen Rollnick's books on MI (1991, 2002, and 2013) in order to understand and apply the concepts and skills discussed in this book. Should you wish to strengthen your understanding and learning more about MI, we recommend that you turn to *Motivational Interviewing: Helping People Change* (3rd ed.).

Motivational Interviewing: A Guide for Medical Trainees covers the fundamental concepts, skills, and techniques of MI. It also focuses on specific applications of MI in medical settings and diverse populations. The chapters do not follow the tradition of including scientific citations in the narrative; our view is that doing so would interfere with the flow of the text. Instead, we focused on consolidating and summarizing research findings. Throughout this guide, we have used "trainee" as generic for trainees from all medical specialties and levels of training in the U.S. and the United Kingdom (medical students, residents, and fellows; "final med", "intern," "Senior House Officer," and "registrar") who provide patient care. A detailed list of references and resources may be found at the end of the book. As physicians-in-training, we identified several key features that we believe make this guide particularly useful for you:

- High-yield, practical, and concise guide
- Diverse case examples from our clinical encounters across many medical disciplines
- Figures, tables, key points, and helpful tips
- Videos clips
- Personal reflections from trainees
- Self-assessment quizzes designed to support the learning process
- Quick guide to MI
- References and resources

We, the Medical Trainees, believe the collaboration between educators and trainees has produced a unique guide. Of course, we do not find this particularly surprising, as collaboration and partnering are central to the success of the MI approach. As you'll soon learn, building self-efficacy and empowering your patients is another key to effecting successful behavior change; similarly, our teachers and mentors have helped us change how we interact with our patients. Together, we extend this book to you in the true sense of the collaborative spirit of MI. This guide will not only teach you the concepts and skills of MI, but it will empower you, as a physician trainee, to find the most effective ways of integrating MI into your training—and eventually into your medical practice.

Acknowledgments

First of all, I want to express my gratitude and appreciation to my coeditors and collaborators Thomas Kelly, Melanie Gold, and Joshua Morra and all contributors for their work, encouragement, guidance, and wisdom in helping shape and refine this project. I have been privileged to learn and contribute to the learning experience of medical trainees who have provided me intellectual engagement and inspiration. I am also deeply indebted to my patients of diverse backgrounds, whose sharing of their struggles with me has significantly strengthened my appreciation of suffering. A special word of appreciation goes to Dennis Daley. As a mentor, collaborator, and friend, Dennis has played a major role in the development of my personal and professional identity. I wish to acknowledge my indebtedness to my former mentors, Paula Trief, Tony Vinciquerra, and Ihsan Salloum, for their commitment to my professional development. This book was made possible because of the work and influence of many pioneers of motivational interviewing who developed and researched the practical approaches in this guide, including Bill Miller, Stephen Rollnick, Terri Moyers, and many others. In the preparation of this work, the members of the Motivational Interviewing Network of Trainers (MINT) have contributed tremendously to systematically consolidating my perspectives and publishing them. My appreciation goes to my great MINT colleagues Fran Dannenberg and Steve Feinstein. Warm thanks are also due to Allan Zuckoff for his support in building my clinical experience and training in motivational interviewing. I also thank Janis McDonald for her attention to detail and all the work she did in helping to organize and edit the manuscript. Many people have supported me, in one way or another, in the writing of the book, and I owe special thanks, particularly to Cindy Hurney and Kimberly Smith. Kimberly Smith was invaluable in providing crucial editorial input to assure organization and clarity of the text. Also, special acknowledgement goes to Steve Martino for his review of the manuscript and invaluable feedback. Finally, this manuscript could not have been completed without the help and wonderful support of Craig Allen Panner and Christopher Reid of Oxford University Press. The preparation of this manuscript was supported in part by NIDA's Clinical Trials Network, Appalachian Tri-State Node, grant 5U10DA020036-08.

Antoine Douaihy

First, I acknowledge my coeditors, Antoine Douaihy and Melanie Gold. This work was created because of Antoine's vision of its significance for the field, and I thank him for persuading me of its importance. Melanie's breadth and depth of experience brought an enlightened perspective to every chapter. Second, the group of trainees involved in writing this volume provided most of the inspiration for its content and worked continuously despite heavy workloads associated with their status as medical students and resident physicians. A subgroup of them provided exceptional creativity and technical expertise in creating the illustrations and videos.

I want to thank Dennis Daley for mentoring me and for the ongoing support he has provided me as a faculty member, clinician, and as a specialist in applied addiction research. John E. Donovan was also instrumental in my postdoctoral training as a clinician-researcher. My early training in individual and family therapy was critical because I was taught by an outstanding group of clinicians, especially Tom Saunders. Later, at Western Psychiatric Institute and Clinic, Carol Anderson helped me to recognize the overarching influence of the family system as a model for diagnosing and addressing problems in family therapy. The late William Cohen widened my knowledge of psychotherapy. Under his tutelage I came to recognize that each patient, or family, requires both a treatment plan and an individualized, therapeutic strategy. Paul Soloff helped me to understand the critical integration of intrapsychic and interpersonal dynamics that exist in the treatment of all patients.

These are the influences that I try to combine with the relational style that is the core of motivational interviewing. I have learned that a strong therapeutic alliance provides the best opportunity for treating psychological and behavioral maladies, and that motivational interviewing is the best way to establish such an alliance. My hope is that the perspectives expressed in this volume will stimulate medical trainees to integrate the content of their medical training with William Miller's and Stephen Rollnick's invaluable process for establishing truly therapeutic relationships.

Thomas M. Kelly

Editing a book is never a solitary effort. This guide would have been impossible without the hard work, support, and collaboration of my two amazing coeditors and colleagues, Antoine Douaihy and Thomas Kelly. This guide was inspired by *and* written by medical trainees, including medical students, residents, and fellows in various fields of medicine. Their collaboration on this guide makes it a true reflection of the "MI spirit." First and foremost, thanks go to my mother, Rona Beth Fisher of Albuquerque, New Mexico, who taught me from the time I could speak, the importance of listening to language, of communication skills, of respect for people and their different perspectives, and of all the other key aspects of MI.

It was not until my early years as a faculty person in 1998, when I realized that what my mother had taught me was called MI. I also must thank my friend, colleague, and co-investigator, Allan Zuckoff, who taught me MI and provided me with the numerous hours of one-on-one supervision when I was first learning. Allan was a demanding supervisor, and I benefited from his expertise and skill. Allan was also the co-investigator who helped me train and supervise my staff for my NIH R01, using MI to help female adolescents prevent unintended pregnancy and STDs.

Finally, over the last 3 years, I had the honor of receiving supervision again from Allan when I was a telephone interventionist for Mary Amanda Dew, for her study on MI and decision making around organ transplant donation. There is no one who has taught me more about MI than Allan. I would also like to express my appreciation to Bill Miller and Terri Moyers for many years of support in learning and doing research on MI, and especially to Bill Miller and Stephen Rollnick for reviewing this guide and for agreeing to write the foreword for it. Others I wish to acknowledge, who played critical roles in my learning to use, teach, and study MI include Carlo DiClemente, Christopher

Ryan, and Bill Cohen. Each one played a unique and important role in my development. Finally, I wish to thank all the numerous patients, medical students, residents, fellows, as well as my research and clinical staff from whom I always learned new ways to listen and reflect, thus enhancing both the quality of my MI skill and my interpersonal relationships. Special thanks also go to Nasuh Malas, for his groundbreaking work on integrating MI into pediatric residency training, to my co-trainers Dana Rofey and Anne Marie Kuchera, and to Dena Hofkosh, for supporting Nasuh's passion for integrating MI into the pediatric residency program at the Children's Hospital of Pittsburgh.

Melanie A. Gold

About the Editors

Antoine Douaihy, MD, is an associate professor of psychiatry at the University of Pittsburgh School of Medicine. He also serves as the medical director of Addiction Medicine Services and director of the Addiction Psychiatry Fellowship at the Western Psychiatric Institute and Clinic of the University of Pittsburgh Medical Center. Throughout his career he has been actively involved in patient care, teaching, and mentoring medical trainees. Dr. Douaihy has been a member of the *Motivational Interviewing Network of Trainers (MINT)* since 2002. Dr. Douaihy is also a co-editor of the Practice section of the journal Motivational Interviewing: Treatment, Research, Integration, Practice (MITRIP), a MINT online publication. He has focused his career on patient care, education, training, and research in the areas of motivational interviewing, substance use disorders, and HIV/AIDS. In recognition for his dedication to education and training, Dr. Douaihy has been the recipient of multiple teaching awards, including the Leonard Tow Humanism in Medicine Award and The Charles Watson Teaching Award, recognizing him for the qualities of a masterful clinician, academician, caretaker of his patients, educator, mentor, and contributor to the medical school community and community at large.

Thomas M. Kelly, PhD, is an associate professor of psychiatry at the University of Pittsburgh School of Medicine. He is a licensed clinical social worker who has been in practice at the Western Psychiatric Institute and Clinic and the University of Pittsburgh Medical Center since 1982. Dr. Kelly received his doctoral degree in social work from the University of Pittsburgh and is currently the director of the Adolescent Substance Abuse Treatment Service. Dr. Kelly's other work focuses on teaching, consultation, and research. He is a co-investigator with the National Institute on Drug Abuse Clinical Trials Network, and he has over 50 peer-reviewed publications. Dr. Kelly has been a member of the Motivational Interviewing Network of Trainers since 2005, and he routinely conducts training workshops, lectures, and seminars, locally and nationally.

Melanie A. Gold, DO, is a clinical professor in the Department of Pediatrics, Division of Adolescent Medicine at the University of Pittsburgh School of Medicine and in the Department of Behavioral and Community Health Sciences at the Graduate School of Public Health. She is also a staff physician at the University of Pittsburgh Wellness Center's Student Health Service. She is a certified specialist in pediatrics with subspecialty certification in adolescent medicine by the American Board of Pediatrics. Dr. Gold has been a Motivational Interviewing Network Trainer since 2000 and has conducted numerous trainings on motivational interviewing and behavior change counseling for health care professionals across multiple disciplines. Her research interests lie in the areas of adolescent sexuality, contraceptive behaviors, tobacco cessation in adolescents, and motivational interviewing to facilitate health behavior change. Dr. Gold has received funding from the National Institute of Child Health and Human Development to conduct a randomized efficacy trial studying the effectiveness of motivational interviewing for reducing sexual risk-taking behaviors that lead to unintended pregnancy and sexually transmitted diseases among female adolescents. Dr. Gold is the president and founder of Renaissance Research and Educational Consulting, Inc. (RRECI), a consulting firm dedicated to offering health care professionals training, mentoring, and research consultation for a variety of current lifestyle- and health-related issues in order to facilitate the health and well-being of the people they serve.

ASSOCIATE EDITOR

Joshua T. Morra, MD, PhD is a Post Graduate Year II resident physician in the General Psychiatry Program and a candidate for the Psychiatry Research Pathway at the Western Psychiatric Institute and Clinic of the University of Pittsburgh Medical Center. He also actively serves on the American Academy of Addiction Psychiatry (AAAP) Education Committee. Dr. Morra's research and publications have focused on furthering our understanding of addiction neurophysiology through the use of animal models for addiction-related behaviors. During his clinical training, Dr. Morra has developed a special interest in education and motivational interviewing within the field of Addiction Psychiatry. Dr. Morra has been the recipient of multiple national training awards from the AAAP, American Psychological Association (APA), National Institute on Alcohol Abuse and Alcoholism (NIAAA) and National Institute on Drug Abuse (NIDA), including the Ruth L. Kirschstein National Research Service Award, in recognition of his promise as a physician scientist and future leader in the field of Addiction Psychiatry.

Contributors

Carson Adams
University of Pittsburgh
School of Medicine
Pittsburgh, Pennsylvania

Abigail Chua
Department of Medicine
Albert Einstein/Montefiore Medical
    Center
Bronx, New York

Daniel Cohen
Western Psychiatric Institute and Clinic
University of Pittsburgh Medical Center
Pittsburgh, Pennsylvania

Colby Croft
Department of Psychiatry
University of California at San Francisco
San Francisco, California

Byron Doepker
Family Medicine
Group Health Cooperative
Seattle, Washington

Antoine Douaihy
Western Psychiatric Institute and Clinic
Addiction Medicine Services
Addiction Psychiatry Fellowship
Psychiatry Residency Training
University of Pittsburgh Medical Center
Pittsburgh, Pennsylvania

Patrick Henry C. Driscoll
Western Psychiatric Institute and Clinic
University of Pittsburgh Medical Center
Pittsburgh, Pennsylvania

Sarah Faeder
Western Psychiatric Institute and Clinic
University of Pittsburgh Medical Center
Pittsburgh, Pennsylvania

Inti Flores
Department of Psychiatry
University of California at San Francisco
San Francisco, California

Melanie A. Gold
Division of Adolescent Medicine
University of Pittsburgh School of
    Medicine
Graduate School of Public Health
University of Pittsburgh
    Staff Physician
University of Pittsburgh Student Health
    Services, Wellness Center
Pittsburgh, Pennsylvania

Rachel Grubbs
Lake Erie College of Osteopathic
    Medicine
Erie, Pennsylvania

Aaron M. Gusdon
Department of Neurology and
    Neuroscience
Weill Medical College of Cornell
    University
New York-Presbyterian Hospital
New York, New York

Lindsay Hintz
Department of Medicine
Beth Israel Deaconess Medical Center
Boston, Massachusetts

Thomas M. Kelly
Western Psychiatric Institute
  and Clinic
Adolescent Substance Abuse
  Program
Addiction Medicine Services
University of Pittsburgh
  Medical Center
Pittsburgh, Pennsylvania

Adam W. Kowalsky
University of Pittsburgh School of
  Medicine
Pittsburgh, Pennsylvania

Erik Loraas
Western Psychiatric Institute
  and Clinic
University of Pittsburgh
  Medical Center
Pittsburgh, Pennsylvania

Annie Lu
University of Pittsburgh School of
  Medicine
Pittsburgh, Pennsylvania

Wynne Lundblad
Western Psychiatric Institute
  and Clinic
University of Pittsburgh
  Medical Center
Pittsburgh, Pennsylvania

Nasuh Malas
Western Psychiatric Institute
  and Clinic
Children's Hospital of Pittsburgh
University of Pittsburgh Medical
  Center
Pittsburgh, Pennsylvania

Benjamin S. Mantell
Cincinnati Children's Hospital Medical
  Center
Cincinnati, Ohio

Ryan T. Marino
University of Pittsburgh School of
  Medicine
Pittsburgh, Pennsylvania

Joshua Morra
Western Psychiatric Institute
  and Clinic
University of Pittsburgh
  Medical Center
Pittsburgh, Pennsylvania

Seán Naughton
Mater Misericordiae University
  Hospital
Dublin, Ireland

Jane S. Phelps-Tschang
University of Pittsburgh School of
  Medicine
Pittsburgh, Pennsylvania

Zeina Saliba
Department of Obstetrics &
  Gynecology
George Washington University
Washington, DC; Medical College of
  Virginia
Richmond, VA
VCU School of Medicine
Inova Fairfax Campus
Falls Church, VA
Consultant Psychiatrist and Family
  Medicine Physician
HealthWorks for Northern Virginia
Leesburg & Hendon, VA

Erin Smith
Western Psychiatric Institute
  and Clinic
University of Pittsburgh Medical
  Center
Pittsburgh, Pennsylvania

Kimberly Smith
Independent editor and writer
Vancouver, British Columbia, Canada

Loren Sobel
Western Psychiatric Institute
  and Clinic
University of Pittsburgh Medical
  Center
Pittsburgh, Pennsylvania

Robin Valpey
Western Psychiatric Institute and Clinic
University of Pittsburgh Medical Center
Pittsburgh, Pennsylvania

Peter Veldkamp
Pittsburgh AIDS Center for Treatment
Division of Infectious Diseases
Department of Medicine
University of Pittsburgh Medical Center
Pittsburgh, Pennsylvania

Teresa Walker
Western Psychiatric Institute and Clinic
University of Pittsburgh Medical Center
Pittsburgh, Pennsylvania

Niketa Williams
University of Pittsburgh School of
    Medicine
Pittsburgh, Pennsylvania

Motivational Interviewing

1 Why Include Motivational Interviewing in Medical Training?

Take yourself back to the early days of your medical training, when you were an inexperienced student starting your first clinical rotation. Perhaps you arrived on the ward in a crisp white coat, feeling enthusiastic after an inspiring pre-clerkship pep talk that contained the obligatory reference to the "art and science" of medicine. It probably didn't take very long—just a matter of hours—before you observed that in the real world of medicine, many physicians practice the art of our profession with astonishing clumsiness, even as they pursue the scientific aspects with skill and determination. Here's an example typical of this ineffective approach:

PHYSICIAN: The best way to control the pain in your legs is to have better control of your diabetes. You need to start eating better and losing some weight.

PATIENT: Yeah, I know. It's just that when I get stressed, like at work recently, I get home at the end of the day and I want comfort food to feel good, like a hamburger or mac and cheese. I know it's not healthy, but it makes me feel better.

PHYSICIAN: Comfort food? "Comfort food" is just another excuse to eat unhealthy food.

It doesn't take great emotional sensitivity to recognize that this conversation was frustrating and unproductive for both physician and patient. However, while most trainees can confidently identify what they would *not* have said had they been in this physician's shoes, it is significantly more challenging to come up with what one *would* have said to effectively help this patient change her eating behaviors. As trainees, we all aspire to become as skilled in the art of medicine as we are in the science of it. In order to achieve this balance, we must be able to have productive conversations with our patients, first by eliciting and actively listening to their concerns, and secondly, by effectively communicating information and making recommendations. Remember that one of our primary goals as trainees is to help our patients implement whatever behavior changes will best serve *their* health needs, not ours.

Unfortunately, few medical programs offer a formal curriculum devoted to communication skills. Presumably we will absorb these skills along the way, learning through a patchwork approach of observation, trial, and inevitable error. Without proper guidance and supervision, most of us will adopt an approach characterized by authoritarian, confrontational, or guilt-inducing qualities. Clear evidence demonstrates that such an approach will compromise relationships with our patients and ultimately will contribute to negative behavioral and clinical outcomes. Our role as effective healthcare practitioners must include an understanding of the interpersonal skills required to motivate patients to move toward optimal health. In this regard, we find motivational interviewing (MI) incredibly valuable.

WHAT IS MOTIVATIONAL INTERVIEWING?

MI is an egalitarian and empathic "clinical way of being" with a patient. MI is a therapeutic conversation that employs a guiding style of communication geared toward enhancing behavior change and improving health status outcomes.

The book *Motivational Interviewing: Helping People Change* (3rd ed., Pg 29) offers the following definitions of MI for laypersons and practitioners, along with a more technical definition. MI is:

1. "A collaborative conversation style for strengthening a person's own motivation and commitment to change." (pg. 12)
2. "A person-centered counseling style for addressing the common problems of ambivalence about change." (pg. 24)
3. "A collaborative, goal-oriented style of communication with particular attention to the language of change. It is designed to strengthen personal motivation for, and commitment to, a specific goal by eliciting and exploring the person's own reasons for change within an atmosphere of acceptance and compassion." (pg. 29)

THE ORIGINS OF MOTIVATIONAL INTERVIEWING: FILLING A NEED

Psychologist Dr. William R. Miller stated that developing MI was completely unplanned and unanticipated. It originated initially from an inspiration which came from his own data, whereby he noted that accurate empathy is the therapist skill that best predicts patient reductions in alcohol use. Leaving on a sabbatical from the University of New Mexico, Dr. Miller started working in an alcoholism clinic in Norway lecturing on cognitive-behavioral treatment and teaching a group of Norwegian psychologists about reflective listening through role playing with patients and discussing challenging clinical situations. These experiences helped Miller conceptualize some clinical principles and decision rules. This is how "motivational interviewing" emerged. Miller reasoned that direct argumentation was an ineffective way to change someone else's behavior. Instead, he focused on the principle that any person is more likely to be committed to a position that he or she defends verbally. He pointed out that the patient, not the counselor, argues for change. The MI approach is designed to evoke these arguments. Miller's first description of MI was published in 1983 in the British journal *Behavioural Psychotherapy*. In the period after, Miller began doing research and evaluating the approach. Seven years later, he met Dr. Stephen Rollnick in Australia, who had been teaching motivational interviewing in addiction treatment programs in the United Kingdom. In collaboration with Rollnick, he wrote a more detailed description of MI and its associated clinical processes in the book *Motivational Interviewing: Preparing People to Change Addictive Behavior*, first published in 1991.

THEORETICAL UNDERPINNINGS AND ASSOCIATED MODELS

As mentioned earlier, while on sabbatical in Bergen, Norway (1982), Miller began to formulate his initial clinical description of MI. As opposed to being fundamentally grounded in psychological theory, the concept itself arose from intuitive clinical experience. Nevertheless, Miller drew upon several prevailing theories in his descriptions of MI, including the following:

- Festinger's formulation of cognitive dissonance: that when faced with an internal contradiction, we tend to change our thoughts and beliefs in order to resolve the conflict

> ### KEY POINT
> *Leon Festinger* – Cognitive Dissonance: When faced with internal conflict, we tend to change our thinking.

- Bem's reformulation of self-perception theory: that just as we are influenced by our observations of our own behaviors, so too are we influenced by what we ourselves say aloud

> ### KEY POINT
> *Daryl Bem* – Self Perception Theory: People infer their values from their own behaviors and words.

- Bandura's self-efficacy theory: that the stronger an individual believes he or she will succeed in performing a given task, the more likely he or she will attempt to finish that task

> ### KEY POINT
> *Albert Bandura* – Self-Efficacy Theory: Strong belief in one's ability increases the probability of attempting that behavior.

MI follows Carl Rogers' person-centered approach to therapy that is based upon building empathy, congruence, and the positive regard "necessary and sufficient [to establish] interpersonal conditions [which foster] discussion about behavior change." (Rogers, C.R., 1957)

> ### KEY POINT
> *Carl Rogers* inspired MI with his person-centered approach, based on empathy, congruence, and positive regard.

However, unlike classic Rogerian therapy, MI is more goal driven and directional, meaning that there is a clear, positive behavioral outcome.

More recently, self-determination theory (SDT) has been identified as a de facto model for understanding why and how MI works. SDT postulates that all behaviors may be understood as occurring along a continuum ranging from external regulation to true autonomous or self-regulation. Both SDT and MI view the concept of motivation as theoretically central to each model and emphasize the importance of patients developing "intrinsic" motives in addition to assuming responsibility for change. Another similarity is that both models are person-centered and endorse engaging with patients in a safe atmosphere of genuine empathy and unconditional positive regard as a prerequisite for the success of behavioral interventions. SDT emphasizes the core needs of autonomy, competence, and relatedness as relevant to motivating behavior change. Likewise, autonomy support is central to MI and is promoted though reflective listening, eliciting the patient's perspectives and values, providing a menu of choices, and the marked lack of persuasion throughout a clinical encounter. Clearly, many of the tenets of SDT provide a theoretical framework to guide an MI approach, and in many ways, MI may be considered as "the interventional method of SDT."

> KEY POINT
>
> *Self-Determination Theory* – A theoretical construct for why MI works; patients need to take responsibility for change.

FOSTERING CONSTRUCTIVE PATIENT–DOCTOR RELATIONSHIPS

Miller's model of MI stands in contrast to more conventional models of counseling that involve a directive manner that may seem rather controlling. This style often leads to increased resistance to change and may foster patient passivity. Instead, MI focuses on responding to patients with an empathetic, patient-centered tone that is supportive rather than argumentative and that leads to improved patient–doctor relationships with superior outcomes. Miller's conception of MI devotes special attention to evoking and strengthening a patient's intrinsic and expressed motivations for change. Throughout his years of counseling patients while simultaneously formulating MI, Miller found that arguing against resistance is particularly counterproductive; instead, asking patients to articulate their own motivations for change is much more effective than counselors attempting to do the same. MI prioritizes individual responsibility and operates under the assumption that patients are able to make responsible decisions that will lead to desired outcomes. MI also focuses on internal attribution and espouses that placing responsibility for change on the individual patient rather than on external factors leads to more positive outcomes.

BEHAVIOR CHANGE IN HEALTH CARE SETTINGS: WHY WE SHOULD CARE AND HOW MOTIVATIONAL INTERVIEWING HELPS US

Most medical careers will be spent dealing primarily with chronic illnesses (Table 1.1). Chronic disease now accounts for 70% of deaths in the U.S., consumes some 75% of healthcare spending, and represents the leading cause of disability. Almost half of the U.S. population has at least one major chronic illness. How can a nation that spends so much on healthcare be so unhealthy?

Table 1.1 Preventable Morbidity and Mortality

70	Percent of deaths in the U.S. caused by chronic illness
75	Percent of U.S. healthcare spending on chronic illness
4	Modifiable risk factors that could prevent 80% of chronic illness: lack of physical activity, poor diet, tobacco use, and excessive alcohol use
50	Percent of medications for chronic illness not taken as prescribed
30	Percent of chronic illness prescriptions never filled

The Centers for Disease Control and Prevention (CDC) has identified four modifiable risk factors—lack of physical activity, poor diet, smoking and tobacco use, and excessive alcohol use—that could prevent 80% of all heart disease, stroke, and type 2 diabetes, as well as 40% of all cancers.

As trainees, we spend years in medical training and engage in a tremendous amount of time and effort delivering what we believe will be effective therapies. We read the latest scientific literature concerning the most up-to-date treatment modalities and on the subtle but important differences between complex medications. And yet several studies indicate that approximately 50% of medications prescribed for chronic illness are not taken as indicated. In fact, some 20%–30% of such prescriptions are never even filled. What good are our efforts if they are improperly implemented? Some trainees become bitter in spirit and blame patients. A better response to behavior change is to learn and utilize MI. Far from the haphazard trial-and-error approach by which many of us will learn to "communicate," MI is a deliberate, structured framework designed to make full use of a wide range of effective communication skills. MI guides conversations that truly are more effective in motivating behavior change.

THE EVIDENCE: MOTIVATIONAL INTERVIEWING WORKS

MI is broadly applicable in managing medical conditions in which behavior plays some role. Numerous studies have assessed the effectiveness of MI in comparison with the traditional model of giving advice. MI produced better outcomes in 75% of randomized controlled trials that evaluate parameters such as body mass index, hemoglobin A1C, total cholesterol, systolic blood pressure, cigarette smoking, and blood alcohol concentration (Box 1.1). Psychologists and physicians obtained equal results in about 80% of cases. Even more surprisingly, when MI is used in brief, 15-minute clinical encounters, 64% of studies demonstrated a positive patient outcome. Physicians trained in MI are better able to help patients with type 2 diabetes become motivated to implement behavior change and to better understand the condition and its required treatment. Moreover, MI offers a low-cost intervention within primary care settings that produces meaningful changes in body weight which, if sustained, has the potential to modify the progression to full-blown diabetes. Finally, MI has also been shown to be helpful in patients

---

Box 1.1 Behavioral Targets Ideally Suited to Motivational Interviewing

Body mass index
Hemoglobin A1C, dyslipidemia, hypertension
Tobacco use, alcohol use, illicit drug use
Prescription misuse
Medical follow-up adherence
Dental hygiene
Asthma control

with psychiatric disorders such as anxiety, depression, substance use disorders, and other addictions.

MORE REASONS WHY MOTIVATIONAL INTERVIEWING HELPS

Making Effective Use of Limited Time

On my internal medicine rotation, our team managed a busy and complex inpatient service. Between morning rounds, entering orders, talking with consulting services, discussing plans with social workers, afternoon rounds, writing notes, and formal teaching sessions, there was barely time to sit down for lunch. One of the patients I cared for was Mr. G, a 56-year-old man who had been admitted multiple times over recent months for heart failure exacerbations, each hospitalization having been triggered by cocaine use. This time, he was admitted on a hectic day when we were already running behind schedule, and the last thing I felt compelled to do was sit down and have an in-depth conversation regarding his cocaine use and his motivation to quit. This was an important issue that needed to be addressed at some point, by someone: "But that time is not now, and that someone is not me," I said to myself. However, had I known and been able to make use of the spirit and techniques of MI, I might have optimized how I listened and interacted with Mr. G. I know now that I would have had the confidence to engage him in a brief conversation about his cocaine use; I would have decided that the time to discuss it *was* now, and that the person to do it *was* me.

One of the biggest pressures medical trainees face is time. We are constantly trying to judge how to divide our time fairly and efficiently between the many tasks and people demanding our attention. Many of us believe that time spent speaking with one patient is, in effect, time taken away from other patients, from entering orders and writing notes. At the end of each day, those moments also represent time taken away from our own rest, recreation, and personal lives.

The kind of conversation I hesitated to have with Mr. G has the potential to be time consuming, but I've come to realize that this is not necessarily so. Conversations using MI can be brief *and* meaningful. MI offers both a frame of mind and specific techniques that guide how we listen to patients, what we say, and how we say it, such that even 10–15 minutes has the potential to help patients achieve meaningful change.

We make more effective use of our time by using an MI perspective to understand and decipher what patients actually mean when they engage in *change talk* (speech that favors movement toward change) and *sustain talk* (speech about why they behave in ways that sustain the status quo), and to comprehend and respect each patient's sense of *importance* and *confidence* regarding making change happen.

For example, when Mr. G told me that he had been to "more rehabs than [he could] count in the last few years," it was less important to collect this point as historical information than to recognize his words as an expression of the low confidence he felt in his ability to avoid relapse. In this light, Mr. G's statement is much more than a mere detail in a complex history; instead, it provides valuable insight into where he situates himself along a continuum of changing his drug use behaviors.

Rather than seeking solely to convey medical *knowledge* to patients—for example, in discussing with Mr. G the dangers of cocaine use, explaining how it contributed to heart failure, encouraging him to stop using cocaine, and instructing him to take his medications as prescribed—MI focuses on specific *behaviors* and addresses a patient's ambivalence toward changing those behaviors. This change of emphasis allows us to direct our conversations toward areas that make more effective use of our time, whether, as in the case of Mr. G, identifying his reasons for and against continuing to use cocaine, discussing his perceived barriers to abstinence, or exploring how he might improve his confidence in his ability to avoid using again.

In addition to offering guidance on what to say, MI also offers specific tools that help trainees optimize *how* to say what needs to be said. MI includes a variety of strategies for making statements to elicit significant thought and emotion from our patients without (1) putting words in their mouths, (2) asking questions in a nonjudgmental fashion, (3) reacting to patients' ambivalence to change without inadvertently reinforcing hesitation, and (4) verbally noting inconsistencies without expressing approval or disapproval.

Guarding Against Burnout

Somewhere between starting on the wards as a fresh-faced medical student and dragging through an endless clinic day as a weary senior resident, we will all experience moments in which we wallow in pessimism, doubt, and even contempt toward our patients. Even the most idealistic and compassionate practitioners among us may privately admit to passing harsh judgments on patients: *He's manipulating me—he just wants more medications ... It's her own fault she's so fat, she just doesn't have the will-power to stay away from junk food ... He didn't do anything I told him to do last time— what a waste of my time!* Day after day, these frustrations threaten to displace one's sense of compassion, leaving trainees vulnerable to burnout (see Fig. 1.1).

While MI helps us navigate challenging conversations and make efficient use of our time, the underlying *spirit* of MI is valuable in helping trainees guard against exhaustion. To understand how the spirit and attitudes central to MI can help us protect ourselves, a close examination of our judgments may prove helpful. For instance, harsh evaluations of patients are often rooted in our personal fears and frustrations. A thought like "He's manipulating me; he just wants more medication" may reflect a fear of "being played for a fool" and of having one's trust exploited. As we worry that patients are taking advantage of us, we begin to doubt whether they deserve as much respect as we've extended to them, and we put ourselves at risk of falling into a pattern of reacting to this fear with increasing defensiveness and cynicism. The spirit of MI can help us respond to our concerns without resorting to suspicion. One of the attitudes emphasized in MI is *acceptance*, that is, viewing each person as unconditionally worthy of respect. *Although we may reflexively form personal judgments as to whether*

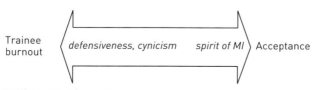

Trainee burnout ⟨ defensiveness, cynicism   spirit of MI ⟩ Acceptance

FIGURE 1.1   Guarding against burnout.

a drug-seeking patient is deserving of respect, an attitude of acceptance reminds us that our judgments do not change each person's inherent worth and potential.

Suppose we worry that an attitude of acceptance doesn't do anything to help patients change. We might think, "He didn't do anything I told him to do last time around—what a waste of my time!" Examining this thought more closely, we may begin to understand it as a reflection of frustration about the sense of futility we sometimes experience in trying to help our patients change their behaviors. The spirit of MI can help trainees avoid responding with distrust by revealing the false premise on which this frustration is founded. An attitude of acceptance promotes respect for our patients' autonomy and rejects the premise that as trainees, we have the power to control and coerce patients into doing something that they do not choose to do. By reminding us to let go of "a power that [we] never had in the first place," Rollnick and Miller note that the essence of MI can free us from the burden of failure and defeat that often accompanies the unpleasant realization that we cannot make our patients change. By fully embracing the spirit of MI, we become intentional in our perceptions of patients and conscious of our role in our relationships with them.

SIMPLY ONE MORE THING?

Amid a seemingly endless number of tasks, responsibilities, and challenges that face medical trainees, MI can seem like yet another unwelcome distraction that delays the completion of each day's duties. Despite this concern, trainees who learn and apply MI have discovered that both the skills and the spirit of MI offer significant practical benefits. MI equips us with a helpful framework for navigating challenging conversations with patients, helps *save* time by guiding our focus toward what's important to say and how to say it effectively, and reminds us to be conscious of our attitudes and perspectives toward both patients and ourselves, and our place within the healthcare system. In the process, MI strengthens our ability to withstand the very real threat of disillusionment and emotional exhaustion during medical training. While the process of learning MI requires a meaningful commitment of time and energy, it is an investment with great potential to bring about better outcomes for patients, and to improve our effectiveness, our time management skills, and the satisfaction we experience in our work as medical trainees.

> **KEY POINT**
> Investing energy into patient conversations using the spirit of MI can actually save time and resources in the long run.

SELF-ASSESSMENT QUIZ

True or False?

1. MI is an evidence-based framework that addresses unhealthy behaviors.
2. MI is a trainee-directed conversation in which trainees assume the role of experts who provide guidance toward a desired behavior change within a patient.
3. Dr. Miller incorporated elements of contemporary psychological theories and adapted them into a goal-driven therapy based on collaboration and respect for patient autonomy.

4. Directly confronting patients regarding their unhealthy behaviors is a cornerstone of MI.
5. Long-term therapy is essential to MI's success as a clinical intervention.
6. An essential element in the spirit of MI is that trainees must relinquish a sense of having the power to change or control patient behavior.

Answers

1. *True.* There is an expanding body of scientific literature validating the effectiveness and efficacy of MI for numerous health-related behaviors. Research continues on the use of MI for numerous health-related behaviors. Research continues on the use of MI among patients with substance use, anxiety, depression, eating disorders, and chronic medical conditions such as diabetes, heart disease, HIV/AIDS, and obesity.

2. *False.* MI is a collaborative conversation between trainees and patients, rooted in the principles of egalitarianism and empathy. It is patient-centered and oriented toward strengthening a patient's motivation and commitment to targeted behavior change.

3. *True.* In the 1980s, Dr. Miller was inspired by Festinger's formulation of cognitive dissonance, Bem's reformation of self-perception theory, Bandura's self-efficacy theory, and Roger's person-centered approach.

4. *False.* MI is based on the observation that argumentative and confrontational approaches compromise trainee–patient relationships and lead to poor outcomes. MI-based interactions are defined by a patient-centered focus, empathy, and support, which have been demonstrated to improve outcomes.

5. *False.* While MI is effective over the course of long-term physician–patient relationships, 64% of studies investigating the use of MI in brief encounters demonstrate positive patient outcomes.

6. *True.* The false sense of power that some trainees believe they possess to change a patient's behavior is contrary to the principles of MI. MI encourages patient-centered care and affirms patient autonomy. Unfortunately, trainees are subject to feelings of failure and defeat when they realize they are unable to force patients to change. Consequently, some trainees are at risk for profound cynicism, burnout, and a pervasive sense of therapeutic nihilism. MI reminds trainees that the responsibility for behavior change rests with patients.

2 Motivational Interviewing
An Overview

This chapter will answer the basic question: "So what exactly is motivational interviewing (MI)?" We will define basic terms; give a brief overview of communication skills and styles used in the medical setting; introduce the concepts of the righting reflex and ambivalence; and describe the spirit and skills of MI. Our goal is to (1) prepare you for more in-depth chapters to come and (2) provide you with a concise reference to which you can refer back for a quick refresher. Some questions to ask yourself as you read this book are as follows:

Have you ever. . . .

- *considered* making a behavior change?
- *considered how* you would make a change?
- *attempted* to make a change?
- *struggled* trying to maintain a change?

Your thoughtful answers to these questions will help you empathize with your patients as they respond to your efforts to facilitate their health behavior changes.

As medical trainees, we have good intentions, and we want to help our patients make healthy choices. And, as you may have learned through personal experiences, or when you have tried to convince someone to make a change, helping other people change their behaviors is not easy. Our instincts are to lecture, warn, scold, beg, plead, or even nag. But that doesn't usually work. Here, we offer another way to help your patients make health behavior changes; that way is MI.

WHAT IS MOTIVATIONAL INTERVIEWING?

Miller and Rollnick (2013), in their third edition of *Motivational Interviewing: Helping People Change*, defined MI as "a collaborative conversation style for strengthening a person's own motivation and commitment to change." (pg. 12)

On the most basic level, MI is:

- A way of being with patients and having a conversation about change, which is nonjudgmental and based on compassion, respect, and empathy.
- A set of learnable communication skills.
- Aimed at helping patients change specific behaviors.
- Patient-centered and respectful, while still being directive and goal oriented toward change.
- Brief and, although it may be delivered in 1–4 sessions as a stand-alone intervention, it is mostly a way of relating to people that can be used in almost all patient interactions.
- Evidence-based.

In essence, MI is about "arranging conversations so people talk themselves into change based on their own values and interests" (Miller & Rollnick, 2013, pg. 4).

To accomplish this, medical trainees using MI:

- Act as guides, not as experts, to collaborate and partner with patients.
- Listen actively, reflecting patients' thoughts, emotions, and an understanding of their situations.
- Develop discrepancy between patients' current behaviors and their goals, values, and beliefs.
- Recognize change talk and selectively elicit and strengthen it.
- Support patients' self-efficacy (their belief in their own ability to succeed) and support patients' hope and optimism for successful change.
- Identify and manage discord and status quo talk, recognizing that ambivalence is a natural component of behavior change; patients can get stuck for a long time, ranging from days to years.

CORE COMMUNICATION SKILLS AND STYLES

What Are the Core Communication Skills?

There are three core communication skills that are part of MI, and they are important in *all* medical trainee–patient encounters. They can be used in varying degrees, depending on the type of communication style needed at the time. The first is *informing*. Informing in the medical setting is defined as conveying knowledge about a condition or medical treatment or even the results of a laboratory or radiologic test by providing facts, diagnoses, prognosis, and recommendations to the patient. The second communication skill is *asking*, especially asking questions that develop an understanding of patients' problems and perspectives. This is usually accomplished using open-ended questions. This is a skill that is different than the usual asking of predominantly closed questions (often numerous and consecutively), for the sole purpose of generating a differential diagnosis and treatment plan that is then dictated to the patient. The third communication skill is *listening*, which is an active process beyond just nodding your head and saying, "Uh Huh" or "I see." You demonstrate you are listening and that you understand patients' experiences, feelings, and meanings correctly by using reflections, a skill we will discuss in more detail later in Chapter 4.

KEY POINT

Three Core MI Communication Skills

- Informing
- Asking
- Listening

Communication Styles

There are three core communication styles: directing, following, and guiding. A *directing* communication style communicates that "I know what you should do and here is how to do it." This is a communication style that implies the trainee is the expert and

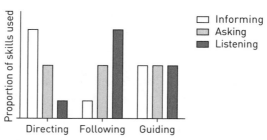

FIGURE 2.1   Communication styles.

will "fix" the patient with his or her knowledge and expertise. A *following* communication style implies that "I trust your own wisdom, I will stay with you, and I will let you work this out in your own way." When you use a following communication style, you listen and demonstrate that you hear patients' perspectives and follow patients wherever their conversations take you, without any push or pull in any particular direction. A following style is often used by psychologists who practice client-centered counseling in the style of Carl Rogers (1965, client-centered therapy). A *guiding* communication style is a combination of being a good listener and offering expertise when needed; it is in between directing and following. MI is an example of a guiding communication style.

KEY POINT

Three Core Communication Styles:

- Directing
- Following
- Guiding

When it comes to communication style, no single one is a particularly good or bad style. All three styles are needed and skillful medical trainees shift flexibly among these styles as appropriate to the patient and situation. For example, when a patient has collapsed in a waiting area, a directing style is most appropriate until you have completed your ABCs (or airway, breathing, circulation) and stabilized the patient. In this situation, you need to take charge and not have a conversation that is following or guiding. Likewise, early on in a mental health evaluation or when a therapist is practicing pure client-centered psychotherapy in a Rogerian style, one might use a following communication style to better understand a patient's experiences and perspective. MI is primarily a guiding style and MI is in between a directing and following style.

When you consider how communication skills and communication styles align (Fig. 2.1), in a directing style one would inform a lot, ask a little, and not listen much. In a following style, one would listen a lot, ask a bit, and not inform much. In MI, which is a guiding style, one would inform, ask, and listen in equal parts. It is important to note that there is still an important role for informing as much as there is for listening and asking in a guiding style.

THE RIGHTING REFLEX

KEY POINT

Learning to curb your righting reflex is fundamental to conducting an MI-adherent encounter.

What is the righting reflex? It is that feeling you have in your gut that you want to desperately help someone, usually your patient, by fixing a problem for the patient or by giving the patient suggestions on how to fix the problem so he or she is no longer ill, in pain, or struggling. It is a natural feeling and a common one for those of us who have entered into the healthcare field. After all, why would we go into medicine if it was not to help people feel better, free of pain and illness?

Unfortunately, although the righting reflex is well intended, following it and trying to step in and "fix" our patients by telling them what to do is not terribly beneficial at helping people feel better or, more importantly, helping them make health-related behavior changes. Part of learning MI is learning to quell your desire to "fix" things for your patients. One needs to learn to rely on alternate approaches that actually have been shown to be effective at helping people make lifestyle behavior changes. It may help to know that, despite your good intentions, telling your patients why and how to make behavior changes will not result in behavior change. It can even damage your therapeutic relationship with them and result in their not returning to see you when they have been unable to make the changes you advised. Furthermore, it might even push them to engage in even more unhealthy behavior because of the pressure you put on them to make changes that they were not ready to make.

AMBIVALENCE

> KEY POINT
>
> Fundamental to the process of MI is recognizing and helping patients to resolve ambivalence.

What is ambivalence? It is when you feel two ways about something, such as whether you should start exercising on a regular basis. On the one hand, you know you should do it for your health because it will help you stay strong and trim, and you will feel better if you do it. On the other hand, you don't feel like going to the gym and getting all sweaty today. You are already dog-tired and you hardly have enough energy to drag yourself home after a day of classes or rotations. You just want to go home, eat something satisfying, veg out in front of the TV, and then go to bed. You feel two ways about it—you are ambivalent about exercising (see Fig. 2.2). It is like having a devil on one shoulder and an angel on the other, each telling you different things to do or think.

Ambivalence is a normal process in behavior change. However, if someone tries to push you one way or another when you are ambivalent, you will naturally push back. If I start to argue with you about why you *really* need to go work out, you will probably counter with how exhausted you are and that I don't understand how hard your day has been. If I agree with you that you had a rough day and you deserve to go home and relax and that exercise isn't really a big deal right now while you are in medical school or residency, you might disagree with me. You might say that you really need to exercise and that you will feel so much better afterward and that it is worth the time to go to the gym. It is important to keep this in mind when it comes to our patients. They are often ambivalent and feel two ways about making health-related behavior changes that we suggest they do, especially lifestyle changes that are hard and require a lot of ongoing effort and commitment. You get to make a decision here—do you

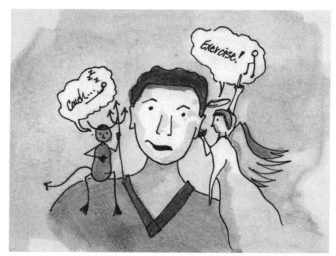

FIGURE 2.2 Ambivalence.

want to push them away from healthy changes by arguing with them or telling them what to do when they are ambivalent, or do you want to help them move toward change by learning to evoke from them their own reasons for commitment to change? You decide.

THE SPIRIT OF MOTIVATIONAL INTERVIEWING

KEY POINT

The Spirit of MI:

PACE

Partnership
Acceptance
Compassion
Evocation

There are four elements of the spirit of MI. Originally there were three identified elements of the spirit of MI: collaboration, autonomy support, and evocation. Chapter 3 will discuss the more recent four elements of the spirit of MI of collaboration/partnering, acceptance, compassion, and evocation. Table 2.1 details the differences between the traditional medical interactions and MI.

SKILLS OF MOTIVATIONAL INTERVIEWING: OARS

There are four critical skills in MI: open-ended questions, affirmations, reflections, and summaries. These are often referred to as OARS. We will describe them briefly here and in more detail in Chapter 4.

Table 2.1 Comparing Traditional Medical Interactions and Motivational Interviewing

	Traditional Medical Interaction	Motivational Interviewing
Medical trainee's role	Provide expertise	Guide
Medical trainee's goals	Explain the problem	Understand patient's perspective on diagnosis, prognosis, treatment
	Diagnosis	Resolve ambivalence
	Prognosis	Strengthen motivation
	Instructing patients on change	Provide information and advice elicit a plan for change
Interview skills	Numerous, consecutive closed-ended questions	OARS
	Give information and advice without permission	Elicit-Provide-Elicit
Response to discord	Arguing	Understanding
	Rationalizing	Roll with resistance
	Convince by providing more information	Reflections
	Directing	Reframing
	Blaming	Reinforcing autonomy
Typical outcome	Mutual frustration	Mutual respect
	Lack of change	Change
	Regression to earlier stage of change	Progression through the stages of change

---

TOOLBOX

OARS

Open-ended questions
Affirmations
Reflections
Summarize

Ask Open-Ended Questions

Questions that are answered with a simple yes or no or single-word answer close the door to elaboration. Instead, ask open-ended questions that encourage patients to expand on their perspective, thoughts, emotions, and concerns in a way that assists the trainee toward a better understanding of patients' specific circumstances.

Examples are as follows:

"What have you noticed after taking your medication?"
"How has having diabetes affected your daily routine?"

"What do you think you will lose if you give up smoking?"

"How would you like things to be different?"

"Tell me more about that."

"Describe for me how drinking fits in with your typical day."

Affirmations: Affirm Patients' Strengths and Past Efforts

Using affirmations to acknowledge patients' personal strengths and/or positive efforts toward change, even when they have not yet been successful, provides support and encouragement.

Examples are as follows:

"You are resilient and persistent; when you set your mind to something, you get it done."

"I appreciate your being so honest with me."

"You are clearly a resourceful, intelligent person."

"That's a good suggestion."

"You did the best you could and learned a tremendous amount from that experience."

Listen Reflectively

Through actively listening and reflecting back the meaning or emotion of what a patient has said, trainees can enhance understanding of patients' perspectives, help clarify patients' thoughts and emotions, and communicate that trainees are engaged and understand patients.

Examples are as follows:

"You're not sure how anyone can help."

"It is hard to imagine not having a cigarette as part of your day."

"You're thinking that now is not the best time to start a new exercise routine."

"It angers you that your family is trying to make you stop drinking."

"You're feeling overwhelmed with work."

"Nothing about being here is useful for you."

Summarize

Summaries provide trainees with an opportunity to reiterate what they hear, highlight important points, and transition to new topics.

Examples are as follows:

"Your blood sugar has been running above 300 in the morning, you feel more tired lately, and with work it has been difficult for you to schedule our appointments together. You're not really sure that taking more medication is something you want to do, and instead you are thinking about cutting out more carbohydrates from your diet."

"You see your drinking as being no different than the people around you. It helps you relax and manage your stress and anger. The only reason you came in is because you are tired of everyone around you complaining about your drinking, even though you don't really see it as an issue. It does worry you a little that you were charged with a driving under the influence (DUI) but only because you cannot work if you cannot drive the truck at your job. You are not really sure you want to do anything about your drinking, at the same time you are willing to hear what kinds of options we have to offer."

The combination of MI skills are used to foster the four processes of MI which are *engaging, focusing, evoking,* and *planning* and will be discussed in Chapter 3.

In summary, ambivalence is a normal part of behavior change and people can be stuck there for a while. Using a directing style and arguing for change when a patient is ambivalent usually results in arguments against change. Since patients present with different levels of motivation, medical trainees would need to learn how to meet their patients where they are, and to adjust their MI skills accordingly. Medical trainees should guard against their desire to give in to their righting reflex and try to "fix" patients by telling them what to do, especially when they are ambivalent about making behavior change. *People are more likely to be persuaded by what they hear themselves say than what you tell them to do.* The overall style of MI is *guiding,* which incorporates elements of *directing* and *following* styles. Medical trainees can more effectively help motivate patients' lifestyle and health behavior changes by learning MI and incorporating the communication skills of informing, asking, and listening into their communication styles of directing, following, and guiding.

SELF-ASSESSMENT QUIZ

True or False?

1. Fundamentally, MI is a collaborative style of therapeutic conversation designed to strengthen a patient's motivation and commitment to change.
2. Essential MI-based communication skills include informing, asking, and listening.
3. MI is a directing style of communication.
4. The righting reflex is a powerful principle utilized in MI.
5. Ambivalence is a normal process in which individuals hold opposing views regarding their behaviors.
6. Four essential skills in MI include open-ended questions, affirmations, reflections, and summaries (OARS).

Answers

1. *True.* MI is a therapeutic exchange between a trainee and a patient with the goal of specific behavioral change. MI is a nonjudgmental approach, based on compassion, respect, and empathy.
2. *True.* Informing fosters patient empowerment by sharing information about a particular condition or medical treatment. Evocative questions and active listening are skills that help trainees understand each patient's experiences and feelings.

3. *False.* MI is a guiding communication style characterized by active listening, attentive questioning, and sharing information as patients permit. MI is based on hypothesizing why patients feel and behave as they do. Thus, MI practitioners delicately balance between asking questions and following up on patient responses in order to test their hypotheses; these are accepted or rejected in response to patient verification or refutation.

4. *False.* The righting reflex is common among both novice and veteran trainees, and it is the desire to help patients by offering solutions and/or telling patients what to do. The righting reflex is fundamentally counter to the MI principle of supporting patient autonomy and, at times, risks damaging a therapeutic relationship.

5. *True.* Nearly everyone who confronts unhealthy behavior will experience ambivalence, in which one holds contradictory views about whether to continue behaving as one has in the past. MI explores patients' ambivalence through a nonjudgmental, supportive, and empathic style.

6. *True.* Open-ended questions are questions that cannot be answered with a simple yes, no, or single word, but rather questions that encourage elaboration and exploration of a patient's experiences and feelings. Affirmations acknowledge a patient's personal strengths and efforts. Reflective listening encourages continued exploration of a patient's experiences and demonstrates to him or her that the trainee is listening closely and trying to understand. Summaries allow trainees to reiterate what has been shared, to highlight important points, and to transition smoothly to other topics of discussion.

3 Spirit and Processes of Motivational Interviewing

Perhaps the most concise way to think about motivational interviewing (MI) is as a person-focused way of engaging people in conversation about changing problematic behaviors. The spirit of MI is not itself behavioral—it is humanistic in the sense of prioritizing the value and agency of individual persons over the purely rational and empirical. It is this quality of humanistic engagement that defines the spirit of MI, the subjective engagement of a trainee working to understand and accept a patient's perspective of the world and his or her health. Each contact or interaction with patients occurs against a backdrop of implicit meaning; in other words, a certain atmosphere shapes the underlying tone of an encounter, which, in turn, affects the disposition of the participants. Generally, this aspect of the doctor–patient interaction is not explored as deeply in medical training as are other parts of an interview; instead, history taking, data gathering, and other so-called *objective* components are accentuated and reinforced. These tasks make up what is commonly referred to as the "traditional" medical interview/assessment. Although they are absolutely indispensable to safe medical practice, these elements are, by themselves, insufficient to engage our patients, focus on the behaviors they wish to change, and motivate behavior change by evoking change talk.

As medical trainees, we receive extensive training concerning the content of questions and methods of gathering information that determine a differential diagnosis and treatment plan. However, we all struggle with competing priorities whenever we encounter opportunities to address the problem behaviors that cause a patient to seek treatment. Should I go back and collect *more* data, or should I tell this person how he or she ought to change? Should I focus on making a diagnosis immediately, or should I listen to this patient discuss the issues that are related, but not essential, to why he or she is here today?

One way to imagine the spirit of MI is as the outer rim and tire on the wheel of a bicycle (Fig. 3.1). The spokes of the MI wheel are the many processes and skills that support this approach. Together, they have the potential to help us engage with our patients, both smoothly and surely. But just as learning to ride a bike takes time, effort, balance, and perhaps a dose of courage, so does learning MI.

Before continuing, let's take a moment to consider another image: that of a skilled and highly experienced mountaineer seeking to guide a novice climber who wishes to scale his or her local peak (see Fig. 3.2).

The seasoned mountaineer has the expertise to climb virtually any summit but has not previously visited this particular hill. The student climber has visited few other mountains but has spent long hours observing the geography and wildlife of the pinnacle they approach together. The student's life has been spent on this hill, yet many of its contours and cornices remain unknown and unmapped. Sometimes the student has ventured beyond the confines of the family settlement, but not often enough to feel confident in the ability to explore further afield; the decision to attempt an ascent now has taken both time and courage.

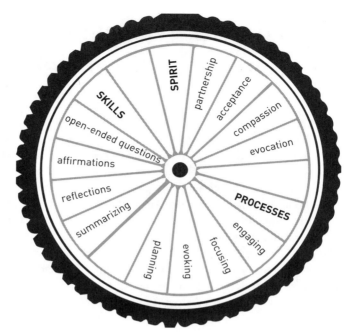

FIGURE 3.1   Conceptualizing motivational interviewing.

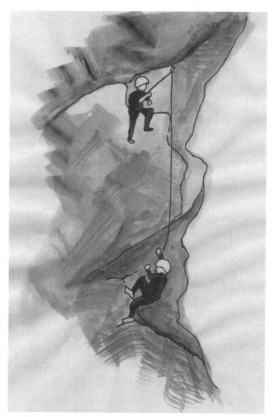

FIGURE 3.2   The spirit of motivational interviewing.

The professional mountaineer works closely with the new climber to uncover two sorts of paths: those that require both climbers' careful attention to small topographic subtleties, and those that are clear to the experienced eyes of the accomplished climber alone, being too well hidden or treacherous for the novice to notice.

Any new ascent is fraught with physical, psychological, and emotional challenges, and so it is on this climb. Despite the inexperienced climber's doubt and uncertainty, the expert actively supports and encourages the beginner in the unfamiliar position of leading the way up the mountain. This in itself is tacit recognition of the worthiness of the journey and acceptance of the new climber's intrinsic value and ability. The mountaineer feels many things: empathy, which arises from an ability to perceive the mountain with the fear and trepidation that the new climber experiences; compassion that comes from understanding the profound vulnerability the new climber must overcome in order to complete the climb, and the willingness to allow the student to chart the course. The mountaineer's goal is to awaken and reinforce the student's inner confidence, strength, and wisdom, and in so doing, increase the prospect of success. As the master shares the skill and finesse gleaned from a lengthy career, so too the novice reveals local secrets known only to one whose life has been spent on *this* hill.

THE SPIRIT OF MOTIVATIONAL INTERVIEWING

The essential spirit of MI is grounded in a sense of genuine interest and curiosity to engage patients with both mind and heart. As the earlier story demonstrates, metaphors provide a useful means to understand one of the great intangibles of medical care: the attitude and mindset that we bring to an encounter, *before* we open the door to greet each patient.

The spirit of MI comprises four key elements: (1) partnership or collaboration, (2) acceptance, (3) compassion, and (4) evocation.

Partnership

A conventional medical interview is hierarchical, even authoritarian. The physician normally assumes the role of expert whose job it is to gather information from the patient in the form of a history, physical exam, and lab and radiology assessments. Privately, physicians analyze the information to determine a diagnosis and treatment plan. Finally, these conclusions are communicated to patients, along with the physician's arguments and medical rationale concerning what the patient should change and how this would best be accomplished. This model confines physicians to the role of feeding advice, information, and directives *into* patients, who are viewed as passive recipients of information and advice (see Fig. 3.3).

Crucially, the relationship between trainee and patient in MI differs in that it is an *equal partnership* focused on whatever behavior change our *patient* wishes to make. Our role as trainees is to explore a patient's experience and perspective in order to understand the circumstances that have caused *this* person to seek care at *this* time and to evoke his or her reasons to change. As partners in the process, we learn to attend to the nuances of our voices and body language, for these elements play a significant role in establishing the tone of the relationship. Interactions based on MI have

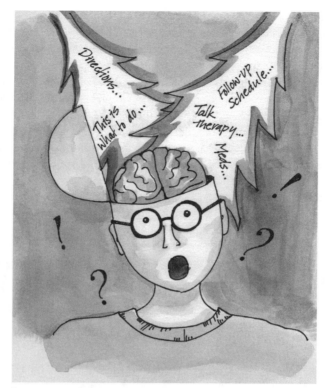

FIGURE 3.3 The conventional medical model.

sometimes been compared to dancing a waltz, in that each partner is highly receptive to the subtlest motions of his or her collaborator in an activity that is demanding but exhilarating.

Imagine that your patient has just expressed concern about a recent diagnosis. You realize that this is not the time for false optimism or a detailed summary of treatment options. Here's how you might reinforce a collaborative style:

- "May I share my perspective on this news? We could discuss the pros and cons of different treatment options based on what makes the most sense for you."
- "You raise very important concerns that we can examine and weigh together. Help me understand more about how you see it."

Remember that one of the assumptions of MI is that we, as trainees, do not have to provide all the answers. Our intent is to help our patients determine which course works best for them.

Acceptance

Accepting our patient means that we recognize and respect all that an individual brings to our encounters. It is profound and unconditional. Acceptance does not, however, require that we approve of our patient's behaviors or choices; but we must accept them.

Acceptance is composed of four elements:

- Absolute worth
- Accurate empathy
- Autonomy support
- Affirmation

Absolute Worth

This aspect of acceptance requires that we acknowledge and respect the absolute value of each patient as an individual human being. The concept of absolute worth assumes that no patient is completely devoid of goodness and trustworthiness, and that uncovering these qualities is a critical element of behavior change. In the absence of this view, therapeutic nihilism—that is, the conviction that a patient is incapable of change—pervades treatment.

Unconditional acceptance commits us to searching for each patient's intrinsic goodness, even in situations when patients believe they lack this quality. In accepting our patients, we resist judging them or their behaviors, realizing that sometimes this will be especially challenging. Although acceptance and behavior change may not seem related, the two do, in fact, form two halves of an exciting dynamic, for when patients feel accepted and learn to accept themselves and their inevitable flaws, they are free to make the changes that help them gain the lives they seek. Philosophers and humanistic psychologists have described this process as one of self-actualization: becoming all that we may be by realizing our full potential. When we model patient acceptance, we facilitate our patient's acceptance of himself or herself, which in turn, facilitates the process of implementing and sustaining change. Keep in mind that acceptance is an *active* process; it is not always easy.

In the following scenario, a patient presents to the emergency department by feigning severe flu symptoms, until he shares, with shame, that he is experiencing acute opioid withdrawal. Some ways of demonstrating acceptance of this patient include the following:

- "You have struggled so much inside yourself that you weren't sure how to be open about that struggle."
- "What is it like for you to share what you've been keeping inside for so long?"
- "You sometimes wonder who could possibly understand all that you've been through and what this has meant for you as a person. Would you share some of your struggle with me?"

Accurate Empathy

Accurate empathy refers to a genuine interest in discovering and understanding how each patient perceives his or her world. We communicate empathy by using thoughtful reflections that demonstrate our belief in the unique value of *this* patient's experiences. Comprehending a patient's frame of reference also acknowledges that person's independence and the validity of his or her point of view. Take care to avoid either over-identifying with your patient's experiences or imposing your own values or perspective on what he or she has shared. Be careful, too, not to dismiss elements of your patient's narrative, however insignificant or irrelevant they may appear at first.

The following patient has suffered much loss and hardship over the course of her illness, but she has yet to share her feelings of this struggle and the changes she wants to make. As she begins to confide in you, here are some ways to empathically elicit more of her story:

- "How was that [experience] for you?"
- "You've really been fighting for your life."
- "What was it like to struggle through that experience on your own?"
- "It surprised you to find out how much you were loved and cherished by so many family members and friends during your last hospitalization."

Another tip regarding accurate empathy is to listen to your own tone of voice and manner of expression: Stay in the moment and attend to the essence of what you hear from your patient. Remember that most patients know when we're "faking" interest in them, should we respond with feeble clichés or forced optimism.

Autonomy Support

We support our patients' autonomy by acknowledging their right to self-determination and their capacity to choose what they will become. Recall that conventional medical models tend to view patients as objective medical conditions, devoid of the independence and volition that are essential to the humanistic view that each individual person is a unique human being. As discussed previously, a traditional medical interview highlights a patient's pathology at the expense of exploring the strengths, resiliencies, and abilities he or she brings to the process of change, and which often determines the success of a treatment plan. A pervasive attitude among some medical practitioners views physicians as authoritarian experts responsible for diagnosing and establishing treatment plans. This attitude assumes that patients are unable to solve problems for themselves. Remember that a key component to the spirit of MI is recognizing, and accepting, that patients themselves *are the agents of change*. This principle is the basis for the self-efficacy that MI fosters and supports.

Many patients have difficulty maintaining prescribed treatment plans. Here are some examples of the questions and statements that reinforce the autonomy of an individual who has successfully maintained sobriety until a recent relapse:

- "What did you draw on from within yourself to maintain your sobriety for so long?"
- "What was it in you that allowed you to manage your stress without drinking for that period of time?"
- "No one can decide for you or force you to change."
- "You know what will work best for you."
- "I'm not here to tell you what to do, or to try to make you do anything you don't wish to do. You'll decide when and if you wish to change anything."

Affirmations

These statements acknowledge our patients' strengths and their past and present efforts to maintain behavior change. Affirmations remind patients that we've listened closely to their experiences, and they are an effective means of communicating acceptance and reinforcing autonomy.

Patients often face major struggles over the course of an illness. Examples of possible responses include the following:

- "Somehow, you've been able to meet the challenges that were once so frightening to you."
- "You've persevered, despite circumstances that many others would not have been able to meet head-on as you have."
- "Sometimes you show a determination that surprises even you."

As we all know, it's easy to forget about past success when we're in the midst of present difficulties. Used appropriately, affirmations help our patients remember the resilience they already possess.

Compassion

Compassion is widely understood as the feeling of being moved by another's suffering, accompanied by a desire to end it. MI holds that compassion is more than an emotional response: It is a stance that places another person's perspective ahead of one's own. While partnership, acceptance, and evocation may be part of many professional relationships, compassion is the principal component that distinguishes *therapeutic* relationships. By definition, then, MI prioritizes a patient's welfare over the practitioner's. MI cannot be used to exploit or take advantage of a patient in any way; such behavior would constitute a serious breach of professional ethics.

The next scenario imagines a patient experiencing significant pain who rudely demands immediate pain relief. An effective way to avoid escalating the situation is to avoid a confrontational reaction and instead respond with compassion:

- "It's frustrating to have to wait even a moment for pain medication when you're suffering like this and you need it *now*. How can we help you be more in control of your pain management?"
- "You have reached your limit, in terms of tolerating the pain, and you can't understand why the nurse didn't respond more quickly when you needed help."

Evocation

MI also diverges from conventional medical interviews in the way that patient information is collected. Instead of relying solely on closed questions, MI uses a process of evocation through which we assist patients to explore how their experiences and perspectives contribute to building motivation to change. In MI, we use collaborative engagement as the means by which a patient's intrinsic motivation is elicited and strengthened.

We have sometimes found ourselves in the role of reluctant and unwilling "expert," stuck in a pattern of asking yes/no questions. One way to break this cycle is by switching to using open-ended questions:

- "Help me better understand [your illness] and how it has affected your life."
- "How has your struggle with [your illness] affected your sense of yourself?"

- "What has changed most for you since you were diagnosed with [this illness]?"
- "What has been the most challenging part of coping with this illness, physically and personally?"
- "Describe for me how you manage to keep your spirits up in the face of [this illness]."

PROCESSES OF MOTIVATIONAL INTERVIEWING

There are four processes within motivational interviewing: (1) engaging, (2) focusing, (3) evoking, and (4) planning. Note that the OARS skills described in Chapter 4 are used in each of these four processes.

Engaging occurs as we establish working partnerships with patients that are collaborative in nature. From the first moment of contact, our goal must be to demonstrate compassion, patience, and acceptance of wherever our patients are in terms of readiness to change their behaviors.

Focusing requires us to identify, develop, and maintain a specific direction in our conversations with patients about change. As with all aspects of MI, the process of establishing an agenda for a discussion must be *shared* with each patient.

Evoking involves eliciting a patient's own motivations and arguments for change. This dialogue is described as "change talk" and refers to the words, phrases, statements, and expressions that are unique to each person. A number of structured questions help elicit change talk, and Table 3.1 links these questions to various phrases that your patients may use to express different aspects of making behavior change. The acronym DARN CAT summarizes these types of preparatory and mobilization change talk (Table 3.1), where the letters represent: Desire, Ability, Reasons for change, Need to change, Commitment to change, Activation language, and Taking steps toward change. Numerous studies find that commitment language is closely correlated to substantive behavior change.

Most people have the capacity to talk themselves into changing behavior, and we are all more likely to succeed in doing so when we express this intention aloud. It takes time to help your patients give voice to their hopes and aspirations for different ways of behaving, but keep in mind that this process has a better chance of achieving long-term, sustainable change than anything *you* might say or do.

The final step of *planning* develops and refines our patients' commitment to change and specific action plans. This may or may not occur over the course of a single conversation; often the planning process requires fine-tuning to the realities of a patient's circumstances, and this can be accomplished through continued contact.

Table 3.1 Change Talk: DARN CAT

Desire	"I really want to find a way."
Ability	"I could do that."
Reasons	"My family is counting on me."
Need	"I just can't keep doing this."
Commitment	"I must—no, I will make a change."
Activation	"I set my quit date."
Taking steps	"I joined a gym last week."

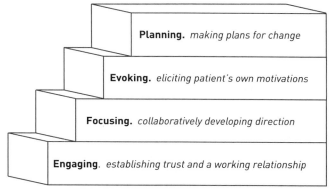

Planning. *making plans for change*

Evoking. *eliciting patient's own motivations*

Focusing. *collaboratively developing direction*

Engaging. *establishing trust and a working relationship*

FIGURE 3.4   The four processes of motivational interviewing.

Much like a flight of stairs, the processes of MI build upon one another, each step relying on the foundation that precedes it (Fig. 3.4). We need to engage each patient to develop the rapport and trust that are essential in assisting him or her to focus attention on whatever target behaviors may be subject to change. Once these are identified, evoking our patient's reasons for change helps build commitment to the process; this is especially important in confronting the inevitable difficulties and challenges that lie ahead. Patients must feel a certain degree of confidence in their ability to succeed before we begin the planning process, in which together, we look ahead to our patient's "new" life that includes a new set of behaviors.

Note that this process does not always follow the tidy, linear course we've used to outline the steps. Sometimes progress will occur in a seemingly horizontal fashion, zigzagging through each phase, and in some situations, we will need to regress to a previous step in order to consolidate what has been discovered and learned. No matter. What is important is that *you and your patient* determine the course you will follow. Whether you move slowly or briskly through the steps is of no consequence whatsoever. What matters is that you and your patients determine the most effective way to promote effective behavior changes that will endure.

PERSONAL REFLECTION

As I progressed through my medical training, I gained confidence in my clinical abilities to gather patient data, analyze relevant elements of the history, and synthesize this data with various test results in order to arrive at a diagnosis. From this point, I would finally determine a treatment plan. But no matter how strong my history-taking skills, no matter how accurate I was at making a diagnosis, I always felt something was missing from my patient encounters. I felt this most acutely whenever the crucial aspect of my recommendations involved helping my patients make lasting behavior change. It was so frustrating to feel stuck in a fruitless attempt to bring about change with patients who were, well, as stuck as I was.

This is what provoked me to learn MI. While medical school had trained me to be adept at collecting and making use of data, it did not teach me how to establish a collaborative or therapeutic relationship. As I worked to understand the true spirit of MI, my patient encounters became more humanistic and less focused on purely rational science. I told myself that I was learning to treat my patients "side by side," instead of "head to head," as I had done previously.

What surprised me most about learning MI was how the spirit of this approach awakened the notion of true patient centeredness within me. Even more surprising was how much more "free" I felt within patient encounters. I discovered that the more capable I became at helping my patients make their own choices about treatment, the better I felt about my ability to provide sound care. Finally, I understood that my choice of words and tone of voice mattered every bit as much as the laboratory tests and medications I ordered. I found it easier to put each patient's needs ahead of my own desire for competence and recognition, and I must say, it felt wonderful!

Another epiphany was learning to view challenging patients with compassion, realizing that these individuals have much to teach me. I know now that when I'm able to stay person centered, I feel more confident in my ability to put my patients first. This has made a huge difference in the way I practice medicine: I feel I'm able to consider *all* of the relevant data now, not simply the obvious physical findings.

I find it highly ironic that through learning to be patient-centered, I feel as though I've given myself the most wonderful gift of my (short) career.

SELF-ASSESSMENT QUIZ

True or False?

1. The four key elements of the spirit of MI are partnership, acceptance, compassion, and evocation.
2. In MI, trainees are seen as experts who provide answers and a clear course for patients to follow in order to achieve change.
3. The four As of acceptance include absolute worth, accurate empathy, autonomy support, and affirmation.
4. The four processes of MI are engaging, focusing, evoking, and planning.
5. DARN CAT represents the dimensions of motivation.

Answers

1. *True.* In a collaborative relationship, trainees do not function as directive sources of advice and information, but rather as equal partners in the behavior changes patients wish to bring about. Trainees accept patients for whom and where they are, with regard to exploring or implementing change. Compassionate medical trainees place patients' perspectives and welfare ahead of their own. Evocation encourages patients to explore how their experiences and perspectives contribute to their motivation for change.
2. *False.* The trainee's role is not to offer or even try to identify all the answers; rather, trainees aim to help patients determine which course of action would work best for *them*.
3. *True.* In MI, acceptance is the ideal standard that implies that trainees accept patients for precisely who they are, regardless of their degree of interest or motivation for changing unhealthy behaviors. Acceptance is embodied by appreciating the absolute value of each patient, expressing genuine interest in understanding

a patient's worldview, supporting each patient's right to self-determination, and acknowledging a patient's strengths and efforts for change.

4. *True.* Engaging with patients is an essential part of establishing sound relationships that allow trainees to understand each patient's experiences and feelings. Focusing involves isolating and recognizing the patient-identified goal that is to be explored, developed, and pursued. Evoking builds upon engagement by describing and elaborating a patient's motivations and arguments for change. Planning is the process that delineates specific goals and actions to bring about, and consolidate, behavior change.

5. *True.* The acronym DARN CAT summarizes the types of preparatory and mobilizing change talk used during the evoking stage of MI. The letters represent Desire, Ability, Reasons, Need, Commitment to change, Activation language, and Taking steps toward change.

4 Building a Toolbox

The concept of building a toolbox comes from the perspective that providing healthcare is an interaction that is both work and a service. The interaction of a medical trainee and a patient is the work, and out of it comes improved or new behaviors that "fix" a problem. However, whether anything gets fixed is reliant on the quality of the service, and the quality of service depends on whether the right tools are used to perform the work. Builders acquire tools as they gain experience. They pick up tools during training and on each job. They learn how to use each tool as it is designed to perform in a particular way. Similarly, medical trainees must also collect techniques or "tools" and learn to use them as part of their interpersonal and clinical skills. They must develop the tools they need to work effectively and then take out each one and use it as needed to fit a particular clinical setting and the individual patients they encounter.

THE WHY AND HOW OF THE THERAPEUTIC APPROACH

Many healthcare–related interactions take place in circumstances where the medical trainee and patient agree about why the patient has asked for treatment and what must be done to achieve a positive outcome. Others occur during circumstances that are unexpected, for example, medical emergencies and accidental injuries. These encounters develop quickly out of circumstances that cannot be foreseen and treatment demands rapid judgment and decision making. As a result, these interactions often include consideration of conditions or behaviors that are occurring coincidently with a "primary problem." Trainees and patients may or may not agree about treatment recommendations in these situations. Finally, some medical interviews occur in situations where the trainee and the patient disagree about many things, including whether there is a need for treatment, the cause of the need for treatment, what condition(s) are in need of treatment, and even the objectives of treatment.

One commonality among all these health-related encounters is that the trainee should maintain the same even-tempered, emotional and behavioral approach. Trainees should relate in a pleasant, conversational manner that includes paying attention to one's own verbal and nonverbal behaviors such as smiling, making eye contact, and showing that one is paying attention to the patient throughout the visit. It also involves responding to the patient's presentation in ways that reduce negative mood and cognitive states, for example, anger, frustration, or confusion. The overarching issue is that trainees work in a service occupation, and most patients have an expectation that their physicians will conduct themselves in ways consistent with what has been referred to as a "good bedside manner." Therefore, failure to approach patients in this way can create discord in the relationship from the very beginning of the evaluation, when the therapeutic alliance develops. Failure to establish a working alliance is especially problematic in clinical situations where the trainee is expected to work with the patient in an ongoing treatment relationship.

You learn to develop your communication style as you become increasingly comfortable with a particular routine of engaging and moving through the interview while still keeping the atmosphere conversational and nonpressured. Using a consistent tone and manner of speaking demonstrates self-assurance and indicates nonverbally that you have experience with interviewing and treatment. It does not mean being arrogant or a know-it-all. Rather, it suggests to the patient that he or she can be assured that your observations and recommendations are based on training and experience. The approach includes admitting openly that you do not know all the answers but that what is not known will be explored in a comprehensive effort with your supervisor to do everything that can be done to collaborate with the patient.

INTEGRATING THE PROCESS AND CONTENT OF INTERVIEWING

All patients have at least one reason why they come in for an evaluation, even if it is only because someone else wants them to be there. Finding out about the reason(s) must be the first order of business because it must be addressed in order to engage the patient. Engaging the patient so he or she wants to talk with you, no matter what brought him or her there initially, is the foundation of the therapeutic alliance. The quintessential example of this can be seen in evaluations of adolescents who are brought to the physician because of drug use. In the vast majority of these cases, the patient is only there because his or her parents want him or her to be seen and "fixed." Therefore, you need to begin by emphasizing that you want what the patient wants, which is for him or her not to have to come for treatment. The rest of treatment then consists of showing the patient that you want to work with him or her toward this objective and the best way to do that is for him or her to participate with you. In this way, his or her parents will agree that there is no need for the treatment. Techniques for doing this are learned through experience and include, among other things, affirming the patient's thinking and behavior when they reflect good judgment, supporting the patient during discussions and negotiations (even when this is contrary to what his or her parents want), and reframing messages so the patient will reframe his or her position and ally with you based on your opinion. However, this is only possible when your patient is engaged with you and not resistant to the process.

Motivation to change begins with motivation to cooperate with an evaluation of the circumstances that brought the patient and the trainee together. As noted earlier, all interactions during the evaluation require paying close attention to patient nonverbal behavior from the outset, especially in circumstances where discord is already created by the situation that brought the patient to the medical trainee. In these interactions, it is important to pay attention to what the patient is saying and even more critical to respond to nonverbal cues. The nonverbal cues often provide information about how the patient is feeling about the evaluation and the trainee. It is necessary to first establish an atmosphere wherein the patient feels comfortable and safe revealing himself or herself without fear of judgment or manipulation. Whether the patient is honest will be based on his or her perception that you are trustworthy and that you want to work with what he or she wants to achieve in his or her interaction with you. It is critical to recognize that the patient will be honest with a medical trainee if he or she believes the medical trainee is being genuine and transparent, even if he or she believes that the trainee does not agree about the focus of treatment.

Here is a clinical example:

TRAINEE: Dr. Jones referred you to me to talk about your use of painkillers. Is that right?

PATIENT: Yeah, he thinks I am using too much. So that's why I am here. I believe in following doctor's orders.

TRAINEE: So you are only here because Dr. Jones said you should call me.

PATIENT (SMILING): Yes, I told him I was taking what I needed to stop the pain but he said that I could overdose and it is too much and that I should talk to you and I thought, well *he is the expert.*

TRAINEE: You didn't think the dose was too much because it stopped the pain, and, at the same time, your doctor said the amount you are taking is dangerous. Have you shared your perspective with him?

PATIENT: I think I tried to once, about 3 months ago. But I remember that he cut me off and said something about getting physical therapy if I still had pain. I remember that was the day he found out I was taking more of the medication than he expected. He seemed angry and I don't remember much of the discussion that day. When I saw him after that visit, I always told him everything was fine because I thought that talking to him about medication would lead to an argument and I don't like arguing, especially with doctors. I mean you guys went to school for all these years so you must be right about these things. Anyway, I just kept taking more of it until last week when he told me that he won't give me any more medication unless I agreed to see you.

TRAINEE: Your doctor suggested a combination of medication and physical therapy about 3 months ago. You are concerned your relationship with him has not been going smoothly and you do not feel as comfortable sharing with him openly about your medication.

PATIENT: Yes, now I remember, his nurse gave me the number of a physical therapy clinic, but I never called them. And yes, I am really frustrated that I cannot have a good conversation with him.

TRAINEE: Before we discuss more, how do you feel about working together to figure out the situation with the medication? We don't have to argue just because we may have a difference of perspective. We can agree to disagree and I won't get angry and I may even end up agreeing with you about some things, if I have enough information to understand your point of view. If we do see something differently, we will talk about it until we better understand each other's perspectives. Usually, when that happens, we can find another way to work on the problem or negotiate a compromise. Most importantly, I believe *you are the expert* on you and your pain. You are the only one who knows what you are experiencing and what you think will work and what won't help you. How does that sound to you?

In this clinical scenario, the patient is giving the trainee a number of inconsistent verbal and nonverbal cues about the history of his treatment. This behavior is due to what had previously been described as "resistance" and is now considered "discord" in the relationship between the patient and the physician. Physician–patient differences regarding perspective on symptoms and coping behaviors have been historically described by physicians as "patient resistance", which connotes pathology that lies within the patient. However, Miller and Rollnick (2013) discuss how an objective view suggests that these differences are more specifically related to discord in the relationship based on prior experiences, views on the objectives of treatment, and patient ambivalence, all of which are "normal." To reduce discord in the relationship with the patient, it must be addressed early on in the encounter. Although it is not clear why the patient is doing so, he has not followed many of the physician's recommendations, despite his statement that he does so or feels he should do so. In fact, the only physician's advice he has taken is following through with the referral. It is possible that he wants to stay on the dose of medication that allows him freedom from pain without needing to attend physical therapy. Therefore, he ignored his physician's earlier recommendations until it was made clear that he would not receive any more medication unless he first sees the trainee to determine whether he is abusing the medication. It is also possible that he does not understand the risks related to staying on high doses of painkillers. The critical issue is that the patient perceives his primary physician as being angry with him and this triggered his unwillingness to talk openly with him about his medication usage. It also signaled the patient to behave in ways that emphasize his deference to your expertise as a way of ingratiating himself in an attempt to get back on his medication. The result is that neither his primary physician nor you understands the reasons for his unwillingness to follow his physician's advice about how to cope with the pain. What is needed is an empathic communication, and it will only occur when you address the patient's misunderstanding that you will become angry with him if he tells you anything that you disagree with. In this encounter, a constructive relationship based on more like a partnership rather than the expert/recipient roles (refraining from persuading and confronting) more likely allows the patient to share openly about his concerns and work collaboratively with you.

ESTABLISHING SAFETY

Establishing safety is primarily related to ensuring that a patient's healthcare information is kept confidential. This means that patients must be interviewed in private, and it is your responsibility to establish a safe environment in which the patient can disclose his or her behaviors, feelings, and opinions. This could involve taking steps to stop patients, for example, from talking about their drug use or any other medical matter in public areas when confidentiality may be compromised. It is often necessary to stop patients from talking in hallways and waiting areas; the medical trainee should always be vigilant when patients can be overheard, and he or she should strongly suggest they delay talking until they are in a more secure place.

Once the setting where the interview will take place is established, you should first explain what will happen during the time he or she and the patient are together. Asking whether the patient has questions at this point is not an efficient use of time, but often patients want to discuss something about their experience before their arrival and, if necessary, you should allow this for up to several minutes. It is important not to show annoyance. Rather, it is best to be patient and empathic through the use of reflections and answer any questions posed at that time. How you handle the first few minutes of the interview and your nonverbal behavior either greatly enhances or detracts from establishing rapport. Occasionally a patient clearly wants to take more time to talk than is permissible prior to starting the evaluation. In these cases you can tactfully say that there will be time to cover such concerns later, and it is necessary now to start the formal evaluation.

THE TRANSTHEORETICAL MODEL OF CHANGE AND ITS RELATIONSHIP TO MOTIVATIONAL INTERVIEWING

Prochaska and DiClemente started their research by observing individuals who had overcome an addiction to nicotine. They noticed that change occurs on a continuum and progresses through different stages. Each individual moves through these stages at his or her own rate that is determined by the individual. The framework is identified as the transtheoretical model (TTM) or stages of change model (SCM). This model provides practitioners a framework for understanding the process of change of problem behaviors and adoption of positive behaviors. The conception of stages of change has had a major impact on the treatment of substance use disorders. Individuals differ in their readiness to change. If we understand change as a process, then we can report positive changes each time an individual progresses from one stage to the next. TTM can be used to match interventions to appropriate stages of change. The TTM can be applied to a broad range of behavior change areas, including drug abuse, eating and weight disorders, gambling, exercise, and condom use.

The TTM views change as a process involving progress through a series of five stages:

- Precontemplation
- Contemplation
- Preparation
- Action
- Maintenance

The change process is cyclical, and individuals typically move back and forth between the stages and cycle through the stages at different rates. Individuals can move through stages quickly or slowly. Sometimes they move so rapidly that it is difficult to pinpoint where they are because change is a dynamic process. However, some individuals may get stuck in the early stages. A person's level of motivation is related to a specific action or outcome. Individuals who use multiple drugs present with different levels of motivation. For example, a patient might be highly motivated (in the action stage) to quit heroin, ambivalent (in the contemplation stage) about reducing alcohol use, and uninterested in quitting marijuana (in the precomtemplation stage).

Motivational interviewing (MI) facilitates behavior change partly by accepting and meeting the patient's current level of readiness for change. This is consistent with the TTM. In fact, MI and TTM share a common heritage. Although TTM is frequently associated with MI, no theory links the two. The stages provided "a logical way to think about the clinical role of MI, and MI in turn provided a clear example of how clinicians could help people to move from pre-contemplation and contemplation to preparation and action" (Miller & Rollnick, 2009, pg. 130). TTM "is intended to provide a comprehensive conceptual model of how and why changes occur, whereas MI is a specific clinical method to enhance personal motivation for change" (Miller & Rollnick, 2009, pg. 130). Using MI does not depend on assigning people to a specific stage of change. Thus, MI is not based on the TTM.

Figure 4.1 contains a brief description of each stage.

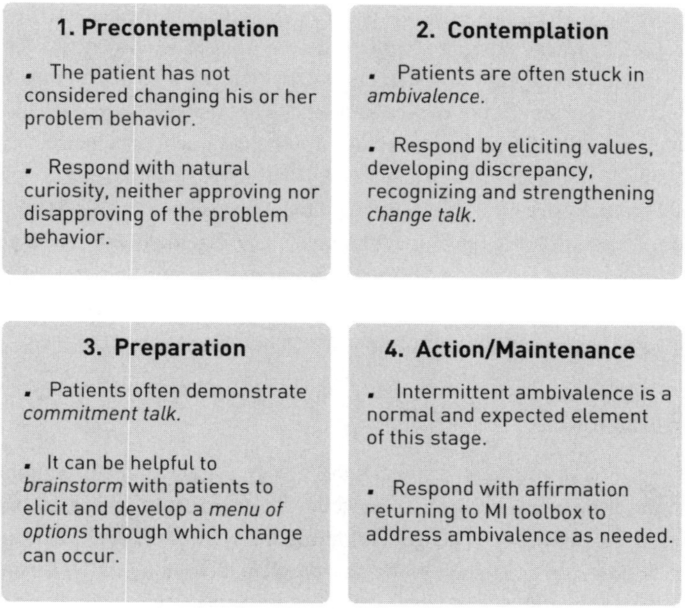

1. Precontemplation	2. Contemplation
• The patient has not considered changing his or her problem behavior. • Respond with natural curiosity, neither approving nor disapproving of the problem behavior.	• Patients are often stuck in *ambivalence*. • Respond by eliciting values, developing discrepancy, recognizing and strengthening *change talk*.

3. Preparation	4. Action/Maintenance
• Patients often demonstrate *commitment talk*. • It can be helpful to *brainstorm* with patients to elicit and develop a *menu of options* through which change can occur.	• Intermittent ambivalence is a normal and expected element of this stage. • Respond with affirmation returning to MI toolbox to address ambivalence as needed.

FIGURE 4.1   Stages of change.

Precontemplation

The patient who is in the precontemplative stage about change may not even see his or her behavior as a problem. An individual in this stage does not usually seek treatment for the specified problem behavior. Sometimes the problem behavior comes up as a related condition when the individual presents for treatment for something else, such as presenting to the emergency room for treatment of abrasions and a head injury sustained when falling down the stairs after drinking too much alcohol. Or the individual may find his or her way into treatment because a loved one has insisted on it, or perhaps as a result of a legal consequence where treatment is mandated by the court. The individual will often use language that suggests change is not a priority. Here are some examples of statements that suggest the individual is in the precontemplative stage:

- "The only problem I have with alcohol is not having enough of it."
- "I feel so creative and free when I smoke marijuana. I get my best grades on it ... I'm not going to change that."
- "Smoking a cigarette is the only time I have for myself all day, and I am not about to give that up with all the stress I have to deal with."
- "I have already heard every reason to stop using pot, but it helps me relax and it helps my pain ... I just don't want to give it up."

Precontemplation is best approached by asking for more information about the patient's thinking at the time of the encounter. As Rollnick stated, it is often important to present yourself as having a "curious or itchy mind" in relation to what patients discuss. It is necessary to proceed with patients in the precontemplation stage in this manner so that you are viewed as neither approving nor disapproving of their behavior. Patients often expect to hear disapproval from physicians, especially if they have encountered it with parents, spouses, friends, or others. The tradition in healthcare has been to immediately attempt to point out and correct what is perceived to be a behavior that is contradictory to a healthy lifestyle. Intense arguments by the trainee for change often undermine the patient's engagement in the change process. As discussed earlier in Chapter 2, this tendency to use direct persuasion and "take up" the argument for change is called the "righting reflex." When trainees engage in the righting reflex with patients who do not view their behavior as problematic, the patient focuses on defending his or her position. This causes several problems, including hampering engagement and creating discord, as well as keeping the trainee away from learning more about how the patient views his or her behavior. It is critical to understand each patient's perspective on his or her behavior before discussing the appropriate interventions.

Contemplation

The contemplation stage of change is characterized by encounters where we hear a patient making ambivalent statements which often follow the form of stating a reason for changing (pro-change argument or change talk), using the word "but," and following with a statement which supports maintaining the problem behavior (counterchange argument or maintaining status quo). The marker of contemplation is *ambivalence* (which is indeed progress compared to the prior precontemplative stage). This individual can be recognized as someone who engages in a certain kind of *self-talk*. He or she articulates reasons for changing problematic behavior (pro-change argument) but then articulates a reason that weighs significantly in favor of continuing it (counterchange argument). The following statements are expressed by patients in the contemplative stage:

- "The biggest problem is how much money pot costs, but without pot I can't function at my job anyway."
- "My gambling has seriously hurt my wife and children, but given all this stress, it is the only outlet that I have for fun."
- "Alcohol may be making me more irritable and anxious, but I am so nervous at parties it is the only way I can have fun when I want to be social."

MI theorists and practitioners have written about the types of techniques that help patients move from the contemplation stage to preparation or action stages. These include focusing on the patient's reasons to change while not ignoring his or her reasons for maintaining the status quo. Exercises such as the readiness rulers and decisional balance are structured ways of doing this. They allow the patient to experience the "big picture" of problematic behavior. These strategies will be reviewed later in the book.

Individuals may ask for more information about interventions as they consider maintaining versus changing a behavior. They are often motivated to seek ways to change that they believe are easier, faster, or that are both evidence-based and seem more expedient compared to ones they have already considered. Here is an example: "My father was able to quit smoking, but I just don't have the same willpower he had. You said that the patch works best if I go to counseling, but will it work if I just want to use it and skip the counseling?"

This clinical example illustrates the patient's thinking processes in the contemplation stage and the use of MI skills to address patient's ambivalence about quitting smoking:

PATIENT: I swear I am going to quit smoking and I make a commitment every night to not smoke the next day, but I want one so badly when I first get up in the morning that I can't control myself. Then I tell myself I'll have one and no more the rest of the day. But once I start, I feel like I have failed and it doesn't matter, so I go back to smoking my usual pack a day.

TRAINEE: I recall you said that you threw away your cigarettes and you don't have any in your home.

PATIENT: Well, I don't, but there is a convenience store across the street and I just go there and get them. They are more expensive there but when I want one, it is so bad that I don't care how much they cost. I just don't have the willpower.

TRAINEE: You give in to a strong impulse with the idea that you'll change your behavior the rest of the day. Smoking even one cigarette causes you to feel as though there is no reason to follow through with your plan not to smoke for the rest of the day. So the most important problem is that your physical urges are stronger than your capacity to resist.

PATIENT: Yes, that's about it. If I just didn't have that first one, I think I would feel so good about having accomplished not smoking first thing in the morning that my commitment not to smoke would be stronger throughout the rest of the day. It's just that when I get up, I start going through the motions and it includes having that first cigarette.

TRAINEE: Having that first cigarette is a major part of your routine. How might you vary your routine?

PATIENT: I don't know. I never really thought about it.

TRAINEE: What's your usual morning routine?

PATIENT: I get up and put coffee on. It takes about 15 minutes to brew. During that time I take a shower and get dressed. Then I get coffee, and I have my first cigarette with it. I have something to eat, and I usually have about 20 minutes to read the paper. I'll have some more coffee and maybe have another cigarette. Then I need to get out the door to work.

TRAINEE: Having a cigarette with coffee is the way you start your morning. How does smoking fit in with your commute to work?

PATIENT: I don't smoke in my car. People complain about it, and I know it lowers the resale value for when I want to trade it in. I won't do that.

TRAINEE: When you have a strong reason to avoid smoking, you are able to stick with it. How does smoking fit in with the rest of your day?

PATIENT: Sometimes I get a chance right before work, but if I don't, it's at my break around 9:30 a.m.

TRAINEE: Your plan to stop smoking could work if you found a way to change your morning routine so you don't have the opportunity at home to smoke when having coffee and breakfast. How could you change that?

PATIENT: Well, I guess I could decide to have coffee out. I could go right to the shower and leave the house right after I get dressed. There are some fast food places I could hit on the way to work.

TRAINEE: You are considering a different strategy to help you not smoke. You could even take the time to read the paper, and you wouldn't be able to smoke because restaurants are smoke-free.

PATIENT: Yes, but I am thinking ahead here. I am thinking that I could just go outside of the restaurant and smoke if I have an urge that is bad enough.

TRAINEE: Well, you are making a valid point that could also apply to many other situations you encounter during the day. But you said if you could get past having that first cigarette when you first get up, you believe it would help your self-confidence for not smoking at other times. You talked about bargaining with yourself—that you will have just one and no more the rest of the day. How would dealing with the urge to smoke in the restaurant be different than dealing with the urge to smoke the first cigarette in the morning?

PATIENT: I would probably think, hey I have made it this far, and I would want to see how much further I could go without smoking. That might work.

Preparation

The individual who is in the preparation stage of change is more likely to utter explicit change talk as well as express behaviors that signal change is imminent. The individual in this stage has made a commitment to change. This individual may buy a dieting book as part of preparing to lose weight or buy a nicotine replacement kit as a step toward quitting smoking.

Action

The individual in this stage believes in his or her ability to change the behavior and to take steps toward change. Individuals may present with specific questions about how to continue to make or maintain the changes they have already determined they want to make. Although much of the new material they present is likely to be positive, because they are moving forward, trainees must be prepared for dealing with negative outcomes or experiences of temporary failure. It is important to remember that even people in the action stage of change will be having new experiences, including challenges and perhaps temporary failures that continue to affect their perspective on the original goals. The critical issue is that change is a dynamic process and ambivalence is "normal," meaning that it is expected to kick in anytime throughout the process of change. Recalling what the patient presented earlier, it is quite possible that the amount of energy expended in accomplishing the goal of not smoking at home in the morning will bring to consciousness how hard the struggle is to stop smoking completely and result in discomfort over that negative emotion after "achieving" his goal, which may lead to even stronger cravings to smoke.

Maintenance

Maintenance involves the individual proactively working to prevent any return to the unhealthy behavior. Individuals in this stage consolidate the change into a lifestyle that can sustain the change.

CORE MOTIVATIONAL INTERVIEWING SKILLS: OARS

As we reviewed earlier, the essence of MI lies in its spirit. Built upon the foundation of the spirit are the four processes we outlined. To carry out the four processes, there are four core therapeutic skills. They are summarized by the acronym OARS (Open questions, Affirmations, Reflections, and Summaries) and are largely derived from the person-centered approach. The primary goal in MI is to elicit change talk, and the skills to be discussed are designed to achieve that purpose. It is important to remember that OARS does not describe a linear process of conducting the clinical encounter. Rather, these communication skills are used throughout a clinical encounter to promote engagement, establish trust, and evoke change.

These are defined and described in the following sections.

Open-Ended Questions

"An open-ended question is like an open door"—one that opens the door of conversation and invites patients to consider their thoughts carefully before answering. When asking an open-ended question, think about it as a request to explore with the patient the issues that he or she finds most important or most emotionally significant. It is an invitation for patients to "tell their stories." And most important, when asking open-ended questions, the trainee must be willing to carefully listen to the patient's response (see Fig. 4.2).

Tips

- Rhythm: start by asking one open-ended question, followed by one or two reflections based on the patient's answer to the question, then follow with another open-ended question. Aim for a 2:1 or 3:1 ratio of reflections to questions.
- Avoid asking several questions in a row. Even when they are open ended, too many questions in a row can lead to patient defensiveness or settling back into a passive role.
- "How" and "what" are the easiest question stems with which to start open-ended questions. They help us avoid asking close-ended questions such as those that start with "can," "do," "have," "will," "when," "could," and "did" (and they help us to avoid using the word "why").
- Ask the patient to elaborate more by saying, "Tell me more about that" or "Describe for me. . ." or "Walk me through a typical day" or "Paint me a picture of. . ." or "Help

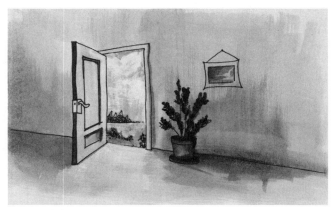

FIGURE 4.2 Open-ended questions.

me understand. . ." These statements function like open-ended questions by inviting the patients to elaborate more about their experiences or perspectives.

- Avoid or limit your use of close-ended questions that close down a conversation or might result in a one- or two-word answer, except for those that ask for permission.

Open-Ended Question Starters

Do use words that invite talking:

- What. . .? For example, What was it like? What will you do. . .? What did you think about. . .? What is your take on . . . ?
- How. . .? For example, How did you feel about. . .? How did you like. . .? How do you plan to. . .?
- Tell me about. . .
- Describe for me. . .

Avoid using words that start close-ended questions:

- Can you? Could you? Do you? Have you? Did you? Will you? Should you? Where did you. . .? How long or how many? When did you. . .? Who?

Except to *ask permission* to give information or advice:

- Is it okay if. . ..? Would you mind if. . .? May I tell you about. . .? Would it be okay if?

Examples of open-ended question stems using "what":

- "What is that like for you?" (a simple, powerful question that suggests that you want to know about another's experience from his or her own frame of reference—an empathic question by definition)
- "What is your understanding of. . ."
  - "What is your understanding of the events that led to your seeking help?"
  - "What is your understanding of what contributed to your not taking medications. . .?"
- "What are your thoughts regarding. . .?"
  - "What are your thoughts regarding your decision to pursue treatment now?"
  - "What are your thoughts regarding your using marijuana?"
  - "What are your thoughts regarding how you managed stress in the past?"
- "What are you like when you (negative behavior)?"
  - "What are you like when you drink?"
  - "What are you like when you. . .?"
- "In what other circumstances do you see yourself . . . (negative behavior)?"
  - "In what other circumstances do you see yourself acting out of anger?"
  - "In what other circumstances do you see yourself not exercising to manage your stress?"

- "What would you need to change in order for you to ... (positive behavior/goal)?"
  - "What would you need to change in order for you to live the life you would like to have?"
  - "What would you need to change in order for you to achieve the goals you have set?"

Examples of open-ended question stems using "how":

- "How do you feel about. . .?"
  - "How do you feel about your weight gain?"
  - "How do you feel about your relationship with alcohol?"
- "How were you able to. . .?"
  - "How were you able to successfully lose weight in the past?"
- "How do you see your ... to be related to your. . .?"
  - "How do you see your depression to be related to your substance use?"
  - "How do you see your eating habits to be related to your lifestyle at home?"
- "How would you like your life to be different?"

There are also some open-ended questions you can ask that direct the patient to acknowledge his or her own sense of agency and autonomy:

- "What was in you that changed?"
- "What did you draw on within yourself to make that different decision?"
- "How were you able to gather the courage to make that change within yourself?"
- "How have your inner strengths helped you in the past in tough situations?"

Examples of open-ended questions in contrast to close-ended questions:

- "I understand you are struggling with your drinking, how has it been affecting you?"

Versus

- "Is your drinking affecting you?"

Another example:

- "What has your relationship with your children been like?"

Versus

- "Do you have a good relationship with your children?"

Affirmations

To affirm is to accentuate the positive by being supportive and encouraging people's personal goals. Affirming overlaps with empathy in two ways: by being genuine and meeting people where they are through understanding their personal frames of reference. Affirmations can comment on an inner strength or personal attribute, a positive past step or behavior, or an attempt to change behavior. A well-formulated affirmation puts into words what you have found is "right" with your patient, rather than what is wrong.

Tips

- Start statements with "you."
- Avoid "I" statements in affirmation (e.g., avoid "I am proud of you"). By placing "I" in statements, it takes the focus away from the patient and makes the statement more about "ingratiating" than affirming.

Examples of affirming statements focusing on a patient's "specific efforts":

- "You have worked hard to do the right thing, despite how hard it is."
- "You have been successful in sharing your thoughts and being truthful about your emotions."
- "You feel proud of yourself for being able to control your diabetes."
- "You are really eager for guidance and treatment; for you, part of recovery is asking for help."

Examples of affirming statements focusing on a patient's "specific qualities":

- "You have had some significant setbacks in following through with your goals. At the same time, you still continue in treatment. You are so determined."
- "You have been through a lot of struggles in your life. You are a survivor."
- "When you set your mind to something, you make it happen."

Examples of affirming statements communicating a "genuine value" of a person:

- "You have shared so many strong feelings with me."
- "Thank you for sharing your struggles with me."

Reflections

Reflective listening is a core component of MI. The goal of reflecting is to make a best guess at the underlying emotion and desires in a patient's statement. It can be conceptualized as a way of testing hypothesis. It is the primary method of building "accurate empathy." Relatedly, reflective listening functions to deepen communication between the trainee and the patient and to deepen the patient's self-understanding of the many aspects of what contributes to his or her struggle with change. It may appear to be misleadingly easy. In fact, it is likely the most difficult MI skill for medical trainees to master. If reflections are not done appropriately and genuinely as statements, they tend to create discord in the therapeutic relationship, making the patient less likely to open up. At the same time, even when reflections are not stating the accurate hypothesis, through the process of correcting the trainee, patients may clarify their perspective and emotions without affecting the therapeutic relationship. Reflections involve different levels of complexity and depth.

Broadly speaking, there are two types of reflections: simple and complex.

Simple Reflections

Repeat or rephrase in different words the same meaning or emotion of a patient's statement.

While useful in establishing rapport with the patient, simple reflections do not add to the content of the conversation, and this tends to yield slower progress within the engagement process.

Complex Reflections

Add to the underlying meaning or unexpressed emotions that the patient might be meaning or feeling.

Reflecting the feelings that were verbally expressed by the patient, such as saying, "You feel ashamed," "You are feeling depressed," after a patient has said, "I feel so embarrassed about this," or "I feel really down." This is a deep form of listening.

Complete the paragraph with what you think the patient would say next.

May reflect two sides of what the patient is feeling or thinking and conveying that the trainee heard the reasons for and against change (double-sided reflection).

Focus and emphasize the underlying emotion and the unspoken content of the conversation.

Can be used to amplify or reinforce desire for change.

They help the patient view his or her effort, even if not resulting in major success, as a positive step forward indicative of a commitment rather than failure. This is an example: "You included working out in the gym as the only physical activity and you excluded walking back and forth to work and working in your yard three times a week."

Accurate complex reflections help to move the therapeutic conversation forward.

Tips

- Start reflections with "you." Reflections beginning with the generic phrases of "it sounds like. . ." or "it seems like. . ." or "what I hear you saying. . ." can be annoying if they are repetitive.
- Name the emotion. Even if you get it wrong, patients appreciate that you are trying to understand them and their perspective.
- Be brief. Reflection should not be longer than the statement it follows.
- Be selective. Emphasize content or process that would be helpful for the patient in self-understanding and evoking change.
- Take risks. Make an educated guess regarding the underlying reasons for their experiences and their current readiness for change.
- Do not be afraid to be wrong in offering the reflection. Choose the reflection from a point of empathy and desire for more understanding. We have found that even when we are wrong, patients will correct us and continue forward. Either way, we understand more and continue to move forward with the patient.
- Establish rhythm: follow reflective statements with an open-ended question. Such as "What do you think about that?" or "What is your perspective?" or "What do you make of that?"

- Watch your tone of voice. A deflection in the tone of the reflection keeps it as a reflection. An inflection in tone is often a question masquerading as a reflection.
- Avoid letting your lack of confidence or certainty about the content of your reflection result in your tone drifting upward at the end of the reflection, which can turn a well-formulated reflection into a question.

Examples of simple reflecting statement stems and how to advance them to complex reflecting statements:

PATIENT: "I am concerned about my diabetes not being well controlled after I got my blood work today. I have changed my diet and I take my medications as I am supposed to, but I am not sure what else I could do."

Possible reflections:

- You are. . .

SIMPLE: "You are worried about your diabetes."
COMPLEX: "You are very frustrated about not being able to have better control over your diabetes despite doing your best."
SIMPLE: "You are not sure what else to do."
COMPLEX: "You are struggling with figuring out what else you could do to improve your diabetes."

- You feel. . .

SIMPLE: "You feel concerned."
COMPLEX: "You feel frustrated about not being able to see your diabetes controlled after you made changes in your diet and you're taking your medications appropriately."

Examples of more complex reflections:

- "On one hand, you feel you have done all you could do to control your diabetes and on the other hand, you want to figure out what else you need to do."
- "You care so much about controlling your diabetes and you want to figure out what else you could work on changing to help you better control it and live a healthier life."

Troubleshooting Related to Reflections

Going Around in Circles
Sometimes it feels like the conversation is going around in circles and getting nowhere. It is likely that the reflections are too simple and not assisting the conversation in moving forward.

Tips

- Use more complex reflecting statements.
- Acknowledge the challenge of opening up and sharing thoughts/emotions.

Overshooting/Undershooting It is common to either overshoot or undershoot when learning how to accurately reflect.

Tips

- Don't get frustrated.
- Be a careful listener. If a patient disagrees with your reflective statement, this is a perfect point to ask for further clarification by saying, "Help me understand this from your perspective."
- It is generally better to undershoot than to overshoot, because undershooting invites correction and more elaboration of a problem while overshooting tends to generate sustain (or status quo) talk. For example, reflecting, "This is becoming a little bit of a problem in your life," or "This is a bit annoying to you," is more likely to evoke a response about how much of a problem a behavior is than to say, "This is a huge problem for you," or "This is the worst thing that ever happened to you."

Summaries

Summarizing is essentially a collection of reflections that pulls together a number of points made during the clinical encounter. They are special applications of reflective listening. The goal of summarizing is to foster the therapeutic relationship, to help the patients organize their thoughts, to expand the ongoing conversation, and to move the conversation forward by setting the stage for evoking change. Essentially, to make a good summary statement, think about conveying to the patient: "I have heard what you have said, here is how I understand it, and I want to continue to understand more."

There are three types of summaries: collecting summaries, linking summaries, and transitional summaries.

Collecting Summaries

Collecting summaries are a list of interrelated items that the patient shared. They usually occur in the midst of a clinical encounter.

"You have shared about a number of issues you would like to work on in your life. You want a better relationship with your children and to be a happier person. You also talked about going back to school and finishing your degree."

Tips

- Simple and complex reflections can be followed by "emptying questions" such as asking, "What else?" repeatedly with alternating reflections until the patient's exploration of the topic is fully exhausted. This serves as an invitation to keep adding to the collecting summary list.
- Collecting summaries can be combined with affirmations by listing personal qualities and attributes as well as past efforts at behavior change that evoke patients' confidence for future change:

"You have talked about yourself as a stubborn person, one who sticks to his guns when it comes to challenges in your life. At the same time, you see yourself as a good person who cares a lot about other people. You are also a hopeful person who sees the positives in others." Collecting summary such as this can be followed by an emptying question, for example, "What other strengths do you see yourself having?"

Linking Summaries

Linking summaries are statements that link the current conversation to something else that the patient has previously said at this or at a prior clinical encounter. Linking summaries further strengthen change talk by finding overarching themes and core values in the patient's path of change.

"You find joy in life's little moments, such as drinking a cup of coffee with your wife. That is not unlike something else that you shared earlier in our conversations; you talked about how much you enjoyed reading a good book. You really value life and you have missed finding satisfactions, great and small, in your life."

Tips

- Anatomy of simple linking summary: Reflect-link-reflect. Begin with a brief reflection of the present conversation, then follow with a linking statement, and then another reflection of a past conversation. Examples of linking statements:

"What you said reminded me of something you had shared earlier."
"The way you feel now about (current topics) is similar to the reaction you had with another experience you shared."

- Can conclude with a statement that synthesizes the overarching theme.
- Can be followed by a statement that emphasizes a patient's core values.
- Can be combined with an open-ended question to evoke further change talk.

Transitional Summaries

Transitional summaries are a collection of statements and reflections that emphasize the key points of the present conversation while signaling a shift to a new framework of conversation. This type of summary promotes therapeutic progress and at the same time provides the patient with the option for further discussion before moving on from current conversation.

Tips

- Anatomy of simple transitional summary: Orient-reflect-empty.
- Begin with an orienting statement/question, signaling/seeking permission to pull things together. "Before we talk about. . ., is it okay if I share with you my understanding of. . .?"

For example, "Before we talk about the next step you might like to take in your treatment, is it okay if I share with you my understanding of your current struggles with smoking?"

- End with an emptying question, inviting the patient to bring up anything that has not been mentioned thus far.

"What else you would you like to talk about before we discuss. . .?"
"What other thoughts do you have regarding what we have talked about thus far?"

Another type of transitional summary can end with a key question to signal a change in direction, perhaps toward change: Orient-reflect-use transitional open-ended question.

- Begin with orienting statement/question, followed by a grand summary of important motivating points and with signaling a change in direction.

"Before we move on to discussing what you might want to do next, I would like to review what I think I heard you say thus far and find out from you whether I have it right. . ." Summarize key points, wait for any response, and then say, "So where do you want to go from here?" or "What is your next step?"

AGENDA MAPPING

Now that we have learned how to engage through using OARS, the next step is to learn another tool, which is the agenda mapping ("What to change?"). Agenda mapping through the process of focusing allows the trainee to enter the patient's world and understand the patient's internal frame of reference while balancing the need for therapeutic progression (Fig. 4.3). While thinking about agenda mapping through the process of focusing, it can be helpful in thinking about the process of agenda mapping as operating via agenda sources, styles of focusing, and focusing scenarios.

Agenda Sources

At any point in a clinical encounter, there are three agenda sources at work. While the focus should always be on the patient, these are sources the medical trainee must take into account in the process.

Patient

The critical content here is that the patient brings his or her own internal frame of reference to all therapeutic encounters, and without exploring and entering into the patient's world, it would be impossible to find common ground for the therapeutic communication. The content often includes a blending of the patient's agenda with his or her feelings about the encounter and the trainee.

Setting

The setting refers to where the interaction is occurring and may depend on the specific pre-determined focus of the setting, such as a smoking cessation or family planning clinic. This includes how the request for service may be affected by agency/clinic policy. For example, parents who take their child to an emergency room to address a child's injury may become concerned about the trainee's decision to report the injury to Child Protective Services.

Clinical

The overt agenda here is that the trainee's expertise may help the patient explore other changes necessary to achieve his or her stated goals. This may also include a blending of the trainee's agenda with his or her feelings about the clinical encounter and the patient.

Styles of Focusing

There are three focusing styles that the medical trainee can use to facilitate agenda mapping.

Directing

- The trainee directs the focus of the conversation by essentially dictating and teaching a therapeutic curriculum, which suggests to the patient that he or she has limited power in this therapeutic interaction and decision making.
- While effective in establishing a focus and particularly effective in establishing a focus consistent with an agency's "agenda," "directing" has limited effectiveness in enhancing a patient's sense of self-efficacy and evoking change. It is best utilized in an emergency medical encounter where the medical trainee needs to take control of the situation to ensure that the patient gets urgent care, such as when a patient loses consciousness or requires an urgent medical procedure or is actively suicidal and safety needs to be assured first.
- This style has a limited role within the MI practice, due to its lack of person-focused empowerment.

Following

- The trainee uses a nondirective therapeutic approach and asks many open-ended questions such as:
  - "What do you think is most important to talk about today?"
  - "What concerns do you have today?"
  - "What is the most important priority you would like to engage about today?"
- The trainee follows the natural movement and momentum of the conversation as directed by the patient's agenda and does not influence the direction.
- This method of focusing yields the slowest progress in therapeutic progression.

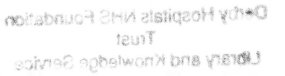

Guiding

This style is the most congruent with the spirit of MI.

Tips

- Tolerate uncertainty and ambivalence.
- Share control with the patient.
- Identify the patient's personal strengths, goals, values, and beliefs.
- Look for and enhance openings for change.

Focusing Scenarios

There are three broad spectrums of the patient's possible perspectives on agenda mapping at any point during the therapeutic encounter.

Clear Direction

- Sometimes the focus and agenda of the therapeutic encounter can be clearly defined by the patient from the onset, and this is the case in a number of scenarios.

The patient is highly motivated and focused on changing a specific behavior and asks for guidance starting at the beginning of treatment.

The therapeutic encounter occurs within a narrowly defined field, such as a smoking cessation clinic or a family planning clinic.

- If the agenda is clearly delineated from the onset, the next step would be to move toward treatment planning and management.

Choices in Direction: Agenda Mapping

- Sometimes there may be a number of possible directions to take a specific therapeutic encounter.

For example: patients may be motivated to find ways to manage their anxiety; however, they might feel overwhelmed by the various facets of anxiety in their lives, such as panic attacks, substance use, deteriorating relationships with family members, and difficulty managing professional life.

- If there are myriad possible directions, the three goals at this point are to assist the patient in structuring thinking, considering options, and choosing a focus.
- Utilizing tools for agenda mapping can be particularly useful in achieving these goals.

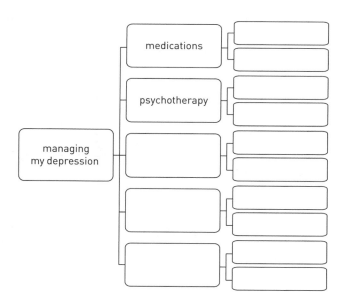

FIGURE 4.3 Agenda mapping. In this example a patient is concerned about managing her depression. She is taking her medications and attending weekly psychotherapy sessions, but she is concerned because she doesn't feel like she is improving and is considering stopping her medicine. She is also wondering what other behaviors she can focus on to better manage her depression. Agenda mapping can help to organize the conversation, to develop behavioral items she would like to focus on, and to expand upon the pros and cons of each item on the agenda.

Tools for Agenda Mapping

Questions to Promote Structured Thinking Start with either, "What makes the most sense for you to focus on right now?" or you can be more directive and ask, "Would it be okay if we talked about. . ." or "Based on what I know about you so far, may I suggest that we talk about some things in your life that relate to your … (e.g., weight, depression, alcohol use, risk of getting pregnant, uncontrolled diabetes)?"

After obtaining permission and giving some suggestions where to focus the discussion, end with "What do you think? You are the best judge of where you want to focus your attention and our discussion."

Tips to Aid in Considering Options Be comfortable with silences. Allow patients time for thought and reflection.
Be generous with summarizing statements.
Invite more options and new ideas by using emptying questions, such as: "What else can you think of?"

Questions to Encourage Choosing a Focus "Of all the things you mentioned that contribute to your … (expressed behavior), what do you think has the biggest influence and in what ways?"

"Of all of the things you listed, what worries you the most?"

"Of the topics you have come up with thus far, which one is the most difficult for you to face?"

It can be useful to use a visual aid such as a chart with circles on it that is either pre-populated with possible topics to discuss, based perhaps on the setting in which the patient is being seen, as well as some open circles in which to enter new, unanticipated topics the patient identifies; or a diagram with all open circles for the patient and medical trainee to fill in as possible topics on which to focus, based on their conversation.

Agenda mapping is particularly helpful when more than one health behavior may benefit from change, because it helps you and the patient to prioritize and focus on the one behavior that the patient agrees to target. It is important to be open and honest about your own agenda while still respecting and understanding the patient's agenda. Whenever possible, it is better to let the patient's agenda take precedence over your own agenda, even when you feel it is in the patient's best interest, because people are more likely to make successful change in the areas that they, not you as the practitioner, are most interested in changing. The goal of agenda mapping is to help the patient select a behavior to discuss and to encourage the patient to decide *what* to talk about, assisted by you. It can be helpful to write on the chart or, better yet, to have the patient fill in circles or cross out items that are not relevant or important to the patient. It is important that you do not use the chart as a checklist or use it to prematurely focus on one behavior at the expense of others.

Introduce the chart, discuss readiness to think about change, and elicit what the patient wishes to discuss.

Example: "On this sheet are some of the topics we can discuss. We could talk about contraception, ways to prevent sexually transmitted diseases, smoking, taking medications, exercising, eating, or drinking alcohol. You will be the best judge of what to consider changing. Which of these do you think we want to talk about?" "These blank spaces are for adding any other topics you think might be of greater concern to you today. What would you include in these spaces?" "What do you think? What would you like to focus on today?"

Other than the chart mentioned earlier, another visual aid that could be particularly helpful in providing a literal overview of the agenda mapping is a drawing of a timeline (Fig. 4.4) for temporal organization.

UNCLEAR DIRECTION

Having a direction first requires patients to identify a number of options from which to choose. Some patients, however, have not yet come to terms with their reasons for seeking treatment or are not yet able to verbalize their own agendas. The medical trainee's role in such an encounter is to help patients clarify their own reasons for coming to treatment as well as their specific goals of treatment. Agenda mapping involves utilizing OARS to engage and listen to the patient's story. As patients verbalize topics for discussion, the trainee can help them come to an understanding as to what, if anything, they wish to pursue in the clinical encounter.

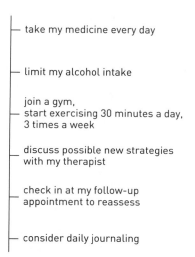

take my medicine every day

limit my alcohol intake

join a gym,
start exercising 30 minutes a day,
3 times a week

discuss possible new strategies
with my therapist

check in at my follow-up
appointment to reassess

consider daily journaling

FIGURE 4.4   Agenda mapping timeline. The patient from Figure 4.3 has now identified a series of behavioral targets she is interested in discussing. To help her prioritize these topics for further discussion, the trainee can guide the patient in developing a timeline, as earlier.

EXCHANGING INFORMATION

The earlier successful studies of MI emphasized the importance of reflective listening during the process of giving personalized feedback of test results. How information is shared with the patient can also affect how it is received. The main reason simple advice does not work is that most people do not like being told what to do, such as "If you continue smoking, you are going to have a heart attack." Rather, most patients would prefer to be engaged in a decision-making process, particularly when they are considering making a choice about changing problematic behaviors. Offering healthcare–related information to the patient should not happen unless the patient gives permission. Remember that some patients may not be interested in having you provide information. When you use scare tactics, lecture, preach, ridicule, moralize, or coerce, they risk creating discord in the relationship and jeopardizing the therapeutic work. A preferred approach to this type of encounter would be to acknowledge and respect the patient's perspective and autonomy: "I respect your decision about not being interested in discussing your behavior, and we can come back to it in the future if you want." Inviting the patient to reflect on the information you shared facilitates the discussion. Bombarding the patient with a barrage of data that we feel pressured to deliver can overwhelm the patient and negatively affect the therapeutic communication.

To share information and recommendations with a patient that is consistent with the guiding style and spirit of MI, the elicit-provide-elicit (E-P-E) is the appropriate framework. E-P-E involves a collaborative mindset when the goal is health behavior change. This approach can also be helpful in working through ambivalence related to change, agenda mapping, and treatment planning.

Elicit-Provide-Elicit (E-P-E)

This framework starts with asking the patients what they know already or are interested in knowing about a specific topic (Elicit). Once the patients share what they already know, you can build on it (Provide). This approach allows you to then reflect on the patient's view of what is offered (Elicit).

Elicit

Explore prior knowledge Examples of question stems:

- "What do you know about. . .?"
- "What is your understanding of. . .?"

Elicit existing emotions Examples of question stems:

- "How do you feel about. . .?"
- "What do you feel when you think about. . .?"

Querying interest Examples of question stems:

- "What are your thoughts about. . .?"
- "How would you describe your interest level in discussing. . .?"

Provide

- Engage first (through first eliciting before providing!).
- Use statements sparingly and keep them short and focused.
- Emphasize personal choice.
- Offer menu of options and add, "You know yourself the best, what do you think?"

Elicit

The goal is to get feedback from the patient on his or her thoughts, questions, interpretation, or understanding of the information just provided. Examples of questions to ask for the second elicit include the following:

- "What do you make of this information or these suggestions?"
- "What is your reaction about the effects of alcohol on your liver?"
- "What do you think about these strategies I shared with you to help you take your medications regularly?"
- "What do you think about what we just talked about?"
- "What do you think is the next step for you?"
- "How might what we just talked about apply to you?"

TRAINEE: What do you know about the effects of drinking alcohol on your liver? (Elicit)

PATIENT: I know it would help to understand how my hepatitis C is affected if I continue to drink.

TRAINEE: You are concerned about how your drinking can affect your liver and your hepatitis C. Would it be ok with you to share what we know about the impact of alcohol on patients with hepatitis C? (Asking permission)

PATIENT: Yeah.

TRAINEE: Drinking alcohol on a liver that is already injured by hepatitis C could damage your liver more and lead to serious consequences such as liver failure. What are you thinking now? (Provide, then Elicit)

PATIENT: So I don't think I should drink at all.

TRAINEE: I wonder if you would be interested in some strategies that other people who have hepatitis C like yourself have used to help them not drink. (Elicit)

PATIENT: I think I don't want to destroy my liver, so yes what are these strategies?

TOOLBOX

Elicit-Provide-Elicit

- Elicit (Engage, Explore)
- Provide (emphasize Personal choice)
- Elicit (Effects of your feedback)

Chunk-Check-Chunk

This is a variation on the E-P-E framework that fits more under the directing style. It is more practical when the trainee must deliver a lot of information, at the same time keeping the patient engaged in the conversation. The trainee starts with providing a "chunk" of information. After delivering the chunk, the trainee stops to check in with the patient about the information. This exchange is followed by another chunk of information. This framework helps you detect and correct misunderstanding that occurs in the clinical encounter. The following is an example of this framework.

TRAINEE: Let me share with you the sort of treatment we will provide for your diabetes. We will discuss your medication regimen and your lifestyle and explore with you the changes you want to make to help you better control your diabetes. You have shared your struggles with remembering to take your medication consistently, and you have been more depressed recently. You have been worried about your high HbA1c. We will get to know you better in the clinic. How does that sound so far? (Chunk)

PATIENT: It makes sense. I know we discussed my concerns about controlling my diabetes. (Check)

TRAINEE: That is not surprising to you.

PATIENT: Not at all.

TRAINEE: And we will also discuss strategies to address your depression and how it affects your ability to manage diabetes. I would like to see if you would be willing to involve your wife in your care. This will help us get a better perspective on your challenges in coping with diabetes. (Chunk)

PATIENT: Clearly it is important to talk about that and sure we can talk with my wife.

TRAINEE: We can figure out how to work together so you are better able to care for yourself.

PATIENT: Yes, sure.

This illustrates the chunk-check-chunk approach, where a lot of information is provided along with periodic short check-ins. The patient's responses are brief and reflected. MI skills are used throughout the exchange. At the end of the exchange, the patient is engaged and willing to work with the trainee.

TOOLBOX

Chunk-Check-Chunk – A more practical variation on E-P-E for providing more information

---

A FINAL THOUGHT

One of the most subtle but powerful skills in the toolbox is "reflection." And one of the most important parts of one's training is learning how to take risks with reflections, even in uncomfortable or emotionally fraught encounters with patients. In fact, the ability to do so can be developed by honing one's skills for reflective listening.

A middle-aged woman who appeared much older than her stated age presented the day after admission to an inpatient psychiatric ward. Not having more refined MI skills, I asked her, "What brought you into the hospital?" She said, "Been out running the streets ... you know." I didn't know. She shared more with me during the session as she told me that she had spent many recent days (and nights) using drugs and foraging in dumpsters for food. She shared with reluctance and appeared ashamed of herself. Then she also told me that she was worried about her health as she also had been prostituting herself with strangers without any protection against sexually transmitted diseases. Uncomfortable, I reassured her that we could order the relevant testing and treat her accordingly, depending on the results. But she was not reassured.

It was still so clear how ashamed she was feeling. And there was silence between us, as it was apparent she had other concerns that were at least as significant as her medical worries. "I have been away from my kids, and I have been whoring myself out for drugs instead," she said, peering up at me from beneath her hanging head. I was startled by her candor, unsure of what to do next. I had an impulse to ask a question or reassure her or even change the subject to something I was more comfortable with. But I had the sense that she wanted to know that I could accept the struggle within her that she was now sharing with me.

Unsure about the sensitive emotions of our engagement, I offered a reflection, but not without having some concerns that it would be too far ahead of ourselves or even too presumptuous on my part: "Some of the decisions you have made have not always led to your being the person you wanted to be." "That's right," she replied, "I never planned to be this person. I'm tired of being this way."

Her having the courage to be open about where she had fallen short of herself let me take the risk of meeting her where she was by using a reflection that was just a bit ahead of where we were together. Of all the issues that were to be part of our agenda during that inpatient engagement, this struggle within her was the central point around which we were able to organize our sessions together and link to other items like spokes to a hub. Even apart from the humanity that I learned from this episode, I learned that while the more technical aspects of MI (like meeting the individual where she is and focusing on an agenda) are important, the basic tools of MI (the OARS) are indispensable. By being able to use them (especially reflections), I feel more confident about facilitating those moments that might otherwise be so emotionally sensitive that I would miss facing them together with the patient who had the courage to share them with me in the first place.

SELF-ASSESSMENT QUIZ

True or False?

1. The transtheoretical model (TTM) or stages of change model (SCM) arose from the early work and development of MI.
2. When working with patients in the precontemplation stage, it is best to confront them directly regarding the negative consequences of their unhealthy behavior(s).
3. A hallmark of the contemplation stage of change is ambivalence.
4. An example of a well-formulated open-ended question is, "Can you tell me how you were able to take your medications in the past month?"
5. A good example of an affirmation is, "I'm very impressed with the work you've done, and it is clear to me that changing this behavior is very important to you."
6. Reflections may be understood as a means to test an hypothesis, and they help trainees make informed deductions regarding the underlying emotions or meanings of a patient's statements.
7. Summaries allow trainees to demonstrate that they have been listening, have understood what patients have shared, and that they are interested in exploring a patient's experiences and perceptions.
8. Three sources for agenda-setting information include patient, trainee, and clinical setting.
9. Of the three key focusing styles, MI is most closely aligned with directing.
10. Elicit-provide-elicit (E-P-E) is a framework that facilitates trainees' ability to offer an expert opinion or clinical information in a way that maintains collaboration with the patient.

Answers

1. *False.* The transtheoretical model or stages of change model was developed by Prochaska and DiClemente through their work with individuals who overcame nicotine and alcohol addiction. They identified five unique stages: precontemplation, contemplation, preparation, action, and maintenance. Although TTM shares a common heritage with MI and provides a conceptual model to understand change, there is no formal theory that links the two together.

2. *False.* A confrontational approach to patients in any stage of change will create problems. Patients often become defensive in response to confrontation, and any therapeutic alliance will be threatened. Instead, a more effective approach is to ask patients for additional information and express genuine curiosity about their present lives and how they understand the behavior of concern.

3. *True.* Ambivalence is a highly-common experience in which patients hold disparate views their behavior(s), and debate the many reasons both for and against change. Ambivalence is a defining feature of the contemplation stage and should be viewed as progress, as compared to precontemplation stage.

4. *False.* Although the second half of this question may be considered open ended, including "can you" at the beginning makes it close ended. Eliminating this restrictive phrase frames the question in an evocative way: "Tell me how you were able to take your medicine over the past month." This is now a fine open-ended question that encourages this patient to elaborate on past successes in following medication routines.

5. *False.* Although this statement may be well intentioned, the use of "I" statements in affirmations is discouraged; they shift focus away from a patient's experience and have the potential to be perceived as ingratiating or patronizing. Remember that MI is patient-centered; affirmations are best when they begin with "you."

6. *True.* Reflections allow trainees to demonstrate active listening, enhance communication, and encourage further exploration of a patient's experiences and feelings.

7. *True.* Summaries confirm active listening and function as helpful transitions. Collecting statements gather and organize interrelated elements that a patient has shared. Linking summaries allow trainees to identify themes within a patient's conversation by linking components in the present conversation with topics or points shared by the patient earlier in the same conversation or perhaps on previous occasions. Transition summaries capture key points within the present conversation and subtly shift focus to a different thread of conversation.

8. *True.* Although a patient always remains at the center of treatment, it is helpful to take into account the setting in which an interaction takes place and a trainee's degree of clinical expertise. Together, these three sources contribute to the creation of an appropriate agenda.

9. *False.* As discussed in Chapter 2, MI is a guiding style that falls between directing and following, when viewed along a continuum of communication styles. With a directing approach, trainees dictate the progress and topic of the exchange, whereas following is a passive approach.

10. *True.* The patient-centered quality of an exchange may easily be compromised when trainees behave as clinical experts. When sharing knowledge and information with patients, the elicit-provide-elicit framework ensures that attention remains where is should be: on the patient. This technique works in three ways: determining what a patient needs or wants to learn about a particular topic; sharing the relevant information; and asking the patient for his or her thoughts and impressions of the material that was shared.

5 Motivational Interviewing in Practice

The fundamental encounter of any healthcare setting occurs between an individual seeking care and the person whose duty it is to alleviate suffering and promote health. Within the context of motivational interviewing (MI), each of these two individuals assumes a significant role within a highly dynamic process directed toward initiating behavior change, while at the same time respecting patient autonomy. MI affirms each patient's capacity to identify problematic behaviors and to select from a range of possibilities those initiatives most likely to bring about and sustain healthy alternatives. This chapter incorporates the core behaviors discussed in previous chapters and expected of MI-experienced trainees: a patient-centered approach, the clear expression of clinical empathy, the use of collaborative language, and the evocation of goal-directed communication.

A PATIENT-CENTERED APPROACH

The concept of patient-centered care assumes that each patient is more than a needy recipient of care: He or she is an individual who lives and works within a context unique to each person's circumstances and existence. Indeed, MI views patients themselves as the true "experts" of their lives, and integrating MI into everyday practice demands that we listen, respect, inform, and involve our patients throughout the course of care. As discussed in earlier chapters, this approach is not without its challenges, particularly in those situations in which we as trainees do not agree with a patient's views or decisions.

Patient-centered care fits perfectly with evidence-based medicine and allows trainees to relinquish the authoritarian style of the past in favor of a more collaborative approach between partners. An essential component is to learn to be mindful of our own subtle verbal and nonverbal cues, as well as those of our patients; equally important is to actively encourage each patient to become a full participant in his or her care.

Sharing information with patients should be designed to facilitate meaningful deliberation and shared decision-making, and it should be tailored to each individual's needs. Although the specific mechanisms by which patient-centered care contributes to improved outcomes are not yet clear, MI has demonstrated significant positive effects with regard to adherence to treatment regimens and self-management plans. Many patients also express reduced anxiety and greater interest in collaboration when MI is used. Some trainees worry that collaborating with patients implies a reduction in the importance of clinical judgment, but this is not the case. Situations remain in which physicians need to, and must assume control, as in any emergency situation. MI allows trainees to use a panoply of therapeutic communication skills that, in combination with clinical judgment, provides for the greatest likelihood of significant and long-lasting behavior change.

Clinical empathy is an essential element of the high-quality care that is associated with improved patient satisfaction and adherence to treatment recommendations; it is a hallmark of a strong physician–patient relationship. Despite some overlap with other caring responses, particularly sympathy, empathy is a unique concept. Sympathy involves the sharing of emotions between an impartial observer and a person who is suffering. In contrast, clinical empathy is defined as the effort of a skilled observer to genuinely understand the world from the perspective of a person who is suffering, which in turn, leads to a sensitive, attuned response from that observer. What differentiates this response from how one might react to family and friends is that it occurs within a therapeutic framework characterized by specific goals and outcomes.

To accurately understand our patients' experiences, we must listen and be present with them in their distress and suffering. "Caring" and "understanding" are among the words most commonly used to describe ideal physicians, and they indicate the high priority most people place upon a physician's bedside manner. We begin to approach this standard of care by expressing genuine curiosity and interest in learning and understanding how our patients have struggled, and this desire to learn is central to an empathic encounter. Active listening enables us to offer astute reflections and, in doing so, demonstrates that we understand not only what our patients express but how they feel. Participants in any meaningful exchange of information—whether between family members, friends, business partners, or romantic partners—are reassured to know that their statements have been validated and understood, and our patients are no different in this regard. Moreover, by creating an atmosphere of empathy and support, we enhance the development of trust with our patients, which in turn fosters increasingly honest and open discussions, even concerning the thoughts, behaviors, and beliefs with which we will disagree.

Most physicians and trainees struggle with identifying and responding to "empathic opportunities" in which negative emotions are expressed. In response to patients with advanced cancer expressing negative emotions such as fear, anger, or depression, for example, "I've got absolutely nothing to look forward to," a group of oncologists responded in an empathetic way only 22% of the time, using "a continuer" allowing the patients to keep expressing their struggles. Rather than acknowledging these challenging emotions, most of the specialists in this sample chose to redirect the discussion to other aspects of medical care, such as potential changes in therapy, using a "terminator" that could make the patient less open about emotional experiences. When oncologists demonstrated improved empathy, patients reported greater satisfaction with individual visits and with the overall patient–doctor relationship.

In any specialty area of medicine, accurate empathic responses in the form of a reflection can direct conversations forward, even in the absence of further questioning. Remember that remaining nonjudgmental is essential to seeing a situation through the eyes of a patient and to understanding how a particular set of behaviors has evolved.

This following exchange is representative of scenarios in which medical trainees either cannot or will not understand a patient's reasons for not taking medications as prescribed. Lacking an accurate comprehension of the patient's struggles makes it almost impossible to identify appropriate interventions.

Scenario 1

TRAINEE: Hi, John, how can I help you today?

PATIENT: Um, I don't know but I've had a hard time breathing, and I can't walk like I used to.

TRAINEE: How long has this been going on?

PATIENT: For the past couple of weeks.

TRAINEE: How long are you able to walk without stopping due to shortness of breath?

PATIENT: Maybe I can go one block or two, but I just can't play with my grandkids like I used to.

TRAINEE: Have you been taking your lung medications?

PATIENT: Well, not really, my schedule has just been so hectic.

TRAINEE: Do you think you could make a commitment to taking those medications since doing so would help with your breathing trouble?

PATIENT: Yeah, I think I could try.

In Scenario 2, reflective listening facilitates empathic understanding of the patient's struggles to adhere to a medication regimen and leads to a negotiated approach concerning recommendations.

Scenario 2

TRAINEE: Hi, John, what made you decide to come in today? (Open-ended question)

PATIENT: Well, doc, I've had a hard time breathing lately, and I can't walk like I used to.

TRAINEE: Your trouble breathing has made it hard for you to do activities that you usually enjoy. (Complex reflection)

PATIENT: Yeah, I mean, I can't even go two blocks like I used to and I can't play with my grandkids for as long.

TRAINEE: Playing with your grandkids is something you really love doing and your trouble breathing is making that hard for you. I understand you were doing better for a while. What are your thoughts about what might be contributing to this now? (Complex reflections followed by an open-ended question)

PATIENT: Well, it's really just been the last two weeks, since I haven't been taking my lung medications.

TRAINEE: You've noticed it is getting worse since you stopped taking your medications. (Complex reflection)

PATIENT: Yes. Everything has just been so hectic at home and I haven't been able to pick them up.

TRAINEE: You've been so busy that remembering to pick up and take your medications has been a challenge. Help me understand what has affected your ability to do so. (Complex reflection followed by an open-ended question)

PATIENT: There's a lot going on, but the main problem is that I lost my job and I just don't have the money to pay for them. Not to mention that I babysit my grandkids, so it's not easy to just find another job. And I love being with the kids, but I just don't have the wind in me anymore.

TRAINEE: You haven't been able to afford your medications and it's been hard to find another job with your grandkids at home. And at the same time, you see the importance of finding a way to get your medications because without them, you're not able to do some of the activities you enjoy. So, you decided to come in so we can figure out a solution together. (Summary)

PATIENT: Exactly, I don't have the money, but I know I need them; otherwise, I can't enjoy the things that mean the most to me.

TRAINEE: You want to be able to participate actively in some aspects of your life that are most important to you. What ideas did you have about getting medications? (Complex reflection followed by an open-ended question)

PATIENT: Well, maybe there's some kind of financial aid, in the short term.

TRAINEE: We do have some options. Would you mind if I share what I think could be helpful? (Asking permission)

PATIENT: No, of course I appreciate your help.

TRAINEE: We have "Option A," which I understand you've tried before. There's also "Option B" and "Option C." What do you think about these possibilities? (Giving information followed by eliciting)

PATIENT: Well, I guess I could probably try "Option B."

TRAINEE: Ok, you know what would work best for you. If you like, we could schedule an appointment for you to see the social worker today to explore more about "Option B." How does that sound? (Autonomy support statement, asking permission, followed by an open-ended question)

COLLABORATIVE LANGUAGE

Naturally, learning to incorporate MI into our usual, everyday approach to patient care takes practice, which requires consciously intending to bring MI skills to patient encounters. This attitude helps us focus our thoughts toward working collaboratively with patients in the moments before we open the door or draw back the curtain prior to our initial contact. Regardless of the considerable knowledge we bring to each encounter, believing solely in our own expertise is an invitation to patient defensiveness and dissonance that will impair our efforts. We cannot overstate the fact that patients themselves are the experts when it comes to their stories and their lives. Patients have insight into what has contributed to their behaviors, and listening closely to these impressions permits us to understand these circumstances and collaboratively formulate an individualized treatment plan. Remember that our goal is to assist our patients in tapping into the knowledge and awareness that they already possess, and that building upon these elements is crucial to maintaining long-term change.

In practice, we have discovered that once a patient permits us to offer treatment suggestions, having a number of available options provides a greater degree of choice. Being open to modifications increased this variety even further. Phrases such as "How do you feel about these suggestions?" or "What do you feel is most important for us to work on?" foster and reinforce a collaborative spirit. By contrast, statements such as "How can I help you today?" or "Let me tell you what I think you should do" restrict an atmosphere of collaboration and trust.

In the early stages of MI training, as trainees we must consciously suppress the urge to impose our own ideas on our patients. Instead, as we learn to elicit our patients' ideas, we discover that these suggestions are much more personalized. While we may sometimes believe that ours are the better ideas, patient-generated input is associated with greater levels of engagement. Moreover, by affirming the value of our patients' collaboration, we reinforce the sense of self-determination.

The following clinical conversation demonstrates the use of collaborative language:

PATIENT: Doc, I just get so anxious. Pot is the only thing that seems to calm me down.

TRAINEE: Your feelings of anxiety can be very overwhelming for you and smoking marijuana makes you find relief and comfort. (Complex reflection)

PATIENT: Yeah, exactly. I've been smoking weed for so long that I really can't remember other ways to deal with the anxiety.

TRAINEE: This has been your lifestyle for quite a while, and imagining any other way is a challenge for you. (Complex reflection)

PATIENT: Yes, it is ... but I'm tired of living this way. I don't have the energy or motivation to be there for my son and to be the role model I want to be for him.

TRAINEE: Deciding to use marijuana has been your way of dealing with your anxiety and comforting yourself; at the same time, you see that it is reducing your motivation and preventing you from being the example you wish to be for your son. You aren't able to be the father you imagined yourself to be, which in turn, increases your anxiety even more. (Summary)

PATIENT: [Becomes tearful; allow a few moments of silence and wait for him to process the information.] I have to; I just have to be there for him.

TRAINEE: You've made the decision to break that cycle. What other strategies could you also think of to help you deal with the anxiety? (Complex reflection followed by an open-ended question)

PATIENT: I don't really know. I just don't know.

TRAINEE: You mentioned to me earlier that you had a period of not using pot in the past. In what ways were you able to cope with your anxious feelings at that time? (Simple reflection followed by an open-ended question)

PATIENT: Well, actually I used to listen to music. I'd go to my car, put the window down, and just listen to some jazz.

TRAINEE: This is a strategy you found useful at that time; how do you feel about using it again? (Complex reflection followed by an open-ended question)

PATIENT: I guess I could do that.

TRAINEE: It was useful before and you're making a decision to give it another try. What other ideas do you have? (Complex reflection followed by an open-ended question)

PATIENT: I just can't think of anything right now.

TRAINEE: Would you mind if I share some other skills that have been useful for other people dealing with these feelings? (Asking permission to give information)

PATIENT: No, not at all, that's why I'm here.

TRAINEE: It can be helpful to understand the sources of your anxiety, identify the thoughts associated with it, how you cope with it, and learn how to control it. This can be done sometimes by writing them in a journal. Other strategies could be helpful in reducing anxiety such as meditation, relaxation, and breathing techniques. How do you feel about considering those suggestions? (Summary followed by an open-ended question)

PATIENT: Journaling is something I've done before; I'd be willing to give it a try.

TRAINEE: There's a "How to Journal Workbook" available; would you like to start working on that together? (Closed-ended question)

Evoking goal-directed communication is a way of encouraging and strengthening our patients' intrinsic motivations to change those behaviors that interfere with optimal health. We accomplish this by establishing rapport with a patient by engaging him or her in a dialogue intended to guide the development of awareness of the problematic behavior and by identifying the discrepancy between that behavior and the goal(s) he or she wishes to achieve.

So, how can you, as a trainee, allow an incongruence of values and behavior to become apparent to patients, without creating a defensive response? Establishing rapport includes engaging patients and providing validation. During this period of engagement, patients often divulge their reasons for change. Even if it is not readily offered, it is appropriate to ask whether they mind sharing this information. Often the reasons are related to their values, which is something that is important to them. When we hear a value expressed, we either pursue it immediately or place it in "our pocket" for the appropriate time. Exploring values often leads to the expression of painful emotion and refocuses attention on the areas of patients' lives that are most important to them. Asking patients what change would mean for them, for their values (e.g., health, autonomy, honesty, self-control, responsibility, family, job, pets, respect), and for their lives often paints a picture of how they see their future. This very naturally leads into a conversation on the ideas they have about how they might reach this goal. This approach leads to less discord compared to other approaches because it is based on eliciting all of their thoughts about what is important to them and how they might address their behaviors. You can imagine if "you told them all the reasons" why they should change, how they might give you the argument opposed to change (i.e., sustain talk). This is because both sides do exist and they are ambivalent.

It is the goal of MI to strengthen change talk. This can be assisted by allowing patients to recognize the discrepancy between present behaviors and future goals. As a patient engages in discussing his or her current problems, we use an array of MI skills to guide the conversation toward future goals and whether the present behaviors are, in effect, obstacles to those goals. This approach helps us avoid sounding, or behaving, judgmentally. For instance, patients will sometimes make statements indicating that their behaviors do not present difficulties, either for themselves or for their families and friends. When used with sensitivity and care, a helpful response is for trainees to offer an amplified, or exaggerated, reflection in order to prompt change talk and potentially to elicit a statement of values. This approach does have its risks, however, and one must attend to subtle inflections of voice and nonverbal cues that might imply judgment or condescencion. Two clinical scenarios follow:

PATIENT: I MEAN, I DON'T TAKE MY DIABETES MEDICATIONS, BUT IT REALLY HASN'T BEEN A BIG DEAL.

TRAINEE: You haven't experienced any problems from your diabetes. (Complex reflection)

PATIENT: Well, I wouldn't say that, I mean, I do have trouble with the nerve pain in my feet and that's affecting my ability to play with my grandkids. (Here the patient makes contradictory statements regarding the effects of nonadherent behavior. Asking about the perspective of a concerned significant other is a helpful way to introduce discrepancy: "What might your wife/husband/children be concerned about?" This has the potential to open a dialogue that evokes values and helps establish patient-determined goals, including strengthening motivation for change.)

PATIENT: I tried to quit smoking but I just can't. I can't deal with all the stress I'm going through.

TRAINEE: You've had a difficult time stopping smoking because you use cigarettes as a way to deal with stressful times. (Complex reflection)

PATIENT: Yes … and I've been doing this for 20 years! And now is just not a good time. My daughter is in and out of the hospital and I've got to have a way to relax.

TRAINEE: That's been tough for you to deal with. I can tell you've been putting in an effort to try to stop. What does your family think about you quitting? (Complex reflections followed by an open-ended question)

PATIENT: My wife quit a long time ago and she really wants me to stop because my daughter keeps having asthma attacks. I know I need to do it; it just seems so hard right now.

TRAINEE: You've seen your wife quit, and your daughter has been having some health problems. You want to stop, and at the same time you're having a hard time doing it. How do you think stopping might affect your family? (Summary followed by an open-ended question)

PATIENT: Well, for one, I'm sure my daughter wouldn't have so many asthma attacks. I have to figure this out, because I just feel so bad that I'm hurting her. Also, my wife would get off my back and quit bugging me.

TRAINEE: It doesn't feel good when you see your daughter suffering or have your wife nagging you. You've been struggling with stopping for a while and, at the same time, you see it important for you to try to improve your daughter's health and have a happy marriage. (Summary)

PATIENT: Yeah, I think I need to try something different. What else could we do, doc?

Early in the conversation about smoking, the patient discusses two aspects of smoking: how it helps him deal with stress, and how it negatively affects his family. Through a series of reflections followed by open-ended questions, the trainee is able to guide this patient to explore his feelings about how smoking has both positive and negative effects on his life. The process demonstrates empathy for the patient's expressed need to choose between the varying effects smoking has on his life; the trainee then explores the patient's ambivalence concerning the behavior without diversion.

The critical element in eliciting change talk is the trainee's selective reflection in the latter part of the exchange. At this point, the trainee has heard the patient say that smoking is his primary way to relax, but that it adversely affects his daughter's recovery from asthma. Instead of asking how smoking helps the patient relax, the trainee affirms the effort the patient has made to stop smoking and then asks the patient to reflect on his family's perspective concerning his smoking. The remaining conversation focuses on the patient expressing various reasons to stop smoking, whereupon the trainee summarizes these reasons. The change talk culminates with the patient's willingness to consider quitting and exploring treatment options.

Putting it all together, we've examined the process of taking a patient-centered approach to behavior change. The approach includes recognizing the patient as an equal partner in identifying changes that will be effective for him or her to lead a healthier lifestyle. The patient-centered approach solidifies the working relationship and allows the patient and trainee to work collaboratively toward goals the patient identifies as he or she resolves ambivalence. Plans to reduce health-related risks are developed as the doctor–patient team uses the same straightforward, collaborative style that led to the patient's original decision to change as a way to improve his or her quality of life.

PERSONAL REFLECTION

Before I learned motivational interviewing, if someone asked me, "Do you listen well to your patients?" I would have confidently answered, "Yes." I was certain that I communicated effectively, and that certainly my patients took my counseling and advice to heart. As a family physician in training, understanding my patients and earning their trust are paramount to what I do. My attitude toward communicating with patients was totally transformed when I began learning and using motivational interviewing. I learned that it is not what we say to our patients but rather how we listen and speak that is essential. It is not important to simply hear what my patient says but rather to listen in such a way so that I can appropriately meet his or her needs. Motivational interviewing opened my eyes to this and helped me to connect with patients more deeply than I realized was possible.

Motivational interviewing is a perfect tool for family medicine. Often patients already know what their ailments are and what needs to be changed to help them get better; they don't need a physician to simply tell them to lose weight or stop smoking. In less than 3 years of medical schooling I have witnessed numerous exasperated patients tell physicians what the physicians wanted to hear, and I have watched as physicians threw their arms up in frustration after the patient left. Both sides knew what needed to change and were annoyed with each other because no change took place; meanwhile, the patient's health did not improve. When I worked with my mentor and practiced motivational interviewing every day in my clinical work with patients with substance use disorders co-occurring with multiple medical problems, I saw a different outcome. Rather than simply telling my patients to stop drinking or to stop smoking, that it was bad for them, and why it was bad for them, I asked them how they felt about their struggles with their drinking and smoking and why they felt it was difficult to stop. I have elicited the change "from within," and from there the patients were willing to discuss and engage in the change process.

Although many physicians believe they are active listeners and good communicators, they are not. This may not necessarily be reprehensible on an individual level, since little time is devoted in most medical curricula toward effective communication. However, many physicians do not even realize they need improvement in this area. While a good physician might accurately diagnose and treat a patient, without listening and communicating well, the physician might miss what the patient truly needs. Likewise, a good treatment plan might help the patient, but if the patient does not understand and cannot follow through, it is meaningless.

Learning and practicing motivational interviewing was a milestone in my medical education and a turning point in my development as a physician.

SELF-ASSESSMENT QUIZ

True or False?

1. The core behaviors expected of experienced MI trainees include: a patient-centered approach, clinical empathy, the use of collaborative language, and the evocation of the reasons in support of change.
2. A patient-centered approach challenges the historically authoritarian style of the trainee–patient relationship.
3. "Clinical empathy" is the sharing of emotions between trainees and suffering patients.
4. "Let me tell you what I think you should do about quitting smoking" is an example of collaborative language.
5. Establishing rapport with a patient and exploring that patient's values lend themselves to conversations about which goals the patient wishes to achieve.

Answers

1. *True.* MI is a collaborative process through which trainees and patients work together to identify problematic behaviors and to explore and strengthen a patient's motivation for change. To this end, a patient-centered approach, clinical empathy, use of collaboration language, and evocation of the reasons for change are vital to effective MI.
2. *True.* Historically, relationships between trainees and patients were defined by a power differential that placed trainees in an authoritative role above their patients and that promoted the sharing of expert advice and opinion to those who were expected to accept it without question. MI challenges such a power differential and views trainee–patient relationships as a collaborative meeting between equal partners.
3. *False.* "Sympathy" is the term used to describe the sharing of emotions between an observer and an individual who is suffering. Clinical empathy requires attention and effort on the part of a skilled observer who wishes to understand the world from the perspective of the patient who is suffering; it is expressed by the use of reflections and a wide variety of subtle nonverbal cues.
4. *False.* This type of statement is the antithesis of collaborative language. By placing "I" at the center of the statement, the speaker references an outdated trainee–patient relationship in which practitioners tell patients what to do. A more collaborative approach is to pose a question, such as "Would you be interested in exploring options that could be helpful as we approach your goal of stopping smoking?"
5. *True.* By exploring a patient's values and aspirations, trainees identify incongruities between the moral and ethical principles a patient upholds vis-à-vis his or her present behavior(s). Highlighting such discrepancies in a nonjudgmental and empathic fashion facilitates a smooth transition into a discussion regarding how maladaptive or unhealthy behaviors might be altered so as to better reflect the patient's sense of integrity.

6 Ambivalence and Discord

We have talked about change talk, but what do you do when patients spend most of the time talking about why change is a terrible idea? Or when, despite your best efforts, patients just won't listen or engage with you? The goal of this chapter is to provide strategies to use when patients express ambivalence about behavior change, when they persist in giving you status quo talk, or when discord exists in your relationship with them.

HOW DO WE RESPOND TO ARGUMENTS *AGAINST* CHANGE?

As Miller and Rollnick observed, ambivalence about change is completely normal and is a part of the process of change. Patients can feel torn between what they consider to be two distasteful options. If we reflect on the term *ambivalence*, we may be reminded of the cliché "stuck between a rock and a hard place." In fact, however, ambivalence is more emotionally intense than that implied by this cliché.

The cliché relates to the perceived need to make a decision when neither option is desirable. Ambivalence, however, is generated by frustration over confrontation with having to choose between one option that is gratifying and at the same time clearly unhealthy, possibly life threatening, and another one that is very difficult to initiate and yet would reduce or eradicate the threat to one's well-being. The "bad" or unhealthy alternative is attractive because it is a behavior that has become ingrained in one's lifestyle as the primary manner of experiencing pleasure or coping with stress. Sustaining an unhealthy behavior also allows the comfort of sameness rather than the anxiety of doing something new with the accompanying worry about the unknown or the possibility of failure. It also allows for continued control over one's own life, rather than responding to or giving into the demands of others. The "better" or healthier alternative is also made up of multiple facets, including better physical health, progress toward achieving an ideal self-image, secure finances, enhanced relationships, and all around improved functioning. However, patients often have little actual experience with the positive aspects of changing their behavior and with success in making change, or it may have been a long time since they experienced a healthy lifestyle. Therefore, implementing a behavior change is difficult because the status quo is so attractive.

The behavioral result of this intense intrapsychic conflict is "sustain talk" (Fig. 6.1), arguments for the status quo; and "change talk," arguments for the need to behave in a different way. The emotional intensity of ambivalence is manifested in the fact that these two types of "talk" will often occur in the same conversation (or even the same sentence). People can talk themselves out of change as easily as they can talk themselves into it. Taking a person-centered empathic approach demands that we recognize both sides of the ambivalence. However, inherent in motivational interviewing (MI) is the expectation of facilitating movement toward the resolution of ambivalence, beyond the realms of thinking and talking about change and in the direction of acting to adopt healthier behaviors.

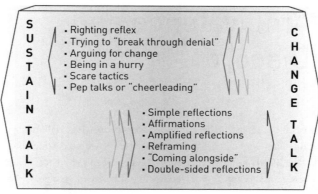

FIGURE 6.1 Resistance and discord.

To engage patients in this process:

1. *Don't overreact to sustain talk by looking for it or fishing for it.* When patients tell you they don't want to change, it is not important to ask or explore why this is so. In fact, it is likely that most patients have already talked about why they are attracted to the status quo. Find an element in patients' statements that allows you to move the discussion toward change talk:

PATIENT: My wife tells me that I have to start paying attention to my cholesterol and triglycerides, but I really don't know what I will eat. I mean, I grew up eating eggs, hamburgers, and pizza five or six times a week, doc. I don't know anything else. Besides, can't I just take one of those "statin" drugs to lower them?

TRAINEE: You developed your eating habits in childhood and it is hard to even think about changing what you eat. While you were describing what you eat just now, you are sharing that you think you must give up *all* the foods you like.

PATIENT: Well, won't I? Everything I see on TV or read online talks about how the American diet is loaded with all the bad stuff, you know, the stuff that clogs our arteries and raises our blood pressure.

TRAINEE: Actually, you'll find that you can make excellent progress improving the health of your heart when you consider making small changes in your eating habits along with other parts of your lifestyle. For example, you probably know that getting regular physical activity helps and, yes, medications can help, too. The idea is to put together a routine that is made up of small changes in whatever areas you feel ready to make and that are really not that hard to live with. What specific changes in your activity level, diet, or medications could you imagine would work successfully for you?

2. *Resist the righting reflex.* Responding to patients' dilemmas or distress with the righting reflex generally involves two elements. The first element is the desire to help. It is almost an instinct to try to correct patients' statements that their behaviors are not damaging. Here are examples of the righting reflex and what *not* to say:

PATIENT: Smoking relaxes me!
TRAINEE: But it's terrible for your health!
PATIENT: I don't think my drinking affects me that much.

TRAINEE: Of course it does. You've been arrested for drunk driving, and you said you've
 gone to work hung over at least several days a week for the past month.

PATIENT: I feel fine. Why should I take my diabetes medications?

TRAINEE: Because you don't want to end up blind and with an amputated leg.

These types of trainee responses are generally counterproductive because they generate anxiety, frustration, or anger in patients. When patients are confronted with an
unwanted reality in this manner, it causes discord in your relationship with them.
These types of responses are not collaborative, empathic, compassionate, or supportive. In fact, they come across as condescending, pushy, and rude. Resistance in these
interactions generally takes the form of "denial." Counter to traditional counseling
lore that highlights the use of stark confrontation to "break through denial," the ironic
truth is that such confrontation actually causes or increases denial. The result of this
process is to put patients in the position of arguing for the status quo, which precludes
any discussion of change. Conversely, the practice of MI assumes that the patient will
be making the arguments for change, and the role of the trainee is to skillfully cultivate
these arguments from patients.

The second element of the righting reflex is for medical trainees to suggest potential answers to problems or to give advice about how to stop engaging in unhealthy
behaviors. Without exploring patients' perspectives and past experiences, we cannot even know what behaviors the patients are willing to change, and whether they
want to try any suggestions we have to offer. Furthermore, it is quite possible that
patients have already tried those suggestions without success. Rather than making
suggestions, it is best to ask patients to tell you about the history of their behavior in
response to the problem, as they define it. In so doing, you will come to understand
the range of behaviors that have been attempted and, more important, the behaviors that have the potential for being successful. This process involves emphasizing
self-efficacy, which entails reviewing past successes each patient has experienced in
addressing the problem, as well as behaviors each patient believes would help, even if
they have not yet been tried.

Reflection can be a powerful strategy. By reflecting sustain talk, patients often
respond with change talk, vocalizing the other side of their ambivalence.

PATIENT: I feel fine. Why should I take my diabetes medications?

TRAINEE: You feel that your diabetes can't be that big of an issue if you don't feel sick.
 (Complex reflection)

OR. . .

TRAINEE: Your health is exactly where you'd like it to be right now, so you see no reason
 to worry about your blood sugar. (Amplified reflection)

Amplified reflections offer a more exaggerated form of a reflective statement. While
the technique is a straightforward reframing of what was said, such a reflection must
be done with particular attention to nonverbal behavior. To avoid coming across as
sarcastic or condescending, it is important to make a statement that implies your
understanding that the patient is simply forming his or her opinion based on how he
or she feels. Your response will come across as sarcasm if your statement is made with
inflection in your voice, implying disbelief that the patient is being honest and that you
assume he or she does not truly believe he or she is at risk simply because he or she

feels fine at the moment. Tone is critical in making amplified reflections, and the tone should be understanding and flat rather than judgmental and questioning.

TRAINEE: You feel you are healthier than you would expect to feel if diabetes were a major problem. At the same time, it is very important to you to stay active and independent, and you would like to take whatever steps are necessary for that to happen. (Double-sided reflection)

Double-sided reflections reflect both sides of the patient's ambivalence. Strategically, these reflections are more effective when you place the part of the ambivalence that supports change last, rather than first.

On a related note, it can sometimes be helpful to "come alongside" by agreeing with patients' arguments for the status quo. Coming alongside can be used when patients argue very strongly for the status quo. Again, however, the effectiveness of the reflection relies on how it is framed. It is, of course, counterproductive to actually agree with patients that they should continue unhealthy or risk-taking behavior. Coming alongside is indicated when unhealthy behavior can be contrasted against another goal that the patient has indicated to be at least as important as continuing the status quo.

PATIENT: I really don't see where it is anyone's business how much weight I gain or how healthy I am. That's my business. That's what I tell my wife when she nags me about eating too much or drinking too much beer. And that's what I am telling you. As long as I am getting to work every day and keeping the roof over our heads and food on the table, I think I have the right to eat and drink whatever I want.

TRAINEE: I agree with you. You work hard because you value providing for the family and you take it very seriously. You work hard and you have the right to decide what you eat and drink.

PATIENT: Yeah, that's the way I see it. I am a responsible guy. Taking care of the family is the most important thing. But after that I should be able to enjoy myself if I want to.

TRAINEE: No argument here. As long as you're not doing anything that hurts your family, you should be able to do as you please.

PATIENT: Yeah, and I know a lot of people who think that way.

TRAINEE: I see here that you were in the hospital last year.

PATIENT: Yeah, I had to have my right knee replaced. The orthopedic guy says the other one isn't as bad. I really only have pain in it in the morning. It's stiff, you know, but once I get going, it loosens up. He's another one who told me I need to lose weight—that's what caused my right knee to give out. When I was in there, I told the guy I was waking up at night with chest pains and they checked my heart, turned out to be acid reflux. I am on medication for that now and haven't had any problems with that. And they told me my blood pressure was high because I am overweight. That's what started my wife on this health kick.

TRAINEE: How long were you laid up with all that?

PATIENT: It was almost 3 months before I could go back to work.

TRAINEE: That must have been hard on you and the family.

PATIENT: Yeah, I got short-term disability but that doesn't pay what I usually get and I missed a lot of overtime. I have three kids. I tell you, it wasn't easy. We almost had to go into our retirement savings, and there isn't much there either.

TRAINEE: What would happen now if you had another episode like that? How would your family get along?

PATIENT: I got to admit, doc, I *did* think about it back then. For 6 weeks all I could do was lay around and so, yeah, I thought about it. I couldn't wait to get back to work and once I did, I got back into the routine of making regular money and it didn't seem like there was any need to worry about that anymore.

TRAINEE: You are really a responsible guy who wants the best for his family. You feel proud of yourself. I see a lot of patients who struggle with taking their responsibilities seriously. So, as you talk about it now, you would want to avoid having another time like that.

PATIENT: Yeah, who wouldn't? I know it would be better if I could be healthier. But I just can't do all those things they told me to do.

TRAINEE: They suggested you do too many things at once and this is so overwhelming to even think about it. What did they suggest?

PATIENT: They gave me this three-page list of all the things I should do. It seemed like they expected me to give up everything I like. And the guy there told me I should start swimming for exercise because it would help me lose weight and be easy on my knees. I can swim, but, hell, I haven't done that since I was a kid. It seemed like a lot. I tried to do some of the things they wanted me to do, but after a while it got too hard to keep up.

TRAINEE: What if we take another look at that list? I think you'll find that you don't have to do *all* those things *all* at once. There is a way we can come up with a few things that you can live with that can help you get healthier. I've done this before and it has worked for many of my patients. Would you want to try?

PATIENT: Sure, when you put it that way, it's worth a shot.

RESISTANCE AND DISCORD

Devon* (*name changed to protect privacy) is a 20-year-old African American man, with a history of end-stage renal disease (ESRD), who requires hemodialysis. He is scheduled for Monday, Wednesday, and Friday hemodialysis sessions. Devon missed a session on a Friday and subsequently presented to the emergency department (ED) the following Sunday with shortness of breath. When he came in the ED, Devon was found to have a systolic blood pressure in the 190s, and he was sent for emergent dialysis with a planned admission to the intensive care unit (ICU) after his dialysis session. After finishing his dialysis session, Devon was transferred to the ICU. Following is an excerpt of the exchange that occurred between the medical resident and Devon during the interview. (Note: Devon is a thin African American man slumped over in bed not making eye contact with the medical resident.)

RESIDENT: (regarding dialysis) Devon, when do you go for dialysis?

PATIENT: [No response]

RESIDENT: Isn't it every Monday, Wednesday, and Friday?

PATIENT: [No response]

RESIDENT: And you missed your dialysis session on Friday, right? What happened?

PATIENT: [No response]

RESIDENT: Come on, Devon, the sooner you answer me, the sooner this will be over.

PATIENT: [No response]

RESIDENT: Now, why did you miss your dialysis session on Friday?

PATIENT: [No response]

RESIDENT: How do you usually get to dialysis?

PATIENT: The bus.

RESIDENT: What happened Friday then? Did you miss your bus?

PATIENT: [No response]

RESIDENT: I know you had some trouble breathing, but we need to make sure you're ok and that nothing else is wrong with you. Was there anything else going on other than the shortness of breath?

PATIENT: [No response]

RESIDENT: How about a headache? Are you having a headache?

PATIENT: [No response]

RESIDENT: [Louder and now pointing to his head] Devon, does your head hurt?

PATIENT: [No response]

RESIDENT: Devon, I need you to answer me. Does your head hurt?

PATIENT: [muttering] No.

RESIDENT: Good. How about your vision? Any blurry vision?

PATIENT: [No response]

RESIDENT: [Louder again] Come on, Devon, is there anything wrong with your vision?

PATIENT: [shakes head no]

RESIDENT: [pointing to chest] Are you having any chest pain?

RESIDENT: Do you know why you are in the ICU?

PATIENT: [No response]

RESIDENT: With you being as hypertensive as you were, you could have a stroke, damage your eyes, or have a heart attack [pointing to each area in turn]. Can you repeat after me so I know you understand what we're concerned about?

PATIENT: [mumbling] Stroke, blindness, and heart attack.

RESIDENT: Good.

This clinical encounter is an example of major discord in the therapeutic relationship that was perpetuated by the trainee's use of a deluge of consecutive closed questions with no intention of allowing the patient to share his perspective.

Historically, the word *resistance* has been used to describe any number of patient characteristics and behaviors that represent an unwillingness to comply with the practitioner's expectations, for example, to come to appointments on time, to accept responsibility for the specific behavior, to follow treatment recommendations, and so on. The construct implies that failure associated with maintaining a therapeutic alliance or making progress in treatment lies with the patient. In MI parlance, the term "discord" was recently chosen as a more accurate term to signify an impasse in the therapeutic relationship. The thinking behind changing the descriptor is that treatment involves the attitudes and behaviors of two people interacting with each other and problems that develop in clinical encounters are related to both the patient *and* the practitioner. It is important to identify the clinical encounters where a patient could have a discordant relationship with a practitioner and still express change talk. Alternatively, a patient could be engaged with a practitioner while expressing sustain talk. A continuing tenet of MI is to keep discord to a minimum in the therapeutic encounter.

Dealing With Discord

The best way to minimize discord is to behave in a manner that prevents it. When you are practicing MI at a high level, your relationships with patients originate from a clear understanding of your responsibilities.

Trainees are responsible for the following:

- Maintaining the structure of treatment so that they meet with patients at the appointed times and allow patients access to them as specified in an agreement made at the beginning of treatment, for example, no contact outside of scheduled appointments; telephone, e-mail contact; and emergency appointments allowed/not allowed, and so on
- Maintaining patient confidentiality as is specified in the treatment agreement
- Offering your best efforts to create an environment where patients can explore their potential for change, including recommendations/referrals to other treatments or interventions according to the trainee's clinical judgment

Implied in these responsibilities is that trainees: (1) make no moral judgments about patient behavior; (2) respect patients' rights to self-determination; (3) recognize that they have no control over patients' behaviors; and (4) are not responsible for "fixing" patients or otherwise solving their problems.

When you approach patients in this neutral, objective manner, you are not engaging in "resistance" toward the patient and, therefore, patients find little to resist or argue against.

Notwithstanding this approach, discord can occur in therapeutic relationships. It may be related to the way you feel about a patient that affects your objectivity (what psychoanalysts call "countertransference"). Sometimes it is due to your reacting overtly to a conflict between your views or priorities and those of the patient. Sometimes patients feel that their autonomy is being impinged upon. Sometimes one or both of you is tired, ill, upset, or distracted by something completely unrelated to the medical encounter.

Your actions can increase or decrease discord. Behaviors that can elicit or enhance discord are as follows:

- Arguing for change or insisting on a single path toward change
- Lecturing, preaching, or presenting yourself as the expert and making rational arguments to "prove" your case as to why patients should change
- Ordering or commanding patients to make specific changes
- Warning, threatening, or using scare tactics to manipulate patients to change
- Failing to allow patients to provide their perspectives and cutting them off
- Shaming, ridiculing, or blaming patients about their beliefs, experiences, behaviors, or health status
- Expressing pessimism about patients' ability to make changes
- Failing to recognize and affirm or, even worse, criticizing patients' efforts
- Being in a hurry
- Giving general reassurances or "pep talks" that everything will be okay

Such behaviors can be an inherent part of treatment in busy clinics or hospitals. The demands made on trainees' time are onerous, and it is normal for these confrontational behaviors to become standard practice in clinical encounters.

When discord arises, pay attention to your emotional responses. It is difficult to not take conflict personally. However, you can learn to stay calm and to think before you react. Consider why the patient is behaving this way. Think about what you may have said or done to evoke this response. Summarize your view of what is happening between you and the patient and ask for his or her point of view. Patients may be reacting to something outside of treatment, and this is important to know. If a patient is concerned about something in the encounter or has taken offense and he or she is expecting an apology, apologize or further explain yourself without hesitation. This is part of the MI focus on a transparent, egalitarian approach that reduces discord. Other strategies that can be of help include reflections as they pertain to sustain talk.

Reflections:

- "You don't want to be here, and you're angry that your wife made you come."
- "You're sick and tired of people telling you what to do. You've been dealing with this for a long time, and you feel that you've heard it all before."

Notice how these statements reflect the content and the feeling that patients may be experiencing. Such reflections of emotion show patients they are understood and you are concerned. As a result, patients feel more comfortable to elaborate on their concerns.

Reframing:

- "It seems like nagging to you because she does it constantly. When people do that, it's often because they are nervous or fearful that something bad will happen to the person they love. It's possible that your wife is worried about you and this is how she expresses it. You know her best. What do you think?"
- "You didn't like that I gave you suggestions about how to cut down on sugar and fat in your diet. It's obvious that you've got your own ideas about how you might approach this. I take responsibility for not asking you about your ideas first. How about discussing how you see it?"

Emphasizing personal choice and control is also important. As you respond to your patients' statements and behaviors, continuously include references to their freedom to choose because it is their responsibility for decisions and what comes out of them. Do this in a matter-of-fact manner without emphasis on the patient being "on an island" without support. You do this by simultaneously reminding patients that your responsibility is to help them as much as possible to make changes toward leading a healthier lifestyle.

Autonomy support statements:

- "You are the best judge about what changes make the most sense to you and how you want to make them. What steps do you see yourself starting with?"
- "I am not here to tell you what to do or try to make you do anything you are not interested in doing. How do you want to proceed from here?"

Affirmations can also make the interaction less adversarial.

Affirmations:

- "I appreciate how hard it must have been to come in here and talk with me about this. You are a strong person to keep working on this."
- "You are making a valid point. You have been very resourceful and thoughtful about what might work best for you to be successful."
- "You worked hard to prevent this from happening and did the best you could."

Shifting focus from the area of contention to a less contentious area that the two of you can agree on can also be helpful. For instance, you might say, "I'm not interested in trying to force you to do something that you don't want to do. What I *am* interested in is how we can work together to keep you healthy." Consider the following exchange:

PATIENT: "I can't ask my boyfriend to start using condoms now—he'll think I am cheating on him or have a disease! I don't know what he will do."

TRAINEE: "You are way ahead of me. I'm not asking you to do something that will jeopardize your safety. Help me better understand your relationship with your boyfriend."

Tailor your statements to the person you're working with. There's no prefabricated phrase that will solve all conflict. Being interested, accepting, and caring goes a long way.

SELF-ASSESSMENT QUIZ

True or False?

1. Sustain talk consists of arguments for the status quo, while change talk argues for the need to behave in a different way.
2. When patients engage in sustain talk, it is helpful to challenge these statements and identify how these views contribute to the unhealthy behaviors in question.
3. The technique of "coming alongside" is used when patients engage in sustain talk.
4. "Discord," the expression that replaces the term "resistance" in MI, is created solely by patients in the clinical encounter.
5. Refraining from moral judgment, respecting patient autonomy, and rejecting the notion that trainees should be able to "fix" their patients allow trainees to approach patients in a neutral and objective manner, which in turn, reduces the potential for discord in their relationships with them.

Answers

1. *True.* Sustain talk and change talk result from the intense intrapsychic conflict patients experience as they work through ambivalence; this process demands that they explore arguments in favor of maintaining the status quo as well as those in favor of change. Patients often engage in sustain talk because they lack experience with either the positive aspects of implementing behavior change or success in doing so. Sometimes patients are far removed from a healthy lifestyle and do not recognize that change is an achievable, viable alternative. The goal of MI is to help guide patients to express more change talk and less sustain talk.

2. *False.* Sustain talk is characteristic of ambivalence and is inevitable among those who are trying to bring about significant behavioral change. Trainees should never belittle sustain talk, try to eliminate it, or explore in any depth why patients might not want to change. Instead, trainees are encouraged to engage, or "dance," with patients by exploring other avenues of discussion, such as clarifying previously discussed change talk, and elaborating patient statements that will shift discussion in the direction of change talk.

3. *True.* Trainees "come alongside" when they acknowledge a patient's arguments for the status quo of maintaining unhealthy behavior; this is contrasted against positive goals and aspirations that the patient has stated as desirable as preserving the status quo.

4. *False.* Historically, *resistance* was used to describe a patient's negative response to the therapist or therapy. The word *discord* was selected by Drs. Miller and Rollnick to signify an impasse in therapeutic relationships. *Discord* reflects the contemporary view that problems arising in treatment are related to both patient and trainee. Several common trainee behaviors have been identified as key contributors to discord.

5. *True.* These principles are fundamental to MI and are essential components in collaborative encounters that help ensure patients feel secure, respected, and confident that they can trust a trainee.

7 Moving Ahead
From Sustain Talk to Change Talk & Evoking to Planning

The assumption underlying the spirit of motivational interviewing (MI) is that each individual has the capacity to change. Our goal, as trainees, is to work collaboratively with our patients to draw out—or *evoke*—their own internal motivations for change and to support their abilities and efforts to resolve ambivalence. Rather than trying to impose change through the use of directive, demanding, or threatening approaches, the process of evoking obliges us to collaborate with our patients as we awaken and inspire each person's intrinsic power to make change a reality.

STRATEGIES TO EVOKE CHANGE TALK

The task of evoking internal motivations for change is often daunting, especially when we consider that many patients struggle with ambivalence for months or years prior to meeting us. On a superficial level, implementing meaningful behavior change should be relatively uncomplicated: One has simply to identify the maladaptive behaviors, determine to address them, and then to set about doing so. Alas, the reality is considerably more complex, and sorting through competing arguments for and against a certain course of action is sufficiently challenging to prevent all but the most determined individuals from achieving anything approaching success. Instead of perceiving change as one single giant step, a more productive approach is to use the following strategies to encourage patients to begin to consider the concept of change and what, in practical terms, this might mean in their lives.

The Importance and the Confidence Rulers

Our first tip in evoking change talk is to elicit our patients' perspectives concerning the significance of making a particular change, and it involves asking patients to rank how important a particular change is for them. This level of interest/disinterest is quantified by referring to a numeric scale ranging from 0 to 10 and asking a patient to choose which number best reflects how important it is that he or she initiate, modify or eliminate a given behavior (see Fig. 7.1). For instance:

TRAINEE: We've been talking about your smoking habits and you've brought up the point that you're thinking about quitting. On a scale of 0 to 10, with 0 being not important at all and 10 being most important, how important is it for you, right now, to quit smoking?
PATIENT: Hmm, I guess ... 6?
TRAINEE: I'm curious ... why would you say it's a 6 and not a 2?

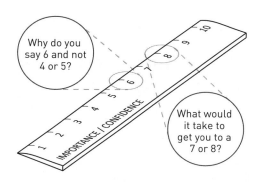

FIGURE 7.1   Importance and confidence rulers.

PATIENT: Well, I guess it's because I realize that smoking affects my health in a bad way, and I'm tired of waking up with this cough every morning. I mean, I know it can cause lung cancer, so I guess that's important, too.

TRAINEE: What are some of the other ways smoking affects you?

PATIENT: Sometimes I notice that my clothes have that stale, smoky smell … it's really pretty awful, now that I think of it.

Note that the focus of this ruler is not upon the actual number that a patient selects as best reflecting his or her present frame of mind, which in this case is 6. By asking the open-ended question, "Why choose that number and not something lower?" we prompt our patient to express his or her perspective regarding why it might be important to change an unhealthy behavior and open up the possibility of discussing it in further detail. It is *critical* to avoid asking the opposite question, that is, "Why did you select a 6 and not a 10?" In all likelihood, this strategy will result in eliciting more sustain talk regarding why the status quo should be maintained and, in doing so, serve only to make the task of behavior change much more difficult.

Even without being asked, some patients tend to focus on why they don't rank the importance of change as closer, or equal, to 10; should this happen, gently redirect your patient to the subject at hand: "I understand there are reasons why the number you selected is less than 10; what I'm curious about is why the number you chose is as high as it is, and not something lower on the scale."

The importance ruler serves as a guide to a patient's perceived longing, need, and justifications for change. Remember that this scale should be used in a nonjudgmental, nonthreatening way that invites your patient to respond with a number of his or her choosing; maintain this neutral and engaged tone throughout your follow-up questions. Should your patient respond by choosing zero, it's fair to ask whether he or she would even consider making a behavior change that seems completely unimportant.

After asking your patient why the number is as high as it is, pursue this line of thought by asking, "What else?" or "Help me understand why the number isn't lower," and reflect what you hear until you sense that all possible reasons have been exhausted. You will recognize that you have reached this point by comments such as "That's it" or "That's really all I can think of." At this juncture, summarize everything you have heard your patient say and then ask, "What would need to happen for the importance level to move up one or two points?" As before, reflect what you hear, asking, "What else?" in order to extend the discussion until its logical conclusion, and finish by summarizing what you've heard and understood.

One scenario in which the importance ruler is especially useful is during patients' discussions of their values and/or goals for the future. Such conversations provide us with opportunities to explore the importance of change as it relates to a patient's values, and how change might affect both short-term and long-term goals:

TRAINEE: As we approach your discharge from the hospital, I'm wondering what some of your goals are after you move on from this part of your treatment.

PATIENT: I think my biggest goal is to stay out of the hospital. I've been in a vicious cycle for a long, long time, and I'm tired of being sick and stuck in a hospital bed for weeks at a time. I want to get back to my life outside this building.

TRAINEE: Staying out of the hospital is really important to you. You've mentioned before that one strategy you believe can help you avoid having to be readmitted is to take your medications as directed once you're discharged.

PATIENT: Oh, definitely! It seems that every time I stop taking medication, I end up back in this place.

TRAINEE: When it comes to staying out of the hospital, how important do you think it is to stay on your medications and take them the way they are prescribed, using a scale of 0 to 10, where 10 is the most important thing for you now and 0 is not at all important?

PATIENT: Probably a 9 or a 10. These medications are meant to keep me as healthy as possible, and whenever I'm taking them, I start feeling better. I need to be more regular and responsible about taking them after I leave so that, hopefully, I won't be back for a while or at all.

TRAINEE: What was it like the last time you had a long stretch without having to come back to the hospital?

PATIENT: It was great! You know, I almost forgot that I had any health problems at all.

The ruler metaphor may also be used to explore a patient's level of confidence in his or her ability to follow through with specific changes in behavior. As with the importance ruler, ask why your patient's confidence level is as high as it is and discuss what would be needed to make it even one or two points higher. Another advantage of this tool is that it may easily be modified to evoke change talk relating to one's readiness, commitment, or hope for sustained change.

When confronted with a pressing demand to make a major life change, we all need to believe it is indeed possible to modify one's behavior; we also need at least a modicum of confidence in our ability to make that change a reality. The confidence ruler helps evoke a patient's level of certainty that he or she will be able to carry through with the proposed changes, and it subtly taps into his or her sense of hope regarding success. Next, we continue the previous exchange:

TRAINEE: You feel that staying on these medications is going to be a vital part of meeting your goal to stay out of the hospital. Using a scale of 0 to 10, 0 means not confident at all and 10 extremely confident, how confident are you that you'll be able to keep taking your medications every day?

PATIENT: Gosh, that's a lot tougher. . .. probably a 7?

TRAINEE: I'm interested to hear why you chose a 7 and not a 3.

PATIENT: Well, I think I've never taken it all that seriously before, and this time I'm approaching it differently. This is my third hospital stay since January, and I'm really sick of being sick. Also, I'm going to try hard to be more organized. The pharmacist gave me a pill organizer and showed me how it can help, and I'm actually going to use it this time. I think it will remind me how to keep all my medications straight, and then I'll be able to take my pills the way you want me to.

TRAINEE: What other strategies have you come up with to help take your medications regularly and strengthen your confidence from 7 to 9, for example?

Encouraging this patient to articulate his or her reasons for confidence provides an opportunity to imagine aloud what success looks and feels like and why this is a reasonable expectation. In turn, the trainee could continue the discussion by validating this patient's other plans to maximize his or her chances of success.

Querying Extremes

> TOOLBOX
> *Querying Extremes* – Explore the highs of change and the lows of sustaining it.

This strategy involves asking your patients to articulate some of the extreme disadvantages of sustaining an unhealthy behavior, as well as the tremendous advantages of changing it.

TRAINEE: If you keep using heroin the way you have been, what are you most worried about?

PATIENT: That I could lose my son. I mean, my ex-husband is already trying to take him away from me.

TRAINEE: If you keep choosing to use drugs in this way, you could lose custody of your child, one of the most important people in your life.

PATIENT: Yes, he is *the* most important person! He's why I need to stop.

TRAINEE: I understand that the worst thing about continuing to use would be for you to lose custody, even visiting rights, to your son. Could we go in the opposite direction for a moment and imagine that you were not using any substances at all for 5 years? What would the best part of that be for you?

PATIENT: I think the best part for me would be becoming the parent I've always wanted to be, and becoming a productive member of society again. You know, having a job, and all that stuff. And I think I would be able to give back, maybe even go to high schools and talk to kids about what heroin did to me and how it affected my life.

By considering extreme examples of possible or certain negative consequences resulting from their behaviors, patients become increasingly aware of the risks of *not* changing. Similarly, by exploring either the potential or real benefits of change, we may evoke meaningful change talk.

In the earlier example, the patient shares her vision of what a new, drug-free life might look like, and she focuses upon relationships with others, including her son and local high school students. When you use this technique, avoid discussing positive and negative outcomes in a general way; instead, ask patients to express the specifics of the best and worst possibilities of either changing or choosing to remain as they are. Thinking about these extremes along a continuum of change often stimulates patients to rank which motivating factors are most salient to their lives and circumstances.

Looking Back and Looking Forward

> TOOLBOX
>
> *Looking Back and Looking Forward* – Examine the pros and cons before and after a targeted change.

Similar to querying extremes, this strategy involves taking a look at an earlier time in your patient's life, before the unhealthy behavior began, and then looking ahead to a future in which either change has been accomplished or, conversely, the unhealthy behavior continues. Let's start with this exchange:

TRAINEE: You mentioned earlier that 5 years ago, you were not using heroin for some 13 months. What was that time like for you?

PATIENT: Honestly, it was pretty awful at first … a real day-to-day grind, I remember, just getting through all the physical stuff. At the same time, I felt like I was doing so much better. I had a steady job for the first time in years, and I was spending time with my family. I even had money in the bank that I could use to buy what I needed, even things I just wanted.

TRAINEE: It was hard at first, and the more you stayed with it, the better you felt because you were doing things that you enjoyed. You felt more independent. Life was easier for you after those first difficult days.

PATIENT: Yeah, easier … it sure was. Things were just more … stable. Everything seems so unstable right now, probably because I'm using again.

Helping your patient reflect back to life before the targeted behavior began, and then exploring the discrepancies between that life and his or her current life often inspires new levels of understanding and insight concerning how the behavior in question is affecting life in the present moment. When we elicit statements such as these, we open up possibilities for discovery that may not have been encountered before.

With a few variations, this technique is also effective in looking ahead toward a life in which change has been implemented. Whether used alone or in conjunction with looking back, projecting one's glance forward allows patients to imagine what life without the unhealthy behavior might be like:

TRAINEE: During our time together, you've mentioned wanting to "get your life back" from alcohol. If you were to stop drinking, what would life without alcohol look like for you?

PATIENT: I don't know … I guess one of the big things is that I'd be able to think straight. I'd be a part of my daughter's life. I'd be there for her, rather than just being a deadbeat dad all the time. And I'd try really, really hard to make the right decisions and become a productive member of society. I used to be like that before I drank, and I want that life again.

As this example illustrates, patients often share extremely difficult and painful aspects of their day-to-day lives that relate directly to the unhealthy behaviors in which they engage. As noted earlier in this book, nonverbal cues play an essential role in maintaining a nonjudgmental atmosphere that supports *realistic*, if cautious, optimism regarding the benefits of change. We know that many, if not most, patients will resist attempts to actively pressure them to change the behavior under discussion; merely itemizing the significant adverse effects of a particular behavior simply isn't effective in bringing about behavior change. A more helpful approach is to reflect back to what the spirit of MI is all about: helping patients formulate and express their *own* arguments for change, using their *own* words.

Exploring Goals and Strategies

TOOLBOX
Exploring Goals and Strategies – Elicit personal values and any discrepancies with behaviors.

Another effective means to evoke change talk is by guiding your patient to explore and to articulate his or her goals and values in life. In many ways, this technique reinforces the first process of MI: engaging. Through our conversations about goals and values, we help patients identify and prioritize the issues of greatest concern to them, those that influence who they are and what they want. From this foundation, we begin to develop discrepancy between these long-standing goals and values vis-à-vis their current behaviors and circumstances. In turn, this discussion often leads naturally into one that evokes change talk.

PATIENT: So I talked to my daughter on the phone last night. She was asking how I'm doing and when I was coming home from the hospital. (Tears in eyes) It all made me miss her so much.

TRAINEE: Your daughter is a really important part of your life, and it's hard being in the hospital away from her.

PATIENT: Yeah ... I just ... I think she's old enough now that she knows why I'm here. She might not know that I'm using and dealing ... but she knows I'm messed up. I have to get my life on track for her.

TRAINEE: You see how your decisions about using drugs are affecting her.

PATIENT: Oh my God, yes! I mean, she doesn't need to see me do it. It affects her, too. I mean ... I was never around and when I was, I was out of it and high. I wasn't even really a parent to her.

TRAINEE: You really want to be a good parent for her, someone who's there for her.

PATIENT: Yeah, I do. I need to stop this cycle for her. She's my number one reason for quitting. I've made this decision for her.

In the first statement of the exchange, this patient makes specific reference to the value he places on family, particularly his daughter. By reflecting this sentiment and acknowledging that the child is an unwitting recipient of impaired parenting, the trainee prompts the patient to identify a prime motivation for behavior change: to become the parent he wishes to be. In this context, the status quo of continued drug use is incompatible with what this patient understands as good parenting. The scene is now set to evoke meaningful change talk in terms of which behavior change(s) would bring this patient's actions closer in line with his values and beliefs.

Another means to evoke internal motivation is to explore a patient's previous experiences in changing his or her behavior. Remember to include both successful and unsuccessful efforts; your goal here is *not* to focus on a particular outcome but to help your patient deconstruct the *process* of change itself: what works for him or her and what doesn't.

TRAINEE: The process of losing weight is really daunting for you. And at the same time, you've mentioned that there was a time, about 6 months ago, when you were losing weight pretty consistently. What strategies were you using at that time that worked for you?

PATIENT: Well, I had a membership to a gym, and one of my friends was going with me three times a week. We made it a planned thing, and that really made it hard to back out. I didn't want to let her down, you know?

TRAINEE: (Nodding) So having someone to exercise with really helped you be consistent with working out. That worked well for you.

PATIENT: Yeah, but then I got that extra project at work and was so stressed out, having to stay late and all that stuff. To cope with everything, I just wanted to nibble all the time and I just didn't have the energy to make it to the gym. I missed a couple of times with my friend, and then it just kind of faded away.

TRAINEE: You're really affected by stress at work, and one of the ways you've dealt with it is by unhealthy eating.

PATIENT: Yes, exactly. I wish I had a better way to deal with it. When I was going to the gym and working out a few times a week, I felt so much better. And it was nice spending time with my friend, too. I really want to get back into that. Maybe I could ask her if she wants to do it again.

Helping patients explore their past experiences with behavior change, particularly in terms of the specific aspects that promoted either successful or disappointing outcomes, often leads to valuable insight. In the earlier exchange, the trainee evokes a positive strategy that yielded significant benefits: planned workouts at the gym, but with a friend, both aspects of which contributed to a sense of good health and well-being. Barriers to this behavior are also identified: high stress levels and time demands at work that interfered with exercising, and an inability to return to regular workout sessions once the habit had been broken.

This conversation provides an ideal starting point from which to brainstorm how these and other, newer strategies might help this patient return to a pattern of exercise that was physically and emotionally gratifying. For instance, how might the work environment/schedule be altered to allow this patient to integrate exercise more easily? Could he or she incorporate walking into his or her daily routine? What conversations could this patient have with his or her exercise buddy to improve accountability? Discussions such as these give our patients opportunities to articulate and reinforce *their* motivations for change, identify specific plans of action, and begin to imagine how these plans might unfold.

Taking the time to explore how change might be implemented is not only helpful in evoking change talk but also an effective transition to the final process of MI: planning.

TOOLBOX
Normalizing Ambivalence – Validate and normalize a patient's conflicting feelings.

As a process, MI is particularly helpful in guiding patients through the difficulties of resolving ambivalence about change. It's worth recalling that not every patient struggles to bring about change; for some individuals, being confronted with the very real consequences of their unhealthy behaviors is sufficient impetus for immediate and sustained behavior change. We have met patients who, having decided once and for all to stop smoking, never smoke another cigarette. Similarly, we have known patients who, in the aftermath of yet another drunken crisis, decide that they will never consume alcohol again.

But as we know, these individuals are in the minority, and most patients experience ambivalence as they come to terms with having to modify their behaviors or make a crucial decision involving their health. One challenge of ambivalence is that many patients feel alone, even isolated, in the experience. To counter this feeling, normalizing ambivalence reduces the sense of isolation. As with every aspect of MI, this strategy requires that first, we establish a therapeutic relationship with our patient before beginning to explore the concept of change and evoke change talk. Patients who are uncertain and/or fearful of change are often reassured to have these feelings validated. For most of us, change *is* difficult; just as attempting to imagine a new way of being in the world *is* both trying and frightening:

PATIENT: (tearfully) I just don't know what to do! My daughter obviously wants me to go to rehab, probably because she thinks I can't do it on my own. But I just want to get out and get back to my life. I want to get on with practicing this stuff outside the hospital, and get my life started again.

TRAINEE: You really are of two minds about all of this. On one hand, you want to be out on your own; on the other hand, you see that your daughter really wants you to go to rehab before coming home because she thinks it would be helpful.

PATIENT: I mean, I think it would be helpful, too. I know it would give me more clean time. But it seems like my daughter expects me to go to rehab just because it's the obvious thing to do. She makes it seem like it's her choice and not mine. But what if I'm not sure? What if I don't want to go to rehab? What if I don't like it?

TRAINEE: I imagine a lot of people in your shoes would struggle with figuring out what's the best thing to do. It can be hard to figure out the next step when you're feeling pulled in different directions.

PATIENT: Yes, exactly, pulled in different directions ... that's how I feel. I want to feel like I'm making the right decision for everybody, both for me and my daughter. But I'm scared!! I've never tried to quit drinking before. I want to think I can do it on my own, but maybe I can't. And that's just ... so scary.

Remember that when discussing change, a patient's arguments are not always logical or based on factual information, and they often include a great deal of emotion and intensity. In these circumstances, we must recognize and appreciate the intense stress that internal struggles present and respond by acknowledging and validating uncertainty with tact and empathy.

In the case described above, note how the trainee subtly reinforces a safe, non-threatening environment by acknowledging and normalizing the patient's fears and uncertainties. Within this supportive setting, the patient is able to express her fear that, should she not be admitted to a rehab center, she may not be able to maintain sobriety. A subtext to this fear is concern that in agreeing to go into rehab, she is submitting to her daughter's coercion. This comment provides an opportunity to explore the patient's feelings of doubt in her own abilities, which may well reflect a long standing negative sense of self. This is *not* a needless diversion; instead, recall that our ability to evoke internal motivations for change requires that our patients believe they have the capacity to bring about, and sustain, meaningful behavior change.

HOW TO RESPOND TO CHANGE TALK: BACK TO OARS

TOOLBOX

Back to OARS When you identify change talk, this is a key time to use your core OARS skills.

As noted earlier in this book, the ratio of change talk to sustain talk is the major indicator of an individual's ability to successfully change unhealthy behaviors. Once we have begun to evoke change talk, our next task is to strengthen and enhance these statements and, at the same time, prompt our patients to articulate further internal motivations for change. This process involves going back to the roots of MI and making use of its core skills: open-ended questions, affirmations, reflections, and summaries (OARS).

Not only do these fundamental tools help strengthen change talk, but they also facilitate our efforts to uncover a patient's internal motivations for change. The MI approach to change talk is founded on the premise that by fully and deeply exploring our patients' internal motivations for change, we guide them to articulate positive aspects of change that they may not have consciously identified in the past. Well-honed communication skills also tap into the level of commitment patients feel toward change, and they help direct an encounter away from a preparatory type of discussion to one that focuses on the practical realities of implementing change.

The essence of responding to change talk is active, reflective listening. When you hear a patient express a wish or longing for change, recognize such comments as the opportunity they are to reflect that patient's hopes for a different future. The art of reflection encourages patients to continue exploring what they have just shared and evokes more change talk in the process.

Keep in mind that MI is a process that involves near-constant feedback. When you respond to change talk and your patient responds with even more change talk, rest assured that you are on the right track. Patients often reply to our reflections with comments such as "Exactly!" or "You're absolutely right," and we've learned to accept these reactions as confirmation that our understanding thus far is correct.

On occasion, patients express change talk that sounds vague, disingenuous, forced, or naïve. At other times, patients seem overconfident or give the impression that they are trying simply to say what they think we want to hear. It's tempting to respond by questioning or challenging these remarks in an effort to nudge the patient out of complacency. Remember that in the spirit of MI, we must take each patient at his or her word and continue the process of evoking change talk, even in these demanding situations.

In terms of particular challenges, we recommend the following responses:

a) *Your patient responds with vague, generalized statements*: This is an opportunity to explore the fine details by asking open-ended questions regarding specific aspects of your patient's remarks.

b) *When your patient's responses seem disingenuous or fraudulent*: Continue to listen closely, reflect statements of change talk, and affirm whatever positive steps he or she is making or has made.

c) *Patients who appear overconfident or exaggerate the extent, magnitude, and speed of the changes they wish to bring about*: Stay focused on the positive and realistic aspects of their comments, taking care to highlight the validity of achievable expectations.

In each of these instances, challenging or confronting your patient may lead to unexpected and unpleasant consequences, especially during the early days of establishing therapeutic rapport. Remember that the latter stage of MI, namely planning, provides ample opportunity to review possible obstacles and barriers to change. Together, you and your patient will have the chance to discuss and review what realistic change looks and feels like. The process of evoking change talk is just that: a *process* that takes time and one that may include unforeseen detours.

STRATEGIES TO RESPOND TO SUSTAIN TALK

Just as *change talk* refers to language that argues in support of making changes in one's behavior, *sustain talk* denotes the words and expressions patients use to explain why things should stay precisely as they are. One of the most accurate predictors of future behavior change is an increase in the ratio of change talk to sustain talk; thus, as patients commit themselves to the process of change, the language they use will reflect this change in perspective. Remember that within the context of a therapeutic relationship, many, if not all, patients are reluctant to relinquish familiar patterns of behavior. If this were not the case, almost everyone would live completely healthy, well-balanced lives.

Let the fundamental spirit of MI guide your response to sustain talk: Respect your patient's autonomy, validate his or her perspective, and aim to collaborate with him or her.

Simple Reflection

The most basic response to sustain talk is a simple, uncomplicated reflection of what your patient has just shared. In some instances, this will evoke an argument *against* your reflection, which in our experience often takes the form of change talk.

PATIENT: I think I'm going to move back in with my boyfriend. Things have been bad in the past, but I think it will get better if I give him another chance.

TRAINEE: You think that by living together again, your relationship will be better.

PATIENT: Well, I don't know if living together will actually help our relationship. The last time we moved in together, it didn't go so well for us. That's when the yelling got really bad.

TRAINEE: Help me better understand your relationship with your boyfriend.

Amplified Reflection

This technique is one step beyond a simple reflection and amplifies or elaborates on what your patient has just said. Let's expand on the earlier example:

PATIENT: I think I'm going to move back in with my boyfriend. Things have been bad in the past, but I think it will get better if I give him another chance.

TRAINEE: You think that by moving in together, the two of you will solve all of your problems and the relationship will be great again.

PATIENT: Well, hold on … I don't think we'll be able to solve *all* of our problems. We have to deal with a lot of stuff … his drinking and all the yelling and screaming, and you know he hits me sometimes, too. Now that I think of it, I really don't know if the relationship was ever "great."

This example demonstrates how a reflection may be enhanced by gently overstating a patient's response in order to evoke an opposing form of ambivalence. In this case, the patient identifies the true nature of her relationship with an abusive boyfriend.

Double-Sided Reflection

Double-sided reflections are used to respond to *sustain* talk by linking such comments to previous expressions of *change* talk. Think of this approach as linking your patient's *present* remarks with those that he or she has articulated in the *past*.

PATIENT: I just don't think I can give up cigarettes … they calm me down when I'm stressed out.

TRAINEE: Your smoking helps you calm down and deal with some of your stress; at the same time, you've mentioned before that continuing to smoke adds to your stress as well.

PATIENT: Yeah, I guess it does. You know, I had that scare last year when the doctors thought they saw a spot on my lung. I was really scared that I had cancer … and that was really stressful. I often think about how awful that was, and then I wonder what sort of damage I'm doing to myself.

A key aspect of using double-sided reflections is that we pay close attention to the conjunction used to link arguments in favor of, and against, change. We're often tempted to insert the word "but" between our statements, yet we've learned that many patients interpret this word as a cue to negate all that has preceded it. Remember that the intent of a double-sided reflection is not to argue with, or dismiss, our patients' sustain talk but to acknowledge and validate it, even as we emphasize opposing aspects of their ambivalence.

So what should you say? We suggest using neutral language that connects conflicting ideas without prioritizing one over the other. Try using "at the same time … " or even "and," both of which reinforce an impartial, unbiased understanding of what you've heard.

Ideally, double-sided reflections should be structured so that sustain talk is reflected first, and change talk is reflected second. Although this may seem trivial, recall that at this point in a therapeutic conversation, the goal is to guide your patient toward change; shaping your reflections in this way mimics a general conversation pattern that typically involves a listener continuing, or picking up on, the speaker's final comment. Thus, by including your patient's change talk in the second half of a double-sided reflection, you provide an opportunity for your patient to respond by expanding upon his or her thoughts concerning change.

Emphasizing Autonomy

The spirit of MI that guides our interactions with patients is founded upon an attitude of partnership and collaboration, and an essential element in these encounters is that we actively encourage and support our patients' autonomy and their ability to choose and enact change. In practical terms, this implies that we must seek out ways to acknowledge our patients' independence, particularly in the sense that it is *they* who are responsible for enacting change, not us. Our role is to awaken, reinforce, and support the motivations that already exist within each patient. The scenario we discussed earlier involving a patient experiencing ambivalence about attending rehab may have taken another direction in the following manner:

PATIENT: I mean, I think it would be helpful, too. I know it would give me more clean time. It seems my daughter expects me to go to rehab just because it's the obvious thing to do. She makes it seem like it's her choice and not mine. But what if I'm not sure? What if I don't want to go to rehab? What if I don't like it?

TRAINEE: This is your treatment and your choice. Even if your daughter has an opinion about the direction she thinks you should go, ultimately, this is *your* decision. You know what is best for you.

Recognizing and validating our patients' autonomy helps reinforce their sense of empowerment and confidence that they do, indeed, possess the capacity to enact meaningful change in their lives.

Reframing

Another way to respond to sustain talk is by reframing a patient's comment, that is, suggesting a different meaning, explanation, or perspective for a given situation or feeling your patient has described. Reframing is one of the hallmarks of cognitive-behavioral therapy (CBT) and is a technique designed to help individuals gain awareness of their thought processes, identify errors in thought, and then consciously replace these maladaptive distortions with thoughts that are more accurate and useful. Let's return once more to the patient who is considering rehab:

PATIENT: My daughter just keeps going on and on about it, and she won't stop bothering me! She's even called some of the rehab places trying to learn more about them ... and then she keeps lecturing me about why I should go.

TRAINEE: I can see how you might take this as meddling. I wonder whether working so hard for your recovery is a way of showing that she really cares for you.

PATIENT: Yeah, you might be right ... she does keep saying that she wants to see me get better.

Maintain a sense of genuine collaboration in your use of reframing. Remember that your goal is to help your patient recognize that a valid, alternate interpretation may exist for the event(s) under discussion; your intent should *not* be to argue or insist that a patient accept your particular explanation. Reframing reminds our patients that sometimes we all experience "blind spots" in our thinking, and that these habits can be changed.

Agreeing With a Twist

This technique begins by reframing a patient's comments, and it continues with a statement of agreement or validation. This combination allows us to align ourselves with a patient's perspective while raising the possibility of a different point of view on the matter.

PATIENT: My father doesn't like me. All he does is yell at me—criticizes whatever I do. I feel like I'm constantly disappointing him. With all this stuff going on, I smoke pot so I don't have to think about it; I can get away from him. It calms me down and cools me off. Is that so bad?

TRAINEE: It's really hard for you to handle your father's negativity and criticism, and you're doing the best you can. I wonder if it's hard for him to deal with his negative feelings, too.

As we know, validating our patients' statements does not require that we agree with what they say; instead, it signifies that we've heard and tried to understand the sentiments our patients express. Although this may seem of little consequence, validating plays an indispensable role in facilitating our patients' readiness to engage with us. Validating with a twist allows us to affirm a genuine interest in our patient's perspectives while gently testing the limits of our relationship by offering new, potentially different ways to interpret a situation. In some instances, our comments will be sufficient to change the direction, content, and tone of the conversation toward a competing argument in favor of change.

Running Head Start

Some patients remain stuck in a pattern of sustain talk and demonstrate little, if any, interest in change talk. In our experience, we find these scenarios especially difficult, for they challenge every aspect of an encounter with a patient. The running head start is designed to prompt movement away from a perspective that sees the current situation as desirable; paradoxically, it works by focusing precisely upon the arguments *in favor* of the status quo (see Fig. 7.2). In practical terms, this means acknowledging that

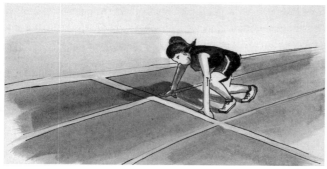

FIGURE 7.2 Running head start.

in some scenarios, changing behavior is too difficult, too demanding, and in short, not worth the effort. Counterintuitive as it appears, this approach has the potential to become a creative—and yes, collaborative—way of inspecting the status quo from a distance, much as one studies a sculpture in an art gallery.

PATIENT: I don't know why my parents made me come here. I don't need to see a doctor.

TRAINEE: There's no reason for you to be here.

PATIENT: That's right! I get into fights, so what? Who cares? It's because those other kids bug me. They make me mad. I'm allowed to be angry, right? That's who I am.

TRAINEE: You like being angry.

PATIENT: You bet I do!

TRAINEE: What do you like about being angry?

PATIENT: I like feeling excited! I like yelling, and I like feeling something rather than nothing.

TRAINEE: So you don't feel numb when you're angry. What else do you feel when you're mad?

PATIENT: It's weird, some of the kids at school are kind of scared of me; they watch what they say and do when I'm around.

TRAINEE: It's good to feel that people respect you. Sometimes it seems that making a big noise and getting into fights is one way to make everyone notice who you are. I wonder if there are any other reasons why kids might notice you, even look up to you.

PATIENT: Well, I'm on the football team. People like me for that.

This strategy has the dual benefit of building engagement while potentially evoking change talk. The trainee acknowledges and accepts the patient's anger, including the possible benefit that being angry causes others to take notice. Instead of being critical of seeking attention in this fashion, the trainee opens an avenue of discussion that may lead away from sustain talk: specifically, what it means to be on the football team, how football players are supposed to act, and whether this young man is likeable.

Coming Alongside

Sometimes simply agreeing with, and validating, a patient's reluctance to change can be an effective response. By joining patients in their struggles with ambivalence and reluctance to change the status quo, we defuse a potential argument and affirm that we are there to help, not to insist or push.

PATIENT: I just really want to keep smoking. I know I should quit, but I just don't want to.

TRAINEE: Your smoking is really important to you right now and you're not ready to quit.

PATIENT: No, I'm not ready. I like smoking, I like the look, I like the taste, I like everything about it.

TRAINEE: You are clearly saying that in spite of the risks, smoking is worth it for you.

MOVING FROM EVOKING TO PLANNING: LOOKING FOR SIGNS AND TESTING THE WATER

After evoking the reasons and benefits of change, you and your patient are ready to take the next step in the MI process: planning for change. The first crucial factor is one of timing: How much change talk is enough to sustain the process? When is a patient ready to move from arguing in favor of change to actually begin brainstorming how to implement change?

Signs of Readiness

Fortunately, there are ways to recognize that a patient is ready to transition to planning. It is important to be aware of these signals and to appreciate them for what they are: indications of our patient's increased willingness to begin the process of planning.

Increased Change Talk

The most obvious sign of readiness is an increase in change talk. In practical terms, patients will demonstrate a rise in both the frequency and amount of change talk, in addition to an increase in the strength, or degree of commitment, reflected in these comments. As suggested earlier, you will note a high ratio of change talk to sustain talk. A second change in language concerns an increase in the ratio between mobilizing and preparatory change talk: Instead of hearing "I can. . .," "I want to. . .," or "I need to. . .," patients begin making comments such as "I will. . .," "I have already. . .," or "I commit to. . .." Note that this is not a hard and fast rule, and in situations in which a patient expresses considerable preparatory change talk, accompanied by other signs of readiness, the lack of mobilizing change talk should not prohibit moving into the planning phase.

Reduced Sustain Talk

As patients commit to the change process, they feel less and less attached to their former arguments against change. Patients who accept the need and advantages of change no longer need to defend the status quo: They're ready to move on to a new state of being.

Small Changes in Behavior

Even before reaching the formal planning stage, many patients begin to take positive action on their own. Admittedly, these may seem to be small steps: An obese patient wanting to lose weight buys new running shoes and takes a walk, or a patient with a history of noncompliance with medications accepts a free medication box from the local pharmacist. Other beginning steps include patients struggling with severe alcohol use who initiate contact with rehab centers, or patients in abusive relationships who visit "safe houses." These actions are key indicators that a patient is not only ready to plan for change but that in fact, he or she has already started the process.

Remember to validate and affirm these accomplishments. For many patients, these actions are the first in a long line toward a new way of living one's life. As you acknowledge these efforts, emphasize their importance as proof of your patient's autonomy and independence, the same qualities that will carry him or her through the challenge of sustaining change.

Relief From Inner Struggles

As patients resolve their internal ambivalence about change, they often experience a dramatic lessening of stress and anxiety. In many cases, we've observed a noticeable relaxation in a patient's face and less tension/greater ease in his or her body movements. Though subtle, these signs suggest that a patient is comfortable with the decision to move ahead.

Envisioning the Future

Another change in speech patterns that reflects the readiness for change is a marked increase in the references patients make regarding a future in which change has occurred. Previously, many of these remarks were prompted by open-ended questions or comments; now, patients volunteer these statements and take the initiative to describe the realities they imagine. Note that the content of these comments may not always be positive; implementing change often provokes some sort of "push-back" from family and friends, and recognizing potential obstacles to continued success is an essential element in the planning process. Of course, unexpected issues may also present along the way, and this possibility highlights the importance of ensuring that your patient has a host of skills and strategies to deal with unwelcome surprises. Part of envisioning the future also involves asking questions and actively seeking more information regarding diagnoses, treatment options, community supports, and so forth.

Jumping In … or Testing the Water

When you sense that a patient is ready to embrace the planning stage, it's time to raise the topic directly, through an open-ended question or another of the communication skills we've discussed. We often use a variation on the following question: "What do you think about moving our discussion into beginning to brainstorm (or plan/identify/outline, etc.) ways to move ahead with (whatever change is to be implemented)?" By the time we arrive at this point, we normally have a solid working relationship with our patients and know whether they are ready to address planning from an honest and realistic frame of reference.

A less direct way to guide a patient toward the planning stage is by "testing the water," which involves summarizing the patient's change talk to date and then posing a key question about how to proceed (see Fig. 7.3). Your summary should include reference to all the essential preparatory and mobilizing change talk that your patient has expressed; in effect, you are providing a transitional bridge to the next logical step in the change process. Keep your question open-ended to ensure that your patient has as much space to respond as possible. Your focus should be on giving your patient the opportunity to choose what to do next. Examples range from a simple, "So … what's next?" to the more complex, "Where would you like to go from here?" Here's an excerpt from one of our interviews:

TRAINEE: Over the past few days, we've talked a lot about your drinking. You've shared how your alcohol use has really affected your relationships with family and friends,

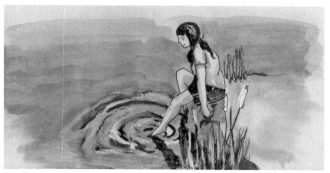

FIGURE 7.3 Testing the water.

and that you'd really like to improve your life. You've talked about wanting to get a good job and participate in society again; these options haven't been available to you because of your drinking. You've also said that you'd like to feel healthy again. And you've told me that you're feeling better, more clear-minded than you have for a long time, now that you haven't had a drink for about a week. What do you make of all this?

PATIENT: Well, for one thing, I've decided to stop drinking. I think I'm ready to turn my life around. I know that I need to go to 12-step programs every day ... and like they tell me, I have to take it one day at a time.

TRAINEE: Going to 12-step programs will be an important part of your recovery, and as you say, on a daily basis. What else do you think will be important for your ongoing treatment?

PATIENT: Well ... I guess I'm not sure. What do you think?

TRAINEE: Perhaps we could work together to brainstorm other treatment options that you could choose to follow in order to stay in recovery. What do you think?

PATIENT: That sounds great. I would really like that.

As always, a discussion that summarizes change talk with the goal of moving toward planning and implementing change must be grounded in the collaborative spirit of MI. Tempting though it may be, refrain from pressuring your patient to take steps that he or she is not fully ready to make. In our eagerness to see our patients thrive, we have sometimes been overly enthusiastic in our recommendations, and we urge you to be aware of this unfortunate hazard. Leave it to your patient to take the leap of faith that is required to move from *thinking* and *speaking* about change to *making change happen*. Remain neutral, but supportive, as you test the water by gently nudging your patient forward. Maintain an unconditionally positive attitude toward your patients, recalling that ultimately, *they* will decide when, and if, they are ready to change.

EQUIPOISE AND COUNSELING WITH NEUTRALITY

In some circumstances, we have little or no sense of which direction to guide our patients toward, as in situations in which a patient needs to make an important decision that does not involve changing unhealthy behaviors. These are known as "equipoise situations" or conditions in which we should counsel with neutrality. In these instances, it is neither appropriate nor ethical for either practitioners or trainees to suggest or direct which course of action a patient takes. Examples of this type of decision include whether to:

- Enroll in a research study
- Stay in or leave a relationship
- Have and raise a child, have an abortion, or choose adoption, especially when trying to decide about an unintended pregnancy
- Donate an organ, such as a kidney or liver segment, to another person who needs it

To counsel with neutrality, from the outset we inform patients of our intention to explore both sides of the decision equitably, and that we will do so from an impartial perspective. Our role in these scenarios is clear: We are there to help patients choose whichever option best suits *them* and their circumstances. Counseling with neutrality may be difficult, especially in those situations in which we may, consciously or unconsciously, be tempted to support one option over another.

One strategy that works well in these situations is to explore the pros and cons of various options by using a "decisional balance." Here is how this tool might be structured to apply to the process of deciding whether to donate a kidney to a relative with severe kidney failure:

Example of Decisional Balance

Advantages of donating a kidney	Advantages of not donating a kidney
Disadvantages of donating a kidney	Disadvantages of not donating a kidney

This grid helps organize and summarize the content of therapeutic conversations concerning any difficult decision. The key point to remember is that your role is to help your patients arrive at *a* decision: not a particular decision, but their decision.

PERSONAL REFLECTION

What I wanted to share about my experience with MI is that, while learning and practicing its skills takes time, effort, and patience, *perfecting* these techniques is another matter altogether. For me, learning to listen—and I mean, *really* listen—to my patients' experiences has been a challenging and sometimes exhausting process. In my "pre-MI days," I don't think I ever realized just how hard it is to truly listen to what another person says. There's so much we need to be aware of: the tone of voice and vocabulary a patient uses, plus his or her body language, and other almost imperceptible cues. And of course, there's the actual content that is expressed and which encompasses the complete range of human emotion, from deepest despair to the most ecstatic joy, and everything in between. Another challenge of moving from sustain talk to change talk is, ironically, my own ability to sustain the attentiveness that is needed to pick up on the subtle signs that indicate that a change of perspective is beginning to occur.

The other point I wanted to emphasize is that despite these challenges, MI has enriched my clinical encounters with patients in ways that I could never have foreseen. I think that most of us as physicians or trainees experience a great deal of satisfaction in making correct diagnoses, ordering and interpreting the most appropriate tests, and prescribing the medications best suited to treat a given problem. Simplistic though it may sound, I think of these as the "tidy" parts of medicine: There are clear questions and clear answers, and everybody goes away happy. But medicine isn't always tidy or straightforward; sometimes it's messy and frustrating. What I find most rewarding about MI is that it has given me the tools to help my patients help themselves and, in so doing, become full participants in maintaining a state of good health and well-being.

SELF-ASSESSMENT QUIZ

True or False?

1. When using the importance ruler, clarifying why a patient chooses 6 out of 10 is more effective than exploring why it isn't 10 out of 10.
2. The confidence ruler can be an important tool for emphasizing hope regarding the future and evoking a patient's internal confidence.
3. "What are you most worried about should you continue to smoke two packs each day?" is an example of "querying extremes."
4. A good example of "looking back" is "You said earlier that 5 years ago you lost 15 pounds and you were able to continue a healthy exercise regimen. How did you manage to gain all that weight back and what happened to your daily exercise schedule?"
5. Exploring a patient's values is a helpful way to evoke change talk and internal motivation for change.
6. Normalizing ambivalence should be avoided because it encourages patients to continue sustain talk.
7. "You see how drinking has negatively affected your relationship with your wife, but at the same time you can't imagine what your anxiety would be like without alcohol" is a good example of a "double-sided" reflection.
8. Reframing helps address sustain talk.
9. MI is a useful approach when trying to convince patients to enroll in research studies.
10. It is never too early to begin the planning stage of the MI process.

Answers

1. *False.* By asking why a patient's ranking is lower than the ideal 10 out of 10, trainees risk eliciting more sustain talk. A more effective approach is to acknowledge and explore why the patient chose 6 out of 10, as opposed to 3 out of 10 (or a similarly lower ranking). This approach fosters change talk and reinforces confidence within the patient.
2. *True.* The confidence ruler is a simple but compelling tool that has potential to nurture confidence in patients as they approach making a major life change.
3. *True. Querying extremes* is a strategy that involves asking patients to explore either the major benefits of changing unhealthy behavior or the possible consequences of sustaining that behavior. Its effectiveness derives from posing questions in a nonthreatening and nonjudgmental manner.
4. *False.* Although the first portion of this question looks back, the second portion emphasizes patient failure rather than previous success. This question would likely be perceived as a discouraging reminder and would not contribute to building patient confidence. In the spirit of MI, a more appropriate question would be: "Five years ago, what changes and strategies did you use to lose 15 pounds?"

5. *True.* Understanding a patient's values is a critical component of successful MI. A clear picture of the people and principles that matter to a patient encourages open discussion of the discrepancies between a patient's values and his or her current behavior.

6. *False.* Ambivalence is a common experience for individuals who confront the process of behavioral change. Validating and normalizing ambivalence helps build engagement with patients and has the potential to evoke change talk. It is another strategy by which trainees create a safe and nonjudgmental space for patients to explore their perspectives.

7. *False.* By following a few basic rules, double-sided reflections are an effective MI tool that helps build discrepancies. The reflection above falls short in two ways: first, the statement is structured so that change talk is reflected in the first half, followed by a reference to sustain talk in the second half; thus, a sense of the status quo lingers. A more compelling phrasing is to reverse this order: Begin the reflection with sustain talk and finish with a reference to change talk. Second, as stated, the reflection includes the word "but," which tends to complicate the meaning and intention of the reflection. More effective choices to link the two halves of double-sided reflections include "at the same time" or even a simple "and." With a few changes, the reflection transforms into a complex statement that invites further change talk: "You can't imagine what your anxiety would be like without alcohol, and at the same time, you see how drinking has negatively affected your relationship with your wife."

8. *True.* Reframing is another useful means of responding to sustain talk that involves presenting a different meaning, explanation, or perspective for a given situation or feeling that a patient describes. Used appropriately, reframing is a gentle way to challenge negative thinking patterns and the emotions they create by positing alternative explanations and new ways of responding. Reframing encourages patients to reevaluate established habits of thought.

9. *False.* There are many situations in which it is neither appropriate nor ethical for trainees to choose the direction of change for a patient. In these equipoise situations, trainees must counsel with neutrality and guide patients toward making decisions, but not a particular decision. These scenarios include whether to enroll in a research study, remain in a relationship, continue a pregnancy or have an abortion, or donate an organ.

10. *False.* Trainees should begin a transition to the planning stage only when patients indicate that they are ready to do so. An early decision to discuss planning risks overwhelming and discouraging patients; another hazard is the discord that may arise when patients feel pushed, rather than guided, to begin planning. A variety of signals indicate a patient's readiness for planning: increased change talk, spontaneously occurring small steps toward change (these should be acknowledged and affirmed), increasing numbers of questions/comments concerning possible change, and statements in which patients describe a future that includes the proposed change(s).

8 Motivational Interviewing in Challenging Encounters

Challenging patient encounters occur across all healthcare settings. From outpatient clinics to inpatient wards, and from operating suites to emergency departments, we cannot imagine a setting in which the potential for patient encounters that unnerve us does not exist. As medical trainees, we are at the forefront of patient engagement, but at times, it seems as though we're also in the direct line of fire of strongly expressed patient emotions. These interactions are difficult in both the moment and long afterward, when the sting of a comment or the memory of having felt woefully underprepared for the barrage of angry words lives on in our minds. Often, the most difficult aspect of engaging with challenging patients is the array of negative feelings that stirs within us regarding our capabilities and our perceived areas of vulnerability. In this chapter, we present a motivational interviewing (MI)–informed therapeutic approach that will help you recognize and manage challenging patient encounters.

A CHALLENGING ENCOUNTER

The following case illustrates many of the features common to challenging patient encounters:

A 38-year-old woman presents with anxiety, type 2 diabetes, alcohol abuse, and ischemic heart disease. She has been prescribed 10 different medications, including insulin. She has not been functioning well. She is managing her diabetes poorly and her hemoglobin A1C is 11 (above the normal range, which suggests poor glycemic control). She does not exercise and drinks alcohol heavily, though intermittently. She is angry with her husband for not understanding her struggles with anxiety. At the outpatient appointment, she demands a benzodiazepine "because nothing else works for my anxiety." When the medical trainee tries to explain the reasons for not prescribing it, she becomes very angry and screams, "I am suffering. You don't understand and you don't care about me! I am not coming back here again!"

We usually expect clinical encounters to conclude with a sense of mutual satisfaction: We anticipate that our treatments will prove effective and, consequently, our patients will feel better. Yet, as we know, this is not always the case, and, as it turns out, the challenge of "difficult" clinical encounters has been discussed in medical literature for decades. In 1949, the *International Journal of Psychoanalysis* published a paper entitled "Hate in the counter-transference," written by the pediatrician D. W. Winnicott. In it, he acknowledged having experienced outright hatred for some patients, under certain circumstances. Later the psychiatrist J. E. Groves wrote extensively about these encounters in his article "Taking care of the hateful patient," in which he notes that in dealing with "difficult" patients, physicians have the capacity to experience intensely "negative feelings, as well as malice and, at times, [a] secret wish that the patient will 'die and get it over with.'" We even attach disparaging labels to patients whose needs we believe we cannot satisfy, such as "heart sink," "train wreck," or "borderline."

Countertransference is the word Freud coined to describe the emotional reactions that an interviewer feels regarding the individual being interviewed. Freud believed that countertransference reactions are caused by a physician's or therapist's own unconscious conflicts; more recently, countertransference has come to be understood as reactions which arise from our own past experiences. Some of the unwanted negative emotional responses that may present in these encounters can range from mild annoyance to frustration, anger, exasperation, helplessness, resignation, disgust, or downright spite and malice. In fact, physicians in the U.S. report 30% of patient encounters to be "troubling," while the Difficult Doctor–Patient Relationship Questionnaire classifies 10% to 20% of all patient encounters as "difficult."

Trainees and practitioners, in general, encounter challenging patients in everyday practice, including the management of common clinical presentations. For instance, an emergency medicine resident may feel annoyed or angry at having been requested to examine a patient described by the triage nurse as a "frequent flier who is always drunk." Similarly, psychiatry residents may experience "heart sink" feelings when dealing with patients who engage in self-mutilation behaviors. Upon graduating from medical school, most of us are very well trained in the straightforward management of patients with diabetes, but we feel lost when dealing with diabetic patients who are demanding, angry, or belligerent. Often, our emotional reactions are accurate reflections of patients' underlying pathologies, complex inner struggles, or conflicts with interpersonal relationships. What is important here is to see our reactions as portals for empathy and understanding, and *not* judgment, labeling, or categorization.

Further evidence suggests that these problems do not lie exclusively with our patients. Some individuals are labeled "difficult" by physicians as a result of frustration with the way in which a patient sought care, or with the relationship itself. Some evidence suggests that patients presenting with multisystem signs and symptoms, and those who physicians perceive as "difficult," are more likely to possess poorer functional status, engage in greater utilization of healthcare services, and have a greater sense of unfulfilled expectations, as compared to a less complicated, more "likeable" cohort.

The notion of "heart sink" has recently been reexamined, with the conclusion that this phenomenon or "difficulty" likely results from ineffective doctor–patient communication that, in turn, leads to discord within the relationship. To understand how this experience occurs, and how it might be avoided, three areas must be considered (Box 8.1): characteristics *we* bring to an encounter; characteristics *patients* bring to the encounter; and factors relating to the healthcare system itself.

The first group of characteristics is familiar to all medical trainees: lack of experience and professional identity, poor communication skills, and an (over-)eagerness to assume the role of expert or authority. Other factors can also come into play at any stage of our careers: fatigue, gaps in knowledge concerning cultural habits and practices, difficulties with time management, a tendency to undermine patient autonomy, failure to trust a patient, and emotional or professional burnout. Important patient characteristics include the following: psychiatric disorders such as depression, anxiety, personality disorders, or impulse control disorders; multiple symptoms involving multiple body functions; failure to adhere to medical advice; and poor response to treatment. Finally, healthcare system features include language and other cultural barriers, time pressures, conflict between patients and staff, and a lack of continuity of care.

Box 8.1 Challenging Patient Encounters

Clinician Factors

Lack of experience
Poor communication skills
Desire to be the expert or authority
Burnout
Overcommitment
Clashes with professional identity
Cultural gaps
Time management
Undermining of patient autonomy
Lack of trust in the patient

Patient Factors

Depression
Anxiety
Personality disorders
Impulse control disorders
Multiple physical symptoms
Nonadherence to medical advice
Poor response to treatments

System Factors

Language and cross-cultural issues
Time pressures during visits
Patient and staff conflict
Lack of continuity of care

Not surprisingly, these three categories often intertwine. For example, the diagnostic process is rife with confusion for patients who present with multiple vague but intense physical symptoms and who are also experiencing anger and despair. If such individuals present for treatment at a time when a physician is feeling pressured, fatigued, and overcommitted, a challenging encounter is more likely to occur. Identifying, understanding, and managing the contributing factors to difficult clinical encounters will lead to more effective and satisfactory experiences for both trainee and patient.

As an egalitarian, empathic therapeutic approach, MI is well suited to fostering a collaborative relationship between patients and trainees that facilitates shared decision-making. This helps in preventing discord in the relationship and resolving difficulties that have already arisen, and it yields higher satisfaction with the encounter for both parties. Remember that your particular interaction with a challenging patient has likely been preceded by other outbursts. Ideally, future encounters will be more positive. Chances are high that many other trainees have been in your shoes. When empathy begins to wane, a helpful response can be to remind oneself of the myriad painful life events and unpleasant circumstances that have contributed to your patient's coping skills, including those that may be perceived as "maladaptive." You may sense that your patient is pushing you away; however, by maintaining the spirit of MI in the encounter and consciously developing compassion, you may succeed in keeping the patient engaged and help break a repetitive cycle of "difficult" encounters. At this point, you may feel that maintaining the spirit of MI is idealistic, if not downright impossible, especially at two o'clock in the morning with a patient who threatens "road rage" if you don't immediately provide *x*, *y*, or *z*. But remember that skillful maintenance of a collaborative, evocative, and person-centered approach will be far more therapeutic and efficient in the long run than an authoritarian and confrontational manner.

STRATEGIES FOR WORKING WITH CHALLENGING PATIENTS

The "Angry" Patient

Key Skills: (a) reflective statements that acknowledge and validate anger; (b) autonomy statements to support a patient's sense of self-efficacy; (c) open-ended questions to explore the situation in greater depth and discover what might be required to resolve the conflict.

Tips: Regulate your affect and be aware of your body language. Stay aware of becoming defensive and resist the need to justify your decision making when it is questioned in a mocking or sarcastic manner. When you feel an impulse to justify a decision under these circumstances, think about framing your perspective such that you clarify your intent to promote adaptive coping behaviors. A communication style geared toward shared decision making is another way to remain person centered.

One morning, one of my colleague's patients stormed into the interview room before we had a chance to call him by name and began an angry tirade, claiming that we had discontinued one of his "as-needed" medications last night and "tricked him." He was yelling, pointing fingers, and at one point, he angrily dismissed the trainee saying, "I don't care what *you* have to say, I need to talk to the *real* doctor." This came out of the blue, in the wake of three or four good MI sessions with the same patient. Here are some examples of my colleague's responses:

- "You're really pissed off right now and feel really disrespected." (Reflection of emotion)
- "It's difficult for you to trust people and you feel like the team has let you down." (Linking past information to the reflection to reinforce rapport)
- "What is anger like for you?" [The patient didn't understand this question] "I mean, what's that like for you?" (An evocative open-ended question. It is very useful to focus on the underlying emotion when you feel stuck)
- "Yesterday you shared with me how you were able to manage your emotions during an argument in the kitchen. How were you able to do that so skillfully?" Or "What made that successful?" Or "What has helped you cope/be effective in the past when you've been really angry? (Supporting and reinforcing self-efficacy)
- "We're not doing anything for you … what is your idea of treatment?" (Repeating patient's last statement, clarifying, and exploring)
- "Anthony, do you mind if I share my perspective with you? [Waited for permission] "You've mentioned that no one listens to you and no one is helping you. Personally, I find it very difficult to hear you and appreciate what you're feeling when you yell.

I wonder if people shut down when you start to yell … communication breaks down and your needs aren't met. What do you think about that?" (Sharing a personal opinion. Always ask permission first and be very careful to adopt an empathic nonjudgmental tone)

> KEY POINT
>
> Reflecting emotion with an angry patient is a key skill the enables *"coming alongside the patient"*.

This particular patient responded very well to my colleague's personal disclosure. He sat down, lowered his voice, and agreed that yelling was not the most effective way to communicate. Later in the interview the patient explored further the roots of his tendency to always think the worst in people and how he could act differently in the future. It's worth emphasizing that the trainee maintained a neutral but concerned affect throughout the encounter. Her body language was relaxed and she did not focus on content (e.g., which medication, why it had been stopped, that he had been told it was going to be discontinued). She focused on the process of interpersonal relatedness while maintaining a person-centered approach using MI skills and strategies and successfully defused what had the potential to be an aggressive exchange.

The "Overwhelmed" Patient

Key Skills: (a) reflections; (b) affirmations; (c) supporting self-efficacy.

Tips: Acknowledge tears. Stay in the emotional moment. Adopt a neutral affect. Choose tones that resonate with the patient's emotions. This approach diminishes discord in the relationship. Evocative questions help patients continue to explore their emotions.

I used to be extremely uncomfortable whenever patients became overwhelmed and began to cry. Do you tend to ignore it? After all, most people seem embarrassed to cry in front of a stranger. Do you offer a supportive moment of silence and then move on with the interview? In one particularly cringe-worthy situation, a patient was sobbing while intermittently apologizing for not being able to "get a hold" of herself. My response was, "Don't be sorry" and was as empathic as it was effective. Following is a transcript in which I found myself in a similar situation:

PATIENT: [Starting to tear up]

TRAINEE: I can see that your eyes are starting to fill with tears … what are the emotions you're feeling right now? (Acknowledge tears, stay in the emotional moment, and explore with an evocative question)

PATIENT: Scared, ashamed … my life is ruined. I can't recover.

TRAINEE: You feel like you've passed the point of no return. (Complex reflection)

PATIENT: Yes. I'm sorry, I need to stop crying and get it together.

TRAINEE: You feel embarrassed. (Reflection of the underlying emotion, instead of responding to the content)

PATIENT: Very embarrassed. I've tried to stop drinking so many times before, but this time is different. I want to recover.

TRAINEE: You want to learn how to start coping with feelings in a different way that doesn't involve alcohol, and you see yourself being determined this time … What does it mean to you to recover? (Transitional summary followed by an evocative question that guides the patient forward)

PATIENT: I believe I can do it ... but I'm scared.

TRAINEE: On one hand, you are afraid to try again, and on the other hand, you're determined in a way you haven't been before. (Double-sided reflection. Always end with the emotion that will mobilize the interview instead of creating a roadblock, which is what might have occurred if the sentence was structured the other way around. Use language that builds self-efficacy) You mentioned earlier that you did not use substances for 8 months. How did *you* successfully stop for those 8 months? (This affirms self-efficacy and continues to move the encounter forward. Also note that, although it is in our common parlance, the word "clean" is judgmental while the term "not using substances" is less so)

By making the effort to acknowledge this patient's obvious emotions, and by exploring what they meant *right now*, this patient and I were able to extend this understanding to the bigger concerns in her life, namely, those related to alcohol abuse.

The "Disengaged or Withdrawn" Patient

Key Skills: (a) acknowledge patient autonomy; (b) astute reflections; (c) affirmations.

Tips: If a patient says he or she doesn't want to talk, it is worth respecting this autonomy and negotiating another time to engage. It may be less convenient for you, but it furthers rapport and provides a good foundation on which to base the next encounter. Consider offering explicitly understanding acceptance as to why it may be too difficult for a patient to engage at this particular time. For example, the patient is experiencing significant withdrawal symptoms from drugs or alcohol, or is exhausted after having just been admitted following a long night in the emergency department. Acknowledge that the patient is struggling and respect his or her wish to meet later. Depending on the context, you could attempt to engage your patient by reflecting that he or she has really been struggling lately and follow this observation with an open-ended question as to how he or she was able to walk into the room and reach out despite these struggles. Try to resist feeling uncomfortable either with silence or with slowing your pace. MI is about meeting patients where they are, both in the content of your reflections and the pace of the encounter. This can be particularly challenging in a medical setting in which we are under intense time pressures. However, slowing down and using carefully chosen effective language will actually save you time and better serve your patient in the end.

An older gentleman with a long history of alcohol abuse was involuntarily committed to our hospital after making homicidal and suicidal statements in front of police officers. He was a small, quiet, gentle man who spoke in one-word replies. At first, I was caught off guard because he did not fit the "usual" patient profile of an involuntarily committed individual who is angry and rebellious. Here is an excerpt from our second session:

TRAINEE: Hi, John. How have you been feeling since we last talked?

JOHN: Fine, I got some rest.

TRAINEE: [pause] Some rest ... (Simple reflection, echoing his words)

JOHN: I've been gathering my thoughts.

TRAINEE: [pause] You have had a chance to rest, to be still, and reflect on what has happened as a result of your actions. (I specifically used the phrase "your actions," instead of "recent events" or "what brought you in," because my goal was to maintain a person-centered approach and place subtle emphasis on the fact that it was *his* actions and not "the alcohol" that led to his admission. Recall that MI aims to evoke a sense of autonomy within patients, rather than implying or assuming passivity)

JOHN: Yes.

TRAINEE: When you say, "gathering your thoughts," what do you mean? (Evoking)

JOHN: I realize that when I'm depressed I shouldn't drink. I should make a phone call instead or try a different vice. (The patient is presenting reasons for change elicited by the open-ended question)

TRAINEE: Drinking is not something you want to do in the future ... you really see a connection between your depression and drinking alcohol. (Reflection emphasizing how depression and substance use are linked)

JOHN: Yes.

TRAINEE: John, how were you able to come to the conclusion that drinking is affecting you? (Open-ended question)

JOHN: Well, take smoking [cigarettes] for example. I can go for 2 days [that is, since admission to the unit] with no nicotine patch, and be fine. Why can't I do that with drinking?

TRAINEE: You're drawing a comparison between smoking and drinking. You realize that you're coping without cigarettes and want to do the same with drinking. John, help me understand, what drives you to drink? (Transitional summary statement followed by an evocative question)

JOHN: Well, sometimes it's the taste, but other times I don't like the taste. I want to drink because I'm pissed off or depressed. Sometimes it's because my friends will be in the bar, playing pool, shooting darts, you know. . .

TRAINEE: There is the social aspect of being out with friends, as well as some of the characteristics of alcohol ... at the same time there are also times where negative emotions drive you to drink. (Double-sided reflection, linking in past information)

JOHN: Yes. Some people blame alcohol for their actions or say it caused their depression, but I know I drink *because* I'm depressed, period.

TRAINEE: John, I really appreciate you sharing this with me; it's not easy to sit in that chair. You pride yourself on being strong for others and you're realizing now that you need to be strong for yourself, too, by being honest and open about your struggles. (Affirmation, encouraging the patient without "cheerleading" responses, such as "That's great," "That shows good insight," or "Good for you")

Looking back on this encounter, I remember how challenged I felt to remain quiet within myself, while remaining fully attentive and present to this patient's reserved, subdued manner of speaking. Had I not been able to respond to his stillness, I wonder now whether I might have missed the remarkable insights we gleaned together over the course of this interview.

The "Manipulative or Entitled" Patient

Key Skills: (a) address thought process rather than content; (b) complex reflections such as amplified and double-sided reflections; (c) autonomy statements and affirmations to communicate that they *are* in control of their emotions and their behaviors, particularly when loss of control is suggested or threatened.

KEY POINT

Stress autonomy with an entitled patient to further establish therapeutic alliance.

Tips: A neutral/relaxed or pleasant/concerned affect is ideal, as is relaxed body language.

During a medical rotation I was called to the floor because a patient on the ward was "freaking out."

TRAINEE: Hi, Jessica. What's going on right now?

JESSICA: I'll tell you what's going on—it's you people and this place. I come here in agony, somehow am able to reach out for help, and then I get nothing in return! Tylenol® isn't going to cut it. I told you this and I'm not stupid, you know! Only Norco® works for my chronic pain!

TRAINEE SAMPLE RESPONSE 1: Well, Jessica, as we spoke about earlier, Norco® is not indicated for your pain as we cannot find a pathological cause of your pain. (Defensive, directly responds to content and intellectualizes)

TRAINEE SAMPLE RESPONSE 2: Jessica, I can see how frustrated you are right now … it took all your energy to come here and you feel that coming here was a waste of time because you're still in excruciating pain. (Complex reflection that addresses thought process and not content)

TRAINEE SAMPLE RESPONSE 3 [SHOULD THE PATIENT CONTINUE TO BE RILED UP]: It's hard to communicate when you're yelling. Would you like me to give you a couple of minutes to cool off? Let's see what's happening right now. I'm a little confused because this morning you were much calmer. (Set limits and also allow the patient a degree of control because internally, the patient feels stripped of it. Acknowledging some personal emotion makes you more of a real person and less of a threat.)

The risk of responding directly to content is that such a stance will likely place you in opposition to your patient, thereby sending you into what I call "interview purgatory," that is, a never-ending debate about your medical management versus their reality versus your credentials versus what they *know* is true, and so on. Direct insults, sarcasm, rhetorical questions, and challenges to medical decision making are situations rife with potential content traps. Addressing your patient's thought process puts the focus back on the patient in a therapeutic and nonconfrontational manner. It is perfectly reasonable to share a personal opinion, similar to sample 1; however, it is better to preface this activity by first seeking permission to do so and then asking for feedback on your opinion after you have shared it. Another useful strategy is to offer the patient a list of available options.

Shea describes seven "core pains" that interviewers should keep in mind when trying to assess and better understand how the "manipulative" behavior, or any form of observable resistance, comes about:

1. Fear of being alone
2. Fear of worthlessness

3. Fear of impending rejection
4. Fear of failure
5. Fear of loss of external control
6. Fear of loss of internal control
7. Fear of the unknown

"Manipulative" or "entitled" patients have learned to fill these voids by manipulating and controlling their environments, thereby also serving to protect their fragile sense of self. How do they achieve this? They attack *your* sense of self . . . along with everyone else's. What a shock it is when you respond in a steady, controlled manner designed to deescalate the situation.

"Manipulative" or "entitled" patients are the patients we struggle with most. Like delirium, manipulation can present in either a quiet fashion or a very obvious one. However, unlike delirium, these interactions seem to pierce right into our core, our very sense of self. They shake us up enough to ruin a morning, a call shift, or even longer. "Flight" is not an option; so instead, we prepare ourselves to "fight." The defense we often use is to put up an emotionless wall that has a two-fold benefit: our countertransference cannot get *out*, and the patient's enraging words or behaviors cannot get *in*. We quickly learn that this is not a sustainable coping mechanism when phrases such as "Who cares if she leaves, I'll be glad!" dare to creep into our minds or when we dread the thought of another challenging patient. This still happens from time to time, when we are tired or having a difficult day. Yet it takes all of 10 seconds to remind ourselves that no one wins this way: it is a lose-lose situation. Remember that when we view our interactions with patients as a battle with winners and losers, then we have the MI approach to use. Once you feel confident about using the strategies we have discussed, your options when dealing with "manipulative" or "entitled" patients will now consist of "fight," "flight," or "use MI."

The "Nonadherent" Patient

Key Skills: (a) explore beliefs and underlying ambivalence; (b) develop discrepancies, that is, how the individual's current behavior or consequences contradict his or her values/beliefs/goals for the future; (c) respond to discord.

Tips: "Why" is a word best avoided when incorporating MI into encounters with our patients. It's subtly judgmental and can limit patient engagement, rather than evoke more change talk. Instead of asking "Why?" pose questions such as "What leads you to. . .?" or "What makes it difficult for you to. . .?" Remember that the dyad formed through MI, the interpersonal process itself, is what helps to bring about motivation for change. Motivation is the behavior itself. Something to ponder, then, is this: Could it be that your patient who has presented to the emergency department with a heart attack, and who hasn't taken her blood pressure and anticholesterol medications, might be intrinsically "unmotivated" or "noncompliant"? How can patients be expected to act out their physician's monologue?

KEY POINT

Avoid questioning a nonadherent patient's behaviors with the pejorative "why?".

Patients with concurrent psychiatric and substance use disorders often sense that these issues get in the way of the person they would like to be, whether mother, father, son, daughter, boyfriend, girlfriend, or perhaps even the person a now-deceased relative had wanted them to be. These feelings are an extremely powerful conduit for change. Religion may also prove very important. Family members of patients who do not adhere to medication or treatment regimens, or who fail to attend medical appointments, are often upset about this behavior and their reactions can also become a stepping-stone to exploring ambivalence and developing discrepancies.

Consider the following summary, in which the arrows mean "leads to":

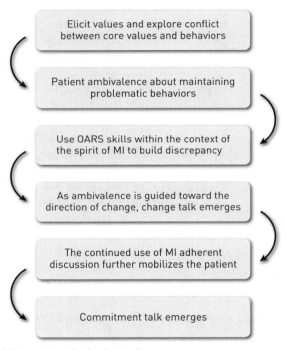

FIGURE 8.1   Mobilizing patients by developing discrepancy.

Discrepancy/conflict between behavior and core values → ambivalence about continued sustained versus changed behavior → through MI, discrepancy increases and ambivalence is guided in the direction of change → the process of change is mobilized and soon the patient is expressing change talk → further mobilize to commitment language (Fig. 8.1).

As mentioned in previous chapters, the process of change is more effective when our patients come up with the reasons for change, and *not* us. Our role is to engage, guide, and evoke reasons for, and commitment to, change.

"Nonadherent" patients are patients we may feel frustrated with, sometimes prompting dramatic statements such as "Mr. Smith is going to die if he doesn't take that medication/make those lifestyle changes/keep those outpatient appointments." More often than not, we as trainees make a grave mistake in thinking that confronting ill patients with the certainty of a negative health consequence, severe pain, or even death will be sufficient to bring about the desired change. It isn't. In fact, we have treated countless individuals in our inpatient psychiatric setting who tell us that their drug/alcohol use or lack of medication adherence actually increases following stern warnings from physicians in starched white coats. In many cases patients' lives may indeed be in jeopardy; but however ardently we tell them this, when we fail—for even a few minutes—to explore the thoughts and feelings that have prevented adherence in the first place, we are much less likely to bring about meaningful change.

THE CHALLENGING ENCOUNTER OF DELIVERING "BAD NEWS"

Breaking bad news is a challenging encounter for any medical trainee. Bad news may be defined as any situation in which "there is either a feeling of no hope, a threat to a person's mental or physical well-being, a risk of upsetting an established lifestyle, or where a message is reality which conveys to an individual fewer choices in his or her life." It is crucial to consider the cultural context of these scenarios since some cultures have different perspectives of delivering, and receiving, bad news. Bad news delivered poorly can negatively affect a patient's responses. Delivering bad news may be very distressing to us because it elicits a profound fear that we will be unable to respond adequately to strong emotional reactions. Taking the time to carefully review the clinical situation, to prepare yourself emotionally, to ensure an unhurried discussion that respects your patient's privacy while encouraging family members to be present as desired by the patient, will help these difficult situations go as smoothly as possible.

Once the consultation is initiated, use the spirit and skills of MI to engage the patient. Using the elicit-provide-elicit (E-P-E) framework, while keeping in mind to ask permission regarding how much information the patient wants to receive, honor his or her autonomy. It is crucial to pay close attention to a patient's emotional reactions when sharing bad news. Support can be offered in an empathic approach by reflecting and validating patients' emotions and experiences, and summarizing the discussion. Discuss the implications of the news, elicit patient questions, offer resources and options as appropriate, negotiate the next steps, and arrange for follow-up.

A CLOSING THOUGHT

We work under extreme time pressures atop many other stresses and strains unique to this time in our lives. The following anecdote from Father Gregory Boyle's book *Tattoos on the Heart, The Power of Boundless Compassion* is a fitting end to this chapter on engaging with challenging patients. The next time you find yourself annoyed by an ill-timed pager or a seemingly difficult individual, it may be helpful to recall this scenario.

This woman in her thirties walks through the door. I immediately glance at the clock hanging on the wall. I check how much time I have left before the baptism and am already lamenting that I most probably won't get to all the mail. I find out later that the woman's name is Carmen.. . .. Carmen is a heroin addict, a gang member, street person, occasional prostitute and … she is often defiantly storming down the street usually shouting at someone.

. . .. Now I have seven minutes until the baptism.. . .

Carmen plops herself into one of the chairs in my office and cuts the fat out of her introductory remarks. "I need help," she launches right in. … "I've been at like fifty rehabs. I'm known all over … nationwide.

. . .. I went to Catholic school all my life. Fact, I graduated from high school even. Fact, right after graduation, is when I started to use heroin." Carmen enters some kind of trance at this point and her speech slows to deliberate and halting.

"And I … have been trying to stop … since … the moment I began."

Then I watch as Carmen tilts her head back until it meets the wall. She stares at the ceiling, and in an instant her eyes become these two ponds, water rising to meet their edges, swollen banks, spilling over. Then, for the first time really, she looks at me and straightens. "I … am … a … disgrace."

Suddenly, her shame meets mine. For when Carmen walked through that door, I had mistaken her for an interruption. (pg. 61)

SELF-ASSESSMENT QUIZ

True or False?

1. MI offers helpful techniques and strategies to challenging clinical encounters.
2. Exploring the emotion behind tears is encouraged in MI.
3. When patients refuse to talk, respecting their autonomy may help build rapport.
4. "Why?" questions are a helpful means to engage patients and evoke change talk.
5. The phenomenon known as "heart sink" or a "difficult" encounter may be understood by examining the characteristics both trainee and patient bring to an interview, in addition to complex factors within healthcare systems.

Answers

1. *True.* The spirit of MI is one of collaboration, absolute acceptance, and compassion, making it an ideal framework to approach challenging encounters. Developing compassion and accepting a patient's perspective helps break the unproductive cycle that often accompanies challenging encounters.
2. *True.* Acknowledging a patient's obvious emotion and exploring the nature of what is being expressed validates the experience and is one way of demonstrating compassion and empathy. Such explorations may lead to meaningful discussions of topics or perspectives that are fundamental to patients' progress toward change.
3. *True.* By respecting a patient's wishes, we affirm autonomy and demonstrate respect. Acknowledge that the patient is uncomfortable, perhaps struggling with emotion, and suggest that you meet at another time to begin a therapeutic conversation.
4. *False.* "Why" should be avoided most of the time in all MI-based encounters; these questions are often perceived as judgmental and limit patient engagement.

More relevant questions include, "What leads you to. . .?" or "What makes it difficult for you. . .?" These questions are value-neutral and more likely to encourage further change talk.

5. *True.* "Heart sink" or "difficult" encounters result from a combination of a practitioner's level of expertise and ability, a patient's previous experience with health services, and factors intrinsic to the healthcare system. Important practitioner characteristics include lack of experience and professional identity, gaps in knowledge, weak communication skills, an inability to manage time effectively, and fatigue. Patient characteristics include mental health issues, personality disorders, a lack of willingness to engage with treatment, and previous experience with ineffective practitioners and treatments. Finally, healthcare system characteristics include language and cultural barriers, time pressures, and lack of continuity of care.

9 Brief Interventions

In this chapter, we examine treatment in clinical settings most suited to a brief intervention as an adaptation of motivational interviewing (MI). These include the emergency department, which is a setting specifically designed for single and time-limited patient encounters. Others include specialist offices, where visits are often short and focused on a particular disease or condition. Primary care practice offers medical trainees rich opportunities to practice and refine an MI approach with or without the guidance of a mentor who is trained and experienced in MI.

BRIEF INTERVENTIONS IN MEDICAL TRAINING

It is common in our role to see well-meaning physicians prematurely push patients to make behavioral or lifestyle changes. As a result, we often see patients become defensive to the point of rejecting advice they might otherwise have considered. Yet the nature of the interaction caused them to focus on defending their position rather than on communicating with their physician about something that directly affects their health and quality of life, possibly their life itself. Later, in an informal hallway debriefing, trainees may offer their own complaints about patients who refuse to take the necessary steps to improve their conditions. Thus, this approach to patient care constitutes the classic doctor–patient relationship. This process of simply dictating "doctors' orders" is perpetuated by the next generation continuing to behave in the same manner as their mentors, even though the approach was just observed to have failed.

This conceptualization of the practitioner's role in healthcare is based on a history of medical professionals treating acute physical conditions which respond to treatment primarily without regard to the patient's experiences. In an inpatient setting, pneumonia may be targeted with antibiotics and acute appendicitis resolved with a simple surgery. Practitioners thereby diagnose, treat, and discharge such patients without giving much attention to any considerations beyond the disease. Meanwhile, patients are unlikely to object to this approach because they share with their doctors the objective of reducing symptoms that are painful or impairing.

Modern medicine, however, has gone through an evolutionary process that has redefined the focus of medical care and the role of the medical practitioner. Chronic disease now dominates the healthcare landscape. This new paradigm recognizes the dire consequences of just four chronic, life-threatening risk factors: tobacco use, unhealthy diet, physical inactivity, and excess alcohol consumption, which cause up to 40% of mortality in the U.S. These chronic conditions can be modified but cannot be remedied by practitioners simply dictating acute care plans. Patients ultimately must be responsible for changing these lifestyle-based behaviors, and practitioners must rely on evidence-based methods for helping them to do so.

Brief interventions (BIs) are considered opportunistic interventions, particularly in healthcare settings where patients are being treated for medical conditions and injuries that are the direct result of risk-related behaviors. Patients are either not aware of the connection between their behaviors and why they are being treated, or more likely, they are not acknowledging how their behaviors are putting them at risk. Given this lack of awareness, they may not be prepared for an intensive examination of their behavior by a primary care physician. In these cases, screening, brief feedback, and advice are potentially the best strategies. For example, a positive screen for heavy drinking would trigger a BI, even though the patient did not intend to talk about her drinking during the medical visit. BI has been used to target substance use, including tobacco, and implemented in a wide range of settings, including primary care, emergency rooms, trauma units, and college health services.

What sets apart behavioral conditions, such as substance use and other risk-related behaviors, is that they have elements which serve some purpose to the patients (e.g., using alcohol to self-medicate anxiety). The risks and benefits from such behaviors ensure the presence of ambivalence about giving them up. This ambivalence is a natural step in the change process, but it creates a challenge to maintaining motivation to change. Trainees who fail to show concern for this internal conflict and who convey an interest in keeping interactions brief often instill in patients a feeling that they are not being heard or understood. This dynamic must be changed if trainees are to be effective in treating behavioral conditions, a realization reflected in the decision by the Accreditation Council for Graduate Medical Education, to designate a focus on patient-centeredness and interpersonal skills as core competencies (ACGME, 2007).

BRIEF INTERVENTION BASED ON MOTIVATIONAL INTERVIEWING

How an evaluation is approached in the earliest stages, including the nonverbal behavior of the trainee, greatly enhances or detracts from the therapeutic alliance. Although more in-depth treatment can be provided for patients who are accepting of it, many patients who benefit from BI are not prepared for an extensive exploration of their behaviors because they have a low level of motivation. Prematurely focusing on problems the trainee perceives but the patient does not, creates defensiveness in the patient and a discord in the clinical encounter. The more a trainee insists on pursuing the nonrecognized problem, the more intense the discord becomes, resulting in an even greater difficulty in engaging the patient in a discussion about it. Most importantly, if patients perceive their treatment experience with one trainee as negative, that experience could influence other treatment encounters. Therefore, subsequent efforts to address these risk-related problems become even more difficult for the trainees who follow. The discord created by prematurely focusing on conditions not acknowledged by the patient is the primary reason for the MI tenet to avoid the "righting reflex." Dramatic efforts to encourage patients to rapidly make major behavioral changes are often misplaced. Small doses of treatment in the form of a BI, with an emphasis on the patient's responsibility for deciding about any change, is often the best strategy, and for some patients it may be all you have time to, or need to, offer.

MI has subsequently been developed into BI, conversations about change that may last only a few minutes or comprise a few simple exchanges. While hesitant at first to consider these BIs as a form of MI, the creators of MI have since embraced them as an extension of the spirit and method of MI applied to a new context. In their framing, MI is a "style of being with people" and its underlying spirit may guide the structure and tone of a single sentence or an intense, multisession therapy. Perhaps more clinically relevant, MI-driven BI has been shown to be more effective than the classic finger-wagging, or simply telling people what to do and why. Unfortunately, this is the approach we observe most frequently from our instructors.

BI becomes even more important in primary and secondary prevention efforts. Overutilization of emergency departments, specialist care, and avoidable procedures adds to human and societal cost from modifiable behavioral disorders. In the absence of a primary care physician with whom the patient has a trusting relationship, emergency departments often act as the first contact; patients may reveal critical health and behavioral issues that have been neglected by the patients themselves and their primary practitioners. Even modest effect sizes with BIs on patients who may be early in a disease course, or who are simply at high risk, could have expanding returns over years of a subsequently avoided or mitigated chronic disease. This view of BI lends itself to a reframing as an "opportunistic intervention," a sometimes unexpected chance for trainees to influence health behavior change.

BI is indicated in the following treatment situations:

- Medical care delivered in which a practitioner has time for only a short interaction with the patient, for example, in an emergency department with a patient whose injury is alcohol related or during a preoperative visit where multiple factors affecting outcome might need to be addressed (e.g., smoking, diet, postoperative care).
- Medical care during which a circumscribed behavior can be targeted, for example, in a primary care office with patients who are not taking medications for hypertension properly or at a dentist's office where poor dental hygiene results in dental and gum disease.
- During routine treatment for another condition where a risk-related behavior is uncovered but is not the focus of treatment, for example, unsafe sexual practices or drug use revealed while obtaining a history and physical. On consultation services where evaluation is generally considered the primary role of the practitioner, for example, a consultation liaison psychiatry visit with a patient who accidently overdosed and judged to be safe for discharge would still benefit from a risk-related intervention.

Each of these situations poses unique challenges and considerations, while sharing a need for patient-centered care that respects the patient's own goals and needs.

- An emergency department offers little continuity and often involves an acute concern which may be distracting or debilitating, such as injury or intoxication. In this case, timing of the intervention and subsequent referral to treatment may have the most significant impact on lasting efficacy; as evidence suggests, the significant effect of BI could otherwise fade without further intervention.
- In primary care settings, time may prove more flexible and the therapeutic alliance may already be more established. In this case, effective counseling may be hindered by inadequate knowledge of effective screening methods and discomfort engaging patients in these discussions, areas where an MI-informed approach can have a significant impact.

An incidentally discovered behavioral risk is often challenging because the patient may not consider it a problem and may take offense to any impression of it becoming the focus of a visit. In these cases, effective skills for minimizing discord are critical, and MI, coupled with personalized feedback, has proven to be a particularly effective style for achieving positive outcomes in more angry and aggressive patients.

- A psychiatric consultant is likely to be the most skilled member of the care team with regard to behavioral intervention. In this case, the major barrier to effective intervention is likely one of expectation. Some practitioners may see their role on a consulting service primarily as that of an evaluator, consistent with the request made by the primary team. Even these highly trained and experienced practitioners would benefit from focusing on the first stage in learning MI, a "willing suspension of disbelief and active curiosity" about both the patient's perspective and the role MI might have in changing the traditional modes of practice.

BI utilizing the MI spirit and skills is not restricted to these settings. Many brief applications of MI have been tested and validated, including its use in the following:

- Hospital settings
- Primary care
- Dental settings
- Prenatal care
- Detoxification and drug use
- Smoking cessation
- Emergency departments
- Trauma centers
- Telephone consultations
- Parental treatment adherence

In short, any situation involving modifiable behavioral risks offers opportunities for trainees to practice their OARS skills, while providing them a significant probability of impacting the health of their patients. It is important to note that this can be done without requiring an order or co-signature from a supervising practitioner, and a potentially liberating sensation for them.

INTERPERSONAL STYLE, THERAPEUTIC RELATIONSHIP, AND MOTIVATION TO CHANGE

While support for BI's efficacy is building, the extent of its effectiveness has not been definitively determined. However, the nature of the therapeutic alliance between patient and practitioner affects a patient's motivation and ability to change, and MI has been well established as a "highly effective psychotherapeutic approach for establishing a therapeutic alliance." Learning to perform BI is critical to learning how to conduct MI, because it challenges trainees to maximize use of MI skills, embracing MI as more of a style than a set of prescribed steps. Reflective listening and affirming positive behavior are at the heart of forging a therapeutic alliance, and more abbreviated interactions with patients are precisely the scenarios where this alliance must be formed most efficiently. The sooner in their careers that medical trainees learn to naturally engage in this style of communication, the more effective they will be as physicians.

Medical care is often delivered in single patient encounters in which a practitioner may have only one short interaction with a patient. In this context, it is unsurprising that some physicians excuse themselves of responsibility regarding major behavioral modifications that will likely require longitudinal attention. This attitude can do a disservice to both the patients and the burdened healthcare system. It has been well documented that a single BI can produce real change, reducing healthcare costs and utilization in high-risk populations.

Deciding not to intervene due to lack of time when a modifiable disease course is uncovered is no different than opting not to treat a patient's pneumonia because the practitioner is busy. It represents a gross violation of the patient-centered principles we have embraced in modern ethical codes of medicine. The methods and principles presented here should enable even early medical trainees to apply MI to abbreviated encounters, precisely the sort of encounters they will experience most frequently. Encouragingly, the literature suggests that level of medical training does not significantly influence outcomes, meaning that MI-guided trainees in any number of healthcare fields have the potential to make a notable impact even early in their careers.

A MODEL OF A BRIEF INTERVENTION

A complete brief intervention is based on three steps (Screening, Brief Intervention, and Referral to Treatment, or SBIRT).

TOOLBOX
SBIRT
Screening
Brief Intervention
Referral to Treatment

Screening

Screening must be guided by knowledge of suggestive conditions and at-risk populations. It would be exceptionally low yield, for example, to screen every patient who presents with a urinary tract infection for alcohol abuse. On the other hand, given the high correlation between drug use and trauma-related visits, it is negligent not to screen injured patients for drug and alcohol use.

Brief Intervention

TOOLBOX
FRAMES
Feedback
Responsibility
Advice
Menu of options
Empathy
Self-Efficacy

In the event of a positive screen, we utilize an approach for BIs described by the mnemonic FRAMES.

We will discuss FRAMES in details in Chapter 13.

Referral to Treatment

It is necessary to provide patients who may be experiencing a boon in their motivation the opportunity to follow through with adequate long-term care and investment. It is helpful to know specific resources of which a patient may not be aware. These exist in the form of the following:

- Patient's preexisting or new primary care physician
- Hotlines
- Web sites
- Organizations/meetings
- Medical specialists
- Therapists, social workers, and case workers

PRINCIPLES OF MOTIVATIONAL INTERVIEWING–BASED BRIEF INTERVENTIONS

The fundamental principles of BIs are consistent with the MI model for stimulating change. Discussions must be:

- *Patient-centered*, focusing on the patient's perspective, priorities, and interests
- *Nonjudgmental* and *empathic*
- *Directive* and *goal-oriented*, with an objective of exploring and discussing ambivalence related to problem behaviors without necessarily resolving them

BI poses the unique challenges related to having:

- *Less time* to establish a strong therapeutic alliance and engage the patient
- *Less detailed knowledge* of a patient's unique biopsychosocial status
- Potential *distractions* for both patient and practitioner (e.g., the high activity level of treatment in an emergency room; patients who are not seeking help)

Modifications must be made to standard MI during BIs. As a result, BIs have a narrower focus that concentrates on the following:

- *Personalized feedback* that is best tailored to reasons for the current admission or visit
- *Realistic goals*, often simply helping patients to view a behavior as a problem or schedule a follow-up appointment to further address problem behavior
- Providing, with permission, *discrete options*, including *appropriate referral*, as warranted

POTENTIAL PITFALLS

Using this framework, BIs can create several pitfalls that must be consciously avoided, most arising directly from the time constraint. The most frequently witnessed by us is the tendency for patients to engage in status quo talk while *we* prematurely urge patients to focus on what *we* consider to be problematic behavior. Other pitfalls might include:

- Limited time, which makes a very direct approach seem reasonable. The trainee often feels an urge to be directive and simply begin dictating to a patient what must be done to reduce health-related risk.
- Application of direct pressure, which induces immediate discord in the encounter in the form of arguing, ignoring, interrupting, and/or being overly compliant.
- Disrespect of the patient's right to self-determination through failure to explore his or her perspective and failure to offer alternatives.
- Arguing when patients express a lack of desire to change or reservations about implementing suggested advice. It is critical to avoid such pitfalls because it may not be possible to establish or recover a therapeutic relationship after the righting reflex is triggered in a short interview. Using autonomy statements frequently can help minimize discord.

Autonomy statements reflect the patient's responsibility for his or her well-being, including the full range of thoughts and behaviors. This essentially means that it is up to the patient whether he or she recognizes or denies a problem, contemplates change, or engages in action behaviors. One way to deliver autonomy statements is to refer to your role as that of a "consultant." In this way you note that you have some experience with medical treatment and problem behaviors and you are offering your observations and recommendations. However, emphasis is placed on the reality that it is up to the patient to decide whether he or she wants to consider it. If appropriate, it is also important to emphasize that you do not necessarily expect the patient to agree with you or use your advice, and that it will not affect your relationship or any other treatment you provide for him or her. This stance makes it clear that your objective is to help the patient, and you will not withhold treatment or otherwise punish the patient because he or she disagrees with you.

Engaging in a successful BI means having a reasonable expectation regarding what can be accomplished in 5 to 60 minutes:

- Establish a realistic goal for the interview based on the patient's current stage of readiness to change and, emotional state.
- For a patient who is not ready to change a behavior, it may be sufficient simply to engage him or her in thinking about the problematic behavior.
- Despite media depiction of behavioral changes occurring after epiphanies, in most cases even a near loss of life is not able to instill unwavering motivation to achieve lasting change.
- These moments nevertheless provide an important window of opportunity to direct a patient's attention toward a hazardous behavior and its repercussions.
- Care must be made to avoid falling into the position of utilizing "scare tactics."

SINGLE ENCOUNTER

Emergency Medicine

Emergency departments provide excellent opportunities for us to use the MI approach. Emergency departments serve as natural capture sites for patients who are engaging in unhealthy and risk-related behavior, and patients at emergency departments and trauma-care sites constitute a medical population in need of MI-based BIs.

Trainees often have more time to engage patients in an emergency department than attending physicians. This enables trainees to address risk-related behaviors at a time when unforeseen consequences lead patients to be more open, creating a high potential for a teachable moment.

Screening Process

The first step toward successful BIs is identifying the patients who might benefit from behavioral change. Efficient screening means having a working knowledge of certain at-risk populations. While dependent on the specific nature of the presentation, the following conditions should often prompt screening as noted:

- Trauma: Substance use or intimate partner violence
- Gynecologic or genitourinary complaints: Risky sexual behaviors or sexual abuse
- Esophageal bleeds: Alcohol use (variceal) or eating disorders (Mallory-Weiss)
- Electrolyte imbalance: Eating disorders/diuretic use, alcohol use, or misuse of other supplements or herbal medications
- Infection: Poor diabetes control, intravenous drug use (IVDU), or inadequate dental care

Utilizing inclusion criteria and clinical judgment is a more conservative treatment approach (i.e., greater sensitivity) than giving emphasis to exclusion criteria, whereby fewer people are screened because they do not meet a particular threshold for risk (i.e., greater specificity). For example, a patient with tricuspid valve vegetation warrants discussion of IVDU, even if preconceived biases regarding age, gender, ethnicity, or socioeconomic status affect a trainee's impression of the low likelihood of a positive screen. Conversely, a 70-year-old woman with a urinary tract infection should receive a more rudimentary investigation of her recent sexual history. Similarly, a male in his twenties with an electrolyte imbalance should be asked one or two general questions about his eating habits and body image. More detailed explorations should be reserved for patients only after brief screening verifies the possible existence of a diagnosable disorder.

The process follows a modified SBIRT format, with a much more lengthy screening or assessment process but otherwise similar BI and referral to treatment components.

- Placing the intervention at the end of the assessment maximizes the time spent on building a therapeutic relationship.
- MI spirit for conveying empathy with reflective listening should be utilized during the entire process of obtaining the history and physical interview or assessment to ensure the quality of both the information and the alliance.

- An appropriate goal is assisting the patient in exploring ambivalence, not necessarily resolving it, regarding whether the identified issue is even concerning or deserving of treatment.
- An effective BI can be the reason a patient follows through with initial outpatient treatment and therefore takes advantage of an opportunity at significant behavioral modification.

EXAMPLES OF BRIEF INTERVENTIONS

The duration of MI-based BI depends on the circumstances and the setting of the clinical encounter. We will present and discuss examples of BIs in diverse clinical settings.

Setting: 5–15 Minute BI in the Emergency Room

TRAINEE: Good morning. I reviewed your chart, and it mentioned your friends brought you in because they had a very hard time waking you up. When you woke up, you were saying things that didn't make sense, telling them you had to get to class because you had a big test. So they brought you here. Do you know where you are?

PATIENT: Yeah, the nurse that just left says I'm in the emergency room. I don't remember any of that other stuff happening.

TRAINEE: What do you remember?

PATIENT: I remember going to the party and starting to play beer pong. I remember that I had to drink a lot of times—those guys on the other side of the table were real good. That's about all I remember until an hour ago. (Looking down) Did I throw up?

TRAINEE: Yes, but we gave you something to settle your stomach so that won't happen again. It's 7:30 a.m. now. Your blood alcohol level (BAL) at 1:30 this morning was 0.32. I was wondering whether you know what it means.

PATIENT: Yeah, I know about BAL; I don't need another lecture about drinking too much. If I want to drink, I'm going to. I'm still carrying a 3.4 in my classes, so it isn't hurting me to drink on the weekends if I want to. And this is the first time I ended up in the emergency room.

TRAINEE: You are working hard in school and it is paying off for you. And I do understand that you want to have some fun now and then. Also, you said this is the first time your drinking has *ever* gotten out of hand.

PATIENT: Well, I have missed a few classes and assignments over the past 2–3 months, and last week I didn't get a paper done on time because I was hung over. But I am a good student and my professors let me make up the work. And I do think I deserve to take some time to kick back.

TRAINEE: Your drinking might have caused a few problems with your class work recently, and your professors have been understanding and *always* let you make up the work.

PATIENT: I wouldn't say they always let me make up work. The one guy said he didn't understand, that it was really unusual for me to miss having my paper done on time. He even asked if everything was alright, or if I needed help or something. When I said no, he seemed annoyed and said from now on I need to make sure

I get things done on time. That worried me a little, and I told him that it won't happen again. I do want to keep my grades up.

TRAINEE: You're saying that you might think about cutting down on your drinking if you thought it was causing your grades to drop.

PATIENT: Well, yeah. I am only a year away from getting my degree, and I am thinking about graduate school. I know I'll have to keep my grades up if I am going to get into a good school.

TRAINEE: You have worked very hard and you're getting tired of all the work and want to relax. And you are very close to graduating and, as you say, it is even more important to keep up with doing good work now. You are sharing with me that you can see where things could get worse when it comes to the effect your drinking has on your grades. I am not saying you have to quit drinking. That isn't up to me; it is your call. And I can share with you some strategies on how to cut down—if you would be interested.

PATIENT: I guess it couldn't hurt.

The trainee does not respond to the discord generated around discussion of BAL. Rather, the trainee provides an affirmation for the patient's statement that he is getting good grades and simply suggests that the patient himself is a responsible person who wants to continue to do well. Without dictating that the patient must choose between drinking and not drinking, the trainee addresses the patient's ambivalence about how drinking may be affecting his grades. Early on in the intervention he understates the consequences by saying that he has never had a problem due to alcohol use, and that his professors will always let him make up work. The patient corrected these perspectives and, in the process, started to recognize that alcohol use is causing him problems. Later in the interview the trainee frames the reflections so as to suggest that they emanate from the patient's own perspective on the problem and then indicates that it is the patient's decision about how to proceed. Finally, the trainee makes it clear that he is not telling the patient that he must stop drinking. Rather, he suggests that this is one alternative among others the patient might consider.

Setting: 20 to 30 Minute BI in Consultation Liaison Psychiatry (Inpatient Hospital Room)

On an inpatient psychiatric consult service, a trainee is called upon to see patients who usually present with other medical concerns.

TRAINEE: Good morning. I was asked by your doctor to come and talk with you. Did your doctor tell you I was consulted?

PATIENT: Yeah, and I'm not too happy about it. I told him I don't like shrinks. I really don't want to talk to you, but he said it was the last thing I need to do for him to sign the papers so I can get out of here. So let's get it over with. But, I'm telling you, I'm not crazy and I'm not going to take whatever pills you're pushing.

TRAINEE: You've had a tough experience so far. I didn't realize you felt so strongly about not wanting to talk with me. If I had known that, I would have told your doctor that you might not be interested in talking with me. We are kind of in a similar situation.

PATIENT: So you don't want to talk to me either!

TRAINEE: No, I really would like to talk with you, but I don't want to cause you to get upset about it. That's not good for you. It works best when we both know we want to talk together. You really don't have to talk with me if you don't want to. When I say we're in similar positions, I mean no one can make you talk with me, and I don't want you to have to talk with me, if you don't want to.

PATIENT: Yeah, that makes sense. Well, you are here now so if you want to ask me anything, go ahead. My father isn't coming until this afternoon to pick me up.

TRAINEE: OK, I appreciate your talking with me. I know you weren't prepared for this. By the way, anything you tell me will stay between you and me. Even with your doctor, I don't necessarily intend to tell him everything you tell me, but I need to be able to talk with him about some things. Also, if there are things you don't want to tell me, that would be OK. It's completely up to you what you talk about and how much. Does that make sense?

PATIENT: Yeah, that sounds fair. If you are talking to me about killing myself or going after someone else, I have already heard it from the social worker here. I was angry when I first came in, but I've been here for 5 days and I have settled down. I'm not going to hurt myself or anyone else.

TRAINEE: What were you going through?

PATIENT: Well, I was driving home from New York and it was snowing real hard and I skidded and hit a guard rail. I totaled the car and got all banged up. I was probably driving too fast because I wanted to get home. And I was singing along with the radio, trying to practice. I have some friends at home who know some guys that are real big in the music business. My friends have heard me singing karaoke and told those guys about me and they wanted to hear me and record some songs. I was really anxious to get home because I think this could be a big break for me. I always have thought I sound a lot like Elvis and I know I am going to be as big as he was—if I get a chance. In fact, I remember, when the ambulance guys came, I told them about this big break and to take me home. But they brought me here anyway. I was real pissed off about that. But I guess it was for the best. I have two broken legs and a concussion.

TRAINEE: I can see why you were in a hurry. This was a big chance for you. You see it more clearly now that you need to be in the hospital.

PATIENT: Yeah, at first I was trying to put up a fight with them. I wanted out of here, but you can't do much with two broken legs. And they gave me some kind of tranquilizer and I settled down.

TRAINEE: How long have you wanted to be a singer?

PATIENT: Since I was a teenager. But I wasn't serious enough then, I guess, and I had to get a job. I work for one of the airlines at the airport.

TRAINEE: How was your life going when you found out about the chance to sing back home?

PATIENT: Fine. I mean money is always a problem, but I am making it. I wasn't having any big problems. I live with a roommate and sometimes he can be a pain, but nothing big.

TRAINEE: How do you feel about missing your chance to sing and record? Does that bother you?

PATIENT: Yeah, some. But what can I do? I may try to call my friends and see what's going on and if I can set something else up.

TRAINEE: If you recall, I said that we will keep things confidential. I saw on your chart where you told the nurse when you came in that you don't take any medications. I was wondering whether you have been drinking alcohol or using any street drugs recently.

PATIENT: Well, I drink, sometimes a little too much, but I am keeping it together. I haven't missed work or gotten into trouble. But the night before I started home my roommate had some cocaine and we snorted it. I never used that stuff before but I felt really good on it. Now, I am worried I can get fired.

TRAINEE: Your medical information is protected by confidentiality laws. Were you drinking the night of your accident?

PATIENT: No, I never drink and drive.

TRAINEE: Has any other drug made you feel the way you did on cocaine?

PATIENT: Well, once before. When I was 16, I ended up in a psych ward for 3 days after I dropped acid at a Prince concert. I remember I felt so great and it looked to me like Prince was waving at me to come up on stage. I started up, but the security guards grabbed me. I fought with them because I was convinced that Prince wanted me up there. But they took me away and sent me to the hospital. That's why I don't like shrinks. I wanted to leave the next day, and there was nothing wrong with me, but that shrink made me stay 3 days. He said it was to make sure that my psychosis had cleared up, but I think it was to bill my old man's insurance.

TRAINEE: And these kinds of episodes never happen to you when you are not using drugs?

PATIENT: Yeah, that's right.

TRAINEE: I realize it wasn't your idea for me to come here but, since we have talked, would you like my opinion about some things that may have contributed to your accident?

PATIENT: OK, go ahead.

TRAINEE: Your behavior after using cocaine and acid suggests that these drugs may be causing you to experience a manic-like state, an elevated mood with hyperactivity and problems with thinking realistically.

PATIENT: What? Are you saying that those drugs made me go crazy? I have a hard time believing that.

TRAINEE: Well, it happens to some people. I have seen it before. I'm just saying that's my opinion. I'm here as a consultant and you may disagree with me. No one is saying that you have to do anything with what I recommend, but I think you could potentially avoid these serious effects if you were to decide not to use cocaine or acid and consider following up with counseling after discharge.

PATIENT: I don't know. It sounds pretty far-fetched to think that little bit of coke could have had that big of an effect on me.

TRAINEE: I am available to discuss more about it if you decide to follow up with us in the outpatient clinic. It is up to you.

PATIENT: I don't know, Doc; I'll have to think about it and I may consider it because I can't afford going crazy like that anymore.

TRAINEE: OK. Thanks for talking with me. I'll let your doctor know that we have discussed and you are ready to leave the hospital.

This evaluation/intervention is one whereby the process is fraught with miscommunication and administrative problems that have contributed to the patient's frustration. This, in addition to his previous negative experience with psychiatric treatment, created an initial discord in the encounter. The consulting trainee pointed out that they shared similar experiences. She also gave the control back to the patient by making it clear that it is up to the patient whether the interview goes any further. It is important to note that allowing self-determination in this manner brings in the possibility that the patient will refuse the consultation. However, the trainee truly believes that it would be better for the patient to refuse to see her rather than to endure the interview feeling angry and unwilling to share. It is the act of pointing this out in a manner that the patient perceives as genuine that results in reducing the discord and the patient deciding to continue the interview. The trainee provided an affirmation for the patient's engagement in the encounter. The patient's openness following the initial encounter provides the trainee with accurate information about the etiology of the patient's psychiatric symptoms and allows her to form an opinion about the role of substance use in triggering a manic episode. She is then able to communicate to the patient the risk related to using substances. The patient is now more open to considering following up with treatment.

Setting: 30 to 45 Minute BI in the Endocrinologist's Office

TRAINEE: How are you feeling today?

PATIENT: I am feeling OK, I guess. I seem to feel tired a lot though. I know it is because of my weight. I am always planning to go on a diet, but I never really seem to get around to it. But often it gets to be too hard to plan my diet, and I end up eating things I shouldn't because it's just easier. I get busy. You know, my daughter has moved back in with me and I watch her two kids during the day—so she can work. I really love having them around. I love making sure they are taken care of properly. I've always been the kind to want to take care of people. That's why I was a nurse for so long.

TRAINEE: I didn't know you had been a nurse. Where did you work?

PATIENT: I was a nurse at the nursing home for 25 years before I retired.

TRAINEE: Your grandchildren and your daughter are lucky to have someone like you taking care of them. You have such a busy schedule that staying on a specific diet would be hard, because you would have to buy special foods or prepare low-fat meals that don't fit in with the kids' diet.

PATIENT: Yes, that's right. And sometimes I think the kids' diet is a big part of the problem. Those kids get wound up and I think it's the sugar in their diet. My daughter gets those little jugs of fruit drinks that are loaded with sugar and they drink them all day. I have to confess that I drink them to, because they are around. But I told my daughter that I think we should get natural juices for them, apple or grape, the ones with no artificial sugar, and keep the sugary ones out of the house.

TRAINEE: You made a valid point! It's one way to cut down on the sugar, and it may help everyone in the house. And that goes along with how important it is for you to be sure your family is well cared for. We could talk about other ways to reduce sugar or fat in the family diet, sort of brainstorm about it. What do you think?

PATIENT: Yes, that makes sense.

TRAINEE: So, keeping sugary drinks out of the house is one thing. What other suggestions do you have?

PATIENT: Well, we usually eat butter, but we could get a butter substitute. And we keep whole milk for the kids and I like milk too, but it wouldn't be too much trouble for me to get skim milk.

TRAINEE: You have shared that you are very good at planning for a healthier lifestyle; it must be your nurse's training and how much you value helping people to stay healthy. In fact, you've hit on something that most people don't think about when it comes to what they eat. Most of the time we talk about "going on a diet," which means we want to change our eating habits for a certain amount of time until we lose weight. Really, the best way to handle this is not to think about losing weight but to make a lifestyle change. Whether it is eating less, or less sugar and fat, or walking for exercise, whatever the method, we need to do it regularly and make it part of our lifestyle, and then weight loss takes care of itself. What do you think?

PATIENT: Yes, I think I see what you mean. I think I can do this.

TRAINEE: You are determined to follow through. We can review together what you can do to make these changes, and any other changes you think of as you consider what will lead to a healthier plan for everyone in the family. We also have literature in the waiting room on healthy diets that may work for you, if you want to look at it. Remember, any changes you make will be a step in the right direction. I'll see you in a month, and we'll see how you are doing with your progress. It's always good to set up time for a review of how things are working with your plan. Also, call me in the meantime, if you have anything you want to discuss or questions, including anything you find that is working well for you. I like it when I can get good ideas from my patients that I can pass on to others.

The trainee shows interest in the patient's statement that she is a nurse because this represents an opportunity to develop discrepancy. The trainee does this by linking her past love for taking care of others with how she might apply her professional values in her life today. As the conversation continues, the trainee now suggests that the helpful ideas she generated to assist herself and others in healthier eating is related to the satisfaction she receives in helping others stay well. The trainee employs the "brainstorming" technique because her patient is willing to move further into the process of change. Finally, the trainee stresses the importance of following up to review progress and to reflect on how significant this is to her and her family. In addition, the trainee discusses with the patient the possible need to modify the plan. By doing this she implies that implementing the changes they have discussed is a dynamic, ongoing process.

Brief interventions are a critical skill for both medical trainees and seasoned practitioners alike. Use of BI removes the excuse we give ourselves for not attempting to intervene when time is short or problems are daunting. It is also the skill which all clinicians have the greatest number of opportunities to practice. It is the rare patient who would not benefit from greater adherence to a treatment regimen. Accordingly, trainees have myriad opportunities to practice their brief intervention skills with patients, and develop them in diverse clinical settings throughout their medical careers.

SELF-ASSESSMENT QUIZ

True or False?

1. Brief interventions are targeted therapeutic conversations in which trainees begin the process of helping patients explore the relationship between unhealthy behavior(s) and current health concerns.
2. As an adaptation of MI, brief interventions have been shown to be beneficial only when addressing substance use.
3. Brief interventions are comprised of three steps: Screening, Brief Intervention, and Referral to Treatment (SBIRT).
4. Since brief interventions are necessarily time limited, trainees should be more direct in their exchanges with patients, especially in terms of suggesting the specific steps that will reduce health-related risks.
5. Emergency rooms, inpatient hospital wards, and outpatient clinics are settings in which brief interventions are appropriate approaches.

Answers

1. *True.* Brief interventions are indicated in those situations in which trainees have time for only short interactions with patients, as in an emergency department with an individual whose injuries are related to alcohol abuse. Another example, from a primary care setting, occurs among patients with hypertension who cannot or will not take medications as prescribed. Brief interventions are also indicated when high-risk behaviors are identified during routine interactions or treatment for another condition, such as discussing high-risk sexual practices during a standard history and physical examination.
2. *False.* Brief applications of MI have been tested and validated in many settings, including acute medical settings, dentistry, drug and alcohol programs, emergency departments, prenatal care, primary care, smoking cessation programs, telephone consultations, and trauma centers.
3. *True.* Screening should occur as a function of trainees knowing about possible conditions and recognizing at-risk individuals or populations; realistically, it is impossible to screen everyone for every health-related risk. A prime example is to screen patients injured in motor vehicle accidents for alcohol use. If the screening for alcohol use is positive, a BI is used and referral to treatment, if indicated, depending on the severity of the patient's substance use problems.
4. *False.* Given the time restrictions associated with brief interventions, using a direct approach may seem reasonable; however, it is not recommended. Maintaining the MI approach, even in short and isolated encounters, is vital to the success of the brief intervention.
5. *True.* Brief interventions based on MI are utilized in a variety of clinical settings.

10 Motivational Interviewing in Primary Care

This chapter reviews the application of motivational interviewing (MI) in primary care settings and highlights how you can use MI as an approach for medical illnesses. For outpatient primary care, we offer examples of using MI to address medication adherence, nutrition and weight loss, hypertension, hyperlipidemia, and diabetes management. For inpatient care, we examine applications of MI in primary care admissions. The goal is to emphasize the broad utility of MI throughout primary care medicine in the hope of maximizing its applications and simultaneously increasing the trainee's experience and comfort with this clinical approach.

MOTIVATIONAL INTERVIEWING AND ITS RELATIONSHIP TO MODELS OF CARE

Comprehensive and empirically informed models of care, such as the chronic care model (CCM), advocate for the use of established medical guidelines within an evidence-based healthcare system that addresses the need for patients with chronic disease. CCM comprises six fundamental components that are hypothesized to affect functional and clinical outcomes associated with illness management. The six components are (1) self-management support (i.e., fostering skills-based learning and patient empowerment); (2) decision support (i.e., providing and adhering to evidence-based practices); (3) delivery system design (i.e., promoting proactive coordinating care processes); (4) clinical information systems (i.e., tracking progress through monitoring and outcomes sharing with patients and practitioners); (5) health system (i.e., promoting a culture shift supported by leadership and removal of barriers to care); and (6) community resources and policies (i.e., sustaining care by using community resources to help bridge care outside of facilities). The CCM suggests healthcare systems must get better at creating "informed and activated patients"—patients who are in charge of managing their illnesses. It requires training patients to become self-managers by arming them with the information, motivation, and the confidence to succeed, and this is achieved through using MI. MI is well suited to addressing patients' needs and establishing a powerful therapeutic alliance with healthcare practitioners for long-term care.

Another model of practice related to CCM is the patient-centered medical home (PCMH) that was proposed in 2004 under the Future of Family Medicine project to align family medicine with the needs of the populations and to meet the goals proposed by the Institute of Medicine to provide safe, timely, and equitable patient-centered care. This model emphasizes evidence-based practices and proactive care. The MI approach fits well with the goals of this model as it does with CCM's goals by promoting healthy lifestyle changes.

ROLE OF MOTIVATIONAL INTERVIEWING IN PRIMARY CARE

Eliciting patient behavior change is a major challenge for today's medical trainees involved in medical management. Yet its importance could not come at a better time. Chronic illnesses such as diabetes, hypertension, and obesity have become major factors contributing to under- or overutilization of resources, including medication adherence, health literacy, lack of physical activity, and unhealthy eating habits. On a national level, more focus has recently been placed on prevention and wellness, and behavior change is at the center of that movement. This is where the MI approach is rapidly proliferating and evolving as highly effective and broadly applicable to medical encounters.

MI has expanded across diverse populations and medical disciplines to become a driving force in helping patients achieve behavior change in healthcare settings (Box 10.1). Fundamentally, MI has shown success in enhancing treatment engagement, in improving emotional well-being, and in increasing motivation and confidence to change. Furthermore, MI has been validated as being comparable, and sometimes superior, to other established treatments for a wide range of behavioral objectives.

A key element of MI is the concept that patients intrinsically know and possess what they need, rather than the classic view that practitioners are "providers" who can give patients what they lack (Miller & Rollnick 2013), for example, insight and problem-solving ability.

Miller and Rollnick (2013) provide an introductory definition of MI as "a collaborative conversation style for strengthening a person's own motivation and commitment to change." (pg. 12) The value of such a style is immediately apparent in modern primary care, where practitioners struggle against a growing burden of chronic physical disease exacerbated by an underpinning of mental health and behavioral disorders.

Box 10.1 Validated Motivational Interviewing Behavioral Targets

Alcohol cessation

Cannabis use

Improving diet

Enhancing exercise

Pedometer use

Weight loss

Problem gambling

Eating disorders

Promoting condom use

Decreasing risky sexual behaviors

Increasing adherence to diabetes care

HIV antiretroviral therapy adherence

Physical therapy adherence

Improved pain management

Reducing children's television watching

Decreasing smoke exposure in asthma

The broad applicability of MI makes it an excellent communication style for addressing a range of conditions and applicable to the diverse patient populations treated by primary care practitioners. In fact, the patient-centered nature of MI results in an inherent flexibility, which is widely accepted, as demonstrated by findings that it is more effective in comparison to other approaches when used with diverse populations.

The value of MI for the work in primary care is underscored by the ease with which its processes, skills, and techniques can be understood and learned. MI has been utilized effectively by a wide range of practitioners, including students, master's-level counselors, psychologists, nurses, physicians, and dieticians. Most encouraging for medical trainees is that research indicates the training background of the practitioner (nursing, social work, psychology, medicine, bachelor's, master's, or doctoral level) is *not* predictive of targeted outcomes such as substance use and health-related behaviors (diet, exercise, and safe sex), while the degree of training in MI is predictive of outcomes. This is important because, at times, medical trainees may find themselves feeling that they are not effective members of their treatment team. Conversely, these findings support the conclusion that those trainees who learn MI at an early stage of medical training will be making an immediate and positive impact on patient health.

OUTPATIENT PRIMARY CARE SETTINGS

We commonly become frustrated with patients who refuse to adhere to recommended treatments, self-monitoring, dietary changes, physical activity, or other lifestyle modifications. For MI to be most effective, the interaction between patient and trainee must be focused on achieving an accurate, mutual understanding of the reasons patients choose to follow, or choose not to follow, recommended health behavior changes. Above all, we must accept that one of the basic tenets of MI is patient self-determination and that only our patients can take responsibility for implementing activities and behaviors associated with maintaining good health practices. Still, there are significant barriers faced by patients that may not be readily appreciated by those providing healthcare advice and recommendations. Discussing these challenges and brainstorming ways to address them may help patients overcome these barriers and also strengthen the therapeutic alliance through which a trainee's advice gains influence. Use open-ended questions and reflections to explore the role of finances, access, and social support as potential barriers to making behavior change. Failure to address these considerations may impede the trainee's ability to help a patient succeed in changing, even if progress was made toward resolving ambivalence about change. Awareness of these challenges, as well as direct inquiry about them and brainstorming with patients, will help make the approaches discussed in the next section more effective.

SPECIAL CONSIDERATIONS: FINANCES, ACCESS, AND SOCIAL SUPPORT

Many patients will not disclose financial hardship unless specifically addressed and in a respectful manner. One can explore this issue by saying, "Many of my patients find the cost of medication or treatment to be a barrier to following healthcare recommendations. How much of a barrier is the cost for you?" or "What role does cost have in your following these recommendations?" A good reflection might be to say: "The cost of this medication gets in the way of your being able to follow through on taking it the way we have discussed taking it. It can be hard to choose between your health and other important things you need to pay for like rent, food, or your family's needs." Limited finances can seriously impact access to medications, nutritious food, or other medical equipment necessary for meaningful health behavior changes. Finances should be addressed with *all* patients when crafting health plans. It is important to maintain a sense of relative cost; even $10 copayments may be prohibitive for some patients. It is useful to be familiar with services that increase affordability or provide assistance to patients of lower economic means.

Many patients lack the luxury of safely and affordably accessing a gym or health club for physical activity. Unsafe neighborhoods may turn low-cost exercising such as walking or running into dangerous activities. In some areas, the lack of sports programs for children and the general public makes options for safe and fun exercise untenable. Patients may not be able to afford fresh fruits and vegetables to enhance their diets. Knowledge of low-cost resources for low-income patients (or knowing who to contact or refer patients to) is critical for helping some patients adopt a healthier lifestyle. Trainees can work with each patient individually to construct a realistic plan that the patient views as feasible before leaving the office.

Social support is an underappreciated consideration when it comes to effective behavior change. Behaviors like smoking cessation can be even more challenging when a partner or family member is not similarly inclined to quit. Weight loss can also be especially difficult when friends and family are overweight because they may sabotage a patient's attempts at weight loss, viewing their loved one's attempts to lose weight as a condemnation of their own weight. An otherwise loving family can become deliberately discouraging and act as an impediment to success by sabotaging efforts to change. When possible, help patients identify partners and concerned significant others who can effectively assist them in behavior change, and help them delineate what each supportive person will be able to do to assist them. It can be useful to help your patient anticipate possible social challenges and plan strategies together to overcome these obstacles.

MEDICATION ADHERENCE

One of the most broadly applicable behaviors in primary care in which motivation plays a dominant role is with medication or treatment adherence. Poor adherence to a medication regimen can be a source of poor health outcomes and potentially lead to significant increases in expense and risk through the need for second-line treatments, which may take the form of more invasive procedures, surgery, or brand-name drugs. This process uses more healthcare resources and drives up costs while positive outcomes lag. Lack of adherence without an understanding of why it is occurring can also lead to discord in the relationship between the patient and the trainee as they expect the patient to make changes that he or she may not wish to make.

Increasing motivation for medication adherence can be difficult for some patients because the rewards are often so far removed from the effort. For example, adequate control of hypertension comes with well-established benefits as risks of stroke or heart failure are reduced. While patients may be aware of these negative outcomes and understand that the point of the medication is to avoid them, the actual negative outcomes are usually decades removed from the act of taking daily medication, some of which must even be taken several times a day. This is particularly true when the disease, such as hypertension, is silent and causes no immediate discomfort or symptoms. Modifying behavior when the activity seems so trivial in relation to an outcome that is very far removed can be challenging for some patients. MI can be helpful for addressing this aspect of treatment because of its emphasis on openly exploring readiness, willingness, and confidence for making behavior changes. During this process, patients may discuss their struggle about understanding how taking medication is important to staying healthy. When this occurs, the trainee can reflect metaphors related to the patient's personal experience to illustrate the importance of taking medication as prescribed. For example, with patients who play sports or music, the trainee can discuss the gradual improvement that comes with daily practice. Consistent practice is necessary in order to perform at optimal levels. Similarly, the quality of our health is the cumulative effect of our daily regimens of avoiding risk-related activities while engaging in exercise, making good dietary choices, and adhering to medication regimens.

Some important points to remember in guiding your patient include assessing reasons for nonadherence. Barriers may be psychological or practical. A patient may be skipping doses because he or she feels unconcerned about the underlying health issue, or he or she may not be following your prescribed plan because he or she has financial difficulties with obtaining the medications or concerns about a side effect. Screening questions for medication nonadherence have very low sensitivity. It is more useful to ask patients about possible side effects of their medications using open-ended questions. Provide information (after asking permission) on side effects if the patient is unaware or has inaccurate information and encourage him or her to contact you or return if problems arise. Using the E-P-E framework can be very helpful to explore adherence challenges.

Do your best to prescribe drugs with the fewest daily doses possible since adherence drops off rapidly when patients are expected to take medications three or more times a day. Discuss costs with the patient while prescribing and balance priorities; long-acting medications require fewer doses but are often more likely to be under patent and may be more expensive. When there are multiple formulations with varying cost, allow patients to choose which formulations they want, as this will enhance adherence. Be familiar with common insurance plans and be comfortable working within that framework. Many plans have limits on drug benefits. Prescription drugs may rapidly deplete this amount, even if the patient is initially paying nothing out of pocket. Learn about local, reduced-price programs and identify lists of discount ($4/$10) medications at major pharmacies. These can save money for both insured and uninsured patients. These lists typically include generic statin medications and antihypertensives. Maintain a sense of the challenges posed to patients on low or fixed incomes. A 90-day prescription may be cheaper to fill over time than three 30-day supplies. A medication with a $10 copayment per month may be discounted to $25 for a 3-month supply. However, patients who struggle financially often prefer to pay $10 each month than to pay $25 at one time, which can be beyond their means. Give the patients options and let their concerns guide your mutual decisions. It can be useful to ask yourself, "Am I retaining a sense of quiet curiosity about what will work best for this person?" (Miller & Rollnick, 2013).

When available, it can be useful to corroborate refill information with the pharmacy's records via an electronic health record (EHR). Address any discrepancies in an even-toned, empathic nonconfrontational manner, such as "I see you did not get the medication we talked about last time. What do you make of that?"

Exchanging Information

Education is an ongoing process and can be achieved in a way that is MI adherent. Key elements include assessing each patient's understanding of which medication(s) addresses which problem(s), as well as his or her understanding of the disease or condition and possible outcomes, both with and without treatment. It is critical that you explore patient expectations and verify that each patient understands and agrees to his or her treatment plan. Establishing a mutual purpose includes collaborating to define clearly stated behavioral goals on which both the trainee and the patient agree. Many healthcare plans now provide tracking information (e.g., feedback on treatment impact, such as test results available) to patients, including electronic access when possible, so patients can personally evaluate their own progress. Trainees should emphasize the value of this resource because it promotes the efficient provision of feedback. Furthermore, self-reliance associated with using Internet-based information reinforces patient responsibility for learning about his or her health status. The use of these resources represents a method beyond following up with the physician for additional feedback and increases the chance that changes will be implemented and will lead to better health-related outcomes.

There are often many opportunities to address inadequate or incorrect information. For example, patients may not consider the impact of calories imbibed through soda, juices, milk, or alcohol. Americans consume on average more than 200 calories per day from sugary drinks, a four-fold increase since 1965. A reduction in daily soda intake or a switch to diet sodas, carbonated water, or unsweetened teas can offer some patients a simple starting point that enables them to envision that change is possible. Often the conception of an appropriate portion size is significantly skewed toward larger amounts, and assessing patient knowledge about portion size and offering information about it can be useful.

Patients may have concerns that are not supported by the literature. As stated by one cola-drinking patient with diabetes when given a recommendation to switch to diet cola, "That stuff will give you cancer." One response might be a reflection such as "You're really concerned about how it could affect your health." Another might be asking permission to educate or advice by asking, "Would it be alright if I shared with you what we now know about diet drinks and cancer?" When permission is granted, you can provide information such as "Some early animal studies raised significant concerns about artificial sweeteners and cancer, but large studies in people haven't found any increased risk. In fact, evidence has linked sugared soda with pancreatic cancer, and there is rapidly growing evidence of increased cancer risks with obesity." After providing this information, it is important to ask for feedback on the provided information by saying: "What's your perspective on that information?" The E-P-E framework is again applicable in exchanging information.

Box 10.2 OARS Skills in the Context of Medication Adherence

Open-Ended Questions

- "What do you find most challenging about getting/taking your medications?"
- "How did you feel when you realized you'd missed a dose of your medication?"
- "What are three things you do to help yourself take your medications?"
- "What ideas do you have for improving your consistency with taking your medications?"
- "What changes can we discuss together that might make it easier to take your medication?"

Affirmations

- "You have a lot of great ideas about how to improve the way you take your medication."
- "You've put an incredible amount of work into trying different methods for taking your medications regularly."
- "Thank you for being so honest about how hard it has been to take your medication."
- "You work very hard to make sure you take your medication regularly despite your mixed feelings about taking them every day."

Reflections

- "You're concerned about the effects that taking multiple medications may have on you."
- "You don't think this approach is going to be affordable for you."
- "It's not easy making changes to your daily routine so you can take your medication."
- "Sometimes it just doesn't seem worth it to take all these medications when you already have (add condition here). The damage is done."

Summarizing

- "You find it difficult to take your medications on time, you're struggling with some side effects, you're being pressured by your family to take them consistently, and you don't want to depend on them."
- "You worry about the costs of your medications and you cannot afford the co-pay, you see the importance of not missing any doses, and you are very much conflicted about how to deal with this situation."

Barriers to Treatment Plan Adherence

Encouraging communication about side effects or cost concerns can prevent patient-initiated discontinuation of a treatment. Ask each patient what might cause him or her to discontinue treatment and problem-solve in advance how to manage such situations. Problem solving should be done in an MI-adherent manner. Ideally, elicit first from the patient his or her own ideas on how to solve problems with medication and affirm his or her resourcefulness. If the patient does not come up with ideas on his or her own, offer, with permission, suggestions such as pill boxes, cell phone alarms, automated e-mail reminders, and selecting particular drugs based on cost or number of doses needed per day. Although trainees should not recommend family involvement if the patient is not allowing it, some patients welcome their families' help with reminders, or even maintaining control of medication.

Importance and Confidence Rulers

The rulers are used to assess and bolster medication adherence using a mixture of OARS skills (see Box 10.3).

WEIGHT MANAGEMENT

Most patients are genuinely interested in discussing their weight or strategies for losing weight, but they may find it difficult to broach the topic for fear of being lectured by the trainee. Similarly, major barriers to trainees discussing weight loss with their patients are the trainees' perceptions and concerns that doing so will offend their patients. A good way to address this issue is to have a discussion with each patient about your perspective on the trainee–patient relationship. You can discuss as much as you believe is important, but the highlights should be on your valuing a partnership between physicians and patients whereby each has something to contribute to developing individualized and effective treatment plans. It is important to point out that you realize you cannot control your patients' behaviors and you will not try. Furthermore, you do not

---

Box 10.3 Importance and Confidence Rulers for Medication Adherence

Adherence Importance Ruler

- "On a scale of zero to ten, how important do you think it is to take your medications?"
- "Why are you at a_____and not a zero?" Reflect and explore by asking, "What else?" until the patient has exhausted all the reasons he or she can think of and says, "That's all," and then summarize what you have heard.
- "What would you need to do to increase the importance 1 or 2 points higher?" Reflect and explore by asking, "What else?" until the patient has exhausted all the reasons and says, "That's all," and then summarize what you have heard.

Confidence Ruler

- "On a scale of zero to ten, how confident are you that you can take your medications the way you have been instructed?"
- "Why are you at a_____and not a (pick a number 3–4 points lower)?" Reflect and explore by asking, "What else?" until the patient has exhausted all the reasons and says, "That's all," and then summarize what you have heard.
- "What would you need to do to increase your confidence 1 or 2 points higher?" Reflect and explore by asking, "What else?" until the patient has exhausted all the reasons and says, "That's all" and then summarize what you have heard.

judge people or become frustrated or angry when your patients do not follow your recommendations. Rather, you view this as an indication that you do not understand the patient's perspective well enough. You want to promote an atmosphere where your patients will be open with you because you want to understand where differences lie and work collaboratively to help them recover from illness and generally improve their health. Following this, ask the patient for his or her perspective if he or she has not already commented on the topic.

It is important to discuss weight loss, given the significant effects on individual patients and the cost of healthcare resources allocated to treating obesity-related health problems. With children, trainees can use growth curves to objectively compare weight and weight trajectory to age-based gender norms, and then invite parents' and children's perspectives on that information. With adults, we often lack such readily available graphics with population norms. A body mass index (BMI) chart can be helpful as long as it is used to facilitate a discussion about healthy weight range and the trainee invites and respects the patient's perspective. Many EHRs allow plotting of weight over time, which may visually demonstrate when a patient's weight has steadily increased, decreased, fluctuated up and down, or remained unchanged. It can be less threatening to focus on the trend in a patient's weight, rather than the patient's actual weight number. Furthermore, the trainee should be observant for opportunities to affirm the patient for any strategies, behaviors, or general indication that he or she has the proper perspective for promoting a healthy lifestyle related to weight, for example, eating healthy and exercising.

The goal is to be directive without being authoritarian. You can directly assess a patient's level of concern about his or her weight by asking any of the following open-ended questions:

- "On a scale of 0 to 10, 0 not concerned at all and 10 extremely concerned, how concerned are you about how your weight is affecting your health?"
- "What concerns do you have about your weight?"
- "How concerned are you about your weight *right now*?"

You could also lead with statements such as "I'm concerned that your weight may cause you some health problems" or "I'd like to talk about how your weight may be affecting your health," as long as the statement is followed with a question such as "Would it be okay if we talk about it at today's visit?" Most patients who are sensitive to such an approach are likely to have been sensitized by past experiences with friends, family, or other practitioners, so addressing the issue may require establishing a more longitudinal working relationship. If a patient refuses or declines to discuss weight at an initial meeting, it is appropriate to back off and resist the urge to pressure for change or even to have the patient talk about it. You can give the patient an autonomy support statement such as "I respect your decision to hold off on addressing your weight. You are the best judge of when it makes sense to discuss this. The door is always open, and I am ready to work with you on this when you are ready. What do you want to focus on for today's visit?" This will help establish that the patient is in charge of the encounter and dictates the priorities, while strengthening the relationship for future interventions.

For patients who are not motivated to change, disinterest in addressing weight may arise from not seeing it as a health issue. In these cases, ask first what the patient knows about the health issues. If there is a lack of information or misconceptions, offer information *after* asking for permission to do so and then assess how the patient receives the information. One way to do this is to ask: "Would it be alright if I told you a little bit about why we focus so much on weight, and you can tell me what you think of it?" Another option is to say: "Perhaps I could share with you one piece of information for you to consider, and you can tell me how it fits, or does not fit, with what you know." The information you provide will be most effective when it is personalized to the patient's current conditions so it can increase resonance either immediately or over time. For example, an overweight patient who has friends or relatives with diabetes would be a reasonable patient to offer information to about the causative relationship between obesity and type 2 diabetes mellitus. Or a patient with complaints of knee pain may be quite interested in learning about the benefits of weight loss in reducing current pain and eventual risk of knee replacement. It is better to focus on the potential to prevent illness rather than on the dangers and negative outcomes of not changing course. People prefer to move toward a healthy, positive goal rather than to move away from a negative health consequence.

For patients who are more motivated to change, providing personalized feedback helps to tie weight issues to associated diagnoses or patient interests. While the trainee's primary concern may be health, social impacts may be a more predominant motivating factor for patients and must be appropriately addressed to help them resolve their ambivalence about change. Patients often say they are prepared to make changes when they still have remaining ambivalence about change. They may have attempted changes in the past and may be inhibited by feeling or believing that they will not be able to succeed at making a change. In this setting, it can be helpful to ask for statements of self-efficacy such as "How have you been successful with doing other things you wanted to do in the past? How could you apply that experience to this one?" Focus on past successes that the patient has had and validate the significance. Establish goals based on the patient's interests, ensuring that they are realistic, time-framed, manageable, and appropriate.

Trainees may perceive nutrition and weight issues as requiring a high burden of education, as patient and community knowledge and understanding may deviate sharply from nutritional information accepted within the medical community. Patients' nutritional beliefs commonly display significant cultural variation, with an obese body habitus at times being perceived as "healthy." Assessing a patient's understanding of nutrition and access to nutritious foods is crucial to understanding barriers to change. Patients who might benefit from more extensive education can be referred to a nutritionist if the patient accepts the offer of the referral.

Discussing Change

Providing a menu of options is key. Success is far more likely when patients see a variety of choices and choose their *own* courses of action. Furthermore, how information is offered is important. Providing choices to patients in a limited, controlling manner reduces patients' subjective sense of choice and compromises patient autonomy. Therefore, it is best to offer it by using an open, informational style. A trainee might say, "Would you like to work on decreasing sugary treats in your diet or work on reducing fat?" giving the patient a choice but suggesting that it must be either one or the other. It is preferable to offer several ideas together and encourage patients to weigh in on which they prefer, rather than to offer suggestions one at a time and sequentially. Offering isolated ideas often elicits sustain talk by inviting the patient to argue against each suggestion in turn. By presenting a selection of a few ideas, the patient can be redirected toward considering which option is the best, rather than why each idea won't work (Miller & Rollnick, 2013). At the same time, it is also important to not offer too many options. Too large of a selection of options can be overwhelming and subsequently unmotivating, reducing a patient's confidence in his or her capacity to make the right choice. It is always useful to finish an offering of several suggestions by saying, "or perhaps you have your own better ideas of what to do."

Weight management is an ongoing series of behaviors toward a common goal. Avoid suggesting or advocating for too many changes at one appointment. Guide patients to pick realistic, interim goals on which to build so they experience repeated successes rather than failures. Weight change requires many behavioral modifications, including changes in activity level, eating behaviors, social interactions, routines, and even daily planning. Discussing the range of ways patients can address weight management can give them optimism that they can succeed by making step-wise changes over time. Focusing on small changes that are achievable will help strengthen a patient's self-efficacy, enabling further changes. Even small weight reductions have been shown to produce significant reductions in health risks. Patients are often unaware that these small changes can have a significant impact on health.

HYPERTENSION AND HYPERLIPIDEMIA

Hypertension (HTN) and hyperlipidemia (HLD) are two staples of primary care that trainees must frequently treat, so it is important to consider improvements to these treatment-related interactions. When discussing these diagnoses with patients, you will find many misconceptions about what the diseases are, which medications are treating them, what the risks are of not treating, and even whether the disease states can been cured by treatment. Medical trainees often treat patients taking two unidentified antihypertensives or treat patients who report no medical conditions despite being on a beta-blocker and a statin medication.

Because these conditions are so prevalent, we often assume patient familiarity with basic information about them. Keep in mind that what is basic to a trainee is rarely basic to patients. Assessing a patient's understanding of his or her condition with open-ended questions is a good first step of every appointment, especially with a patient who is new to you. Use open-ended questions to ask patients what medications they take and what each medication treats. When writing prescriptions, it can be helpful to indicate the purpose of each medication, such as "take one tablet daily for treatment of high blood pressure." This labeling informs patients each time they take a dose or refill a pill box what condition is treated by each medication. Drug names, particularly generics, are practically foreign to many patients and are best learned through repetition. Instead of referring to "your blood pressure medication," try to make it a habit to say, for instance, "lisinopril, your blood pressure medication."

Patients with HTN and HLD are typically asymptomatic until they become severely symptomatic. Understanding the disease course and treatment can help motivate some patients to improve their adherence to inconvenient medication regimens that often have a number of side effects. During office visits, it is useful to assess patients' understanding of their diagnoses and the risks of treatment and nontreatment. Patient-initiated discontinuation of a medication can have serious consequences. With antihypertensives, ask patients what they know about the rebound potential of some drugs, as well as the acute risk of strokes or cardiac issues in the event of discontinuation. Provide information when asked or with permission. Ask patients to envision a future where they do not treat their HTN or HLD and what their lives would be like if they survived a stroke or heart attack. You can ask what goals or activities they want to accomplish, such as missing a child's graduation or wedding, or the birth of grandchildren that might be altered by a serious medical event. Even better, ask them what activities they might participate in or what experiences they might have, if they stay healthy and live longer.

Tailoring the Message

Approaching patients who view themselves as knowledgeable but who are misinformed about their medical problems, such as the long-term health impact of HTN and HLD, can be a challenge. Often patients cite information from Internet sources that provide incorrect information. One response is to note that different sources of information exist and refer patients to sources that offer more objective views, for example, WebMD and the National Institute on Drug Abuse (NIDA). It is important to not argue with such patients because doing so reinforces their views by focusing them on defending their position. It is better to accept what they say without making overt attempts to correct them while looking for inconsistencies between the views they hold and their actual experiences. Using an MI approach that encourages free and open discussion, patients often reveal significant personal problems associated with legal and financial problems, injury, withdrawal, and functional impairment. As this occurs, the trainee can ask the patient to consider how these affect his or her life now and how life could be different without such problems. This is the beginning of the process of "developing discrepancy."

It is important to inquire about each patient's goals, values, and beliefs. Not all patients possess the same fear of a stroke, heart attack, or death. The wide range of goals and expectations for the future results in different levels of intrinsic motivation for positive health behavior change. Attempting to treat a patient who does not desire treatment benefits no one. Approach the patient who declines treatment at that visit respectfully and with understanding. Explore, in a nonjudgmental way, why the patient does not desire treatment rather than approaching the issue in a confrontational or coercive way. Offer personalized feedback but do not push or insist on immediate treatment. Provide autonomy statements that the patient is "the boss and best judge of what he or she needs and wants." Keep further education brief and focused, and provided only when asked for, or with permission from the patient. Encourage the patient to return to revisit this issue in the future since it is clear this is not something he or she wants to address at this point in time. Primary care is a long-term relationship. Tending to the quality of the relationship will make the patient more comfortable, enhance follow-up, and build trust for future attempts. Primary care offers the luxury of future sessions, assuming a patient is not discouraged from returning because he or she does not care for the trainee's attitude. It is important to reduce the trainee's self-imposed pressure to achieve goals immediately, that means, inhibiting the "righting reflex".

Practical challenges to behavior change or difficulties in maintaining change often involve barriers as mundane as lack of transportation. Patients may not have as much problem-solving experience as trainees, so it is important to conduct a comprehensive review of what obstacles exist and the resources available to overcome them. For example, it may be helpful to offer 90-day rather than 30-day prescriptions to reduce trips to the pharmacy and total cost. When patients express difficulty remembering to take medication, assess the patient's own ideas regarding how to enhance his or her memory.

Regarding the treatment of HTN and HLD, behavior change has the greatest potential and is, unfortunately, often the least successful intervention. This is where MI can be especially useful. Patients may not understand how their diet or exercise patterns affect either their blood pressure or cholesterol levels. Ask for permission to discuss these topics. People can be very sensitive about them, especially if they are overweight or obese and have felt confronted or judged before. Start with a broad question to assess understanding and progress to a personalized and behaviorally-oriented inquiry:

- "What sorts of foods have you heard are bad for your blood pressure/cholesterol and why?"
- "Which foods do you feel you eat more of and why?"
- "What successes have you had making changes to your diet so far?"
- "What have you heard about how someone's activity level affects blood pressure/cholesterol?"
- "What successes have you had in increasing your physical activity level?"
- "What challenges have you had with increasing your physical activity level in the past?" or "What activities did you do in the past that you'd like to do again in the future?"

If granted permission, offer patients several options and ask them what they think of those options. However, it is always better to ask patients what ideas they have first. Start small with obtainable goals, like after-dinner walks a few days a week or weaning off adding salt to foods. Let the patient suggest or decide where to start in an area where he or she is confident of a successful outcome. Suggest building the magnitude of goals as each patient accumulates successes. Encourage patients to formulate specific, realistic, and time-framed plans that include frequency, intensity, and other small steps they have crafted with your help. Guide the discussion so they express confidence in the plan and a commitment to implementing it. Use the OARS skills to resolve ambivalence about change and build commitment. You can also use the importance and the confidence rulers to focus on whether the barrier to change lies more in a lack of importance or low confidence. Finally, highlight and reinforce any elicited change talk.

DIABETES MELLITUS TYPE 2

Despite the high prevalence of diabetes in our culture, there is still much misunderstanding. Strong evidence reflects that overwhelming numbers of people with diabetes do not meet guidelines for glycemic control, blood pressure, and lipid levels. These care gaps make it more urgent for trainees to address behavior change across all aspects of diabetes care: diet, physical activity, medication adherence, and self-monitoring of blood glucose. Controlled diabetic conditions result in many patients remaining highly functional, and this can cause patients to underestimate the severity of the disease. The negative outcomes of poor management of diabetes require extensive education and facilitation of motivation. Proper diabetes care includes numerous behaviors such as regular visits to a primary care provider, an ophthalmologist, a podiatrist, a diabetes educator, and a nutritionist, to name a few. Other important behaviors include watching calories and carbohydrates, maintaining hydration, getting exercise, losing weight, checking feet regularly for skin breakdown or ulcers, checking blood sugar, taking medication, and attending appointments.

The research evidence for the effectiveness of MI in diabetes care has been strong. MI as an approach is also particularly useful to facilitate behavior change. Convey risks without resorting to scare tactics and using OARS skills and the spirit of MI to foster collaborative discussion. Diabetes is a leading cause of blindness and amputation in the U.S., but many patients consider these outcomes to be unheard of in the modern era. You can use the E-P-E approach to assess what patients already know about the impact of diabetes on their health and promote a desire to learn about this, without spurring discord in the working relationship. One example is to ask: "What do you know about the possible negative effects of diabetes?" and ask for elaboration until the patient has told you everything he or she knows. Affirm the patient's knowledge and then ask: "Would it be alright if I told you a few of the health risks of diabetes that I am concerned about?" (Wait for agreement before proceeding.) "Poorly controlled diabetes can damage many parts of your body, including your kidneys, eyes, or blood vessels. Diabetes is responsible for much of the kidney failure, blindness, and amputations that still occur in this country. How does hearing about those things affect how you prioritize your own diabetes treatment?"

When a patient declines an offer of information, be prepared to respond. One example is to say, "You are the best judge of what information is useful to you. If there is anything you would like to know that I could tell you, the door is always open. Please ask me." Patients have their own values and may not prioritize treatment at the time of their visit with you. Expressions of low importance to make change often emanate from feelings of fear and inevitability or lack of control. A patient who feels confident in his or her ability to change is more able to entertain the possible necessity of and ability to change. Evoking change talk guides patients in their choices about starting the process of change and increases the likelihood of following through with taking steps toward change.

Because tight control of diabetes dictates outcomes, follow-up is critical. Diabetes care is typically a lifelong endeavor, but frequent appointments are not the same as good follow-up. Engaging in a working relationship with the patient is central to diabetes care. Help patients set priorities for each visit that go beyond checking hemoglobin A1c (HbA1c) or blood glucose, and focus on assessing patients' educational needs and planning longitudinally. Allow patients to choose which behaviors to focus on first, perhaps by doing an agenda-mapping exercise (see Chapter 4 where agenda mapping is described). If changes in diet are overwhelming, assist patients in making small steps and wait to discuss exercise recommendations until progress is made elsewhere. Assess whether each patient knows his or her glycemia, HbA1c numbers and find out whether he or she has goals for maintaining healthy blood glucose goals. Validate even small improvements in behaviors regardless of whether they have had large impacts on HbA1c or glycemia. Remind each patient that every dietary or activity change affects his or her health in many ways and validate the difficulties he or she overcame in achieving success without "cheerleading" his or her progress. Paying attention to how the patients express change talk, commitment language, or sustain talk is important in guiding the conversation about change. Responding collaboratively and strengthening change talk leading to commitment language moves the process toward change.

PATIENT: I am not sure I can fit 30 minutes of swimming into my busy schedule.

TRAINEE: You see swimming as an important activity for you, and at the same time it is challenging to fit it into your schedule. What is your schedule like?

PATIENT: I think I can fit 30 minutes of swimming into my busy schedule.

TRAINEE: You are considering fitting in 30 minutes of swimming. What makes it so important for you to do?

PATIENT: I need to stay active and I don't want to gain weight since it affects my diabetes. I also need to check my blood sugar regularly before I eat, and I have started doing it at work since my wife got a new glucometer to keep at work.

TRAINEE: You made some steps toward better managing your diabetes. What other steps would you like to take regarding your diabetes care?

Diabetes, more than most other largely asymptomatic chronic illnesses, requires a complete lifestyle change for most people. Taken as one goal, it would seem insurmountable to anyone. Broken down into little pieces, ongoing diabetes care can feel like a series of triumphs in the interest of the ultimate goal of better health.

INPATIENT PRIMARY CARE SETTINGS

Any hospital admission becomes an opportunity for medical trainees to dedicate time toward working with patients on behavioral modifications. As a learning ground, the hospital provides rich opportunities for medical trainees to test, refine their skills, and use effective interventions.

Brief Admission

Medical trainees have an excellent opportunity to use MI during brief admissions to the hospital. For most of us, time is typically more limited because of greater patient responsibilities and higher patient load. However, the inpatient setting is an excellent opportunity to use MI-based brief interventions (as discussed in Chapter 9) and to incorporate the spirit, skills, and processes of MI in clinical interactions. Medical trainees on inpatient services have the advantage of time. Trainees may see patients more frequently and for greater durations of time than their supervisors. They are often tasked with obtaining complete histories and physical examinations (H&Ps), meaning they have more time to focus on patients' social histories and assess motivations for change as well as to identify potential areas of important behavior change. Even patients presenting with acute, unrelated complaints provide opportunities, such as a young woman with appendicitis who may benefit from discussing her smoking during this period of required abstinence, or an exploration of risky sexual behaviors during a discussion about her abdominal pain.

A complete H&P often substitutes for screening on inpatient units since time is limited and screening for unrelated illness is not often valued. Even a focused H&P can reveal illness-related behavior, such as smoking in a patient with chest pain or unprotected anal sex in a young man with urinary tract symptoms. In these cases, personalized feedback can be especially powerful because the hospitalization itself provides weight to the necessity for change, your task in guiding the patient to the topic is simplified, and the window of opportunity is wide open. There is also great opportunity to discuss personalized feedback.

Using MI in the inpatient setting goes beyond a simple brief intervention. An inpatient hospitalization is an opportunity akin to an abbreviated, intensive treatment. While an interview may last only a few minutes, a patient can be approached one to two times per day, depending on the nature of the issue, receptivity of the patient, and length of the hospitalization. Each interaction can be considered a stepwise intervention. The first step is to identify the behavior as a topic under consideration. This is best achieved using an agenda-mapping (discussed in Chapter 4) approach or asking open-ended questions and using reflections to engage the patient in a therapeutic conversation and determine what behavior he or she wants to focus on. Next the trainee can ask or evoke why that particular topic is an area of desired or needed change and explore what it is about that behavior that makes it an area that the patient has chosen to tackle now. This encourages the patient to consider the behavior change without pressing for action. This approach helps strengthen the therapeutic alliance and makes it clear to patients that they will be treated respectfully and that they are the ones in control of this aspect of their care. This is critical since they may feel that not much is under their control during the hospitalization.

At the next interaction, the discussion can revolve around the patient's past experiences with behavior change. The trainee can emphasize and reinforce past successes, no matter how limited. If a patient expresses a lack of confidence, a discussion using the confidence ruler may facilitate a discussion about how to increase confidence. When the patient expresses change talk, the trainee should elicit more change talk and commitment language. At each visit, it is helpful to address any pressing concerns first. Inquire about comfort, pain, concerns, and questions before returning to the discussion of behavior changes. One strategy is to raise the issue of behavior change only in the afternoons when returning to check on the patient, or after a patient's concern or question has been addressed.

The transition from the inpatient to the outpatient setting is a critical process, since establishing an effective outpatient care plan is key to patient success. During this transition, therapy changes from intensive and continuous to isolated appointments, often with different practitioners. Patients move into a less controlled setting where they have to take the lead in their self-care, which poses the first major transition for a patient who might be newly motivated for change.

It is important, prior to discharge, to help patients set realistic, interim goals, allowing them to dictate what treatments they believe they will find valuable and those they intend to maintain. It is also useful to ask each patient to anticipate barriers, both psychological and practical (such as transportation to appointments), and discuss solutions before discharge.

PERSONAL REFLECTION

Shortly after being diagnosed with diabetes, my father cooked a meal of sweet potatoes and pasta for the family. Upon my mother's remark that it was not, perhaps, the most diabetes-friendly meal, my father expressed surprise. Though he is a chemistry professor, his perception of what constituted "sugars" was inaccurate. His physician knew my father's intelligence and training and therefore assumed he had a certain level of knowledge about diet that he did not possess; my father had little idea what he should and should not eat to maintain good health.

In using MI, there is always a challenge when it comes to educating our patients. MI suggests offering advice with permission, and yet in many cases patients might benefit from both information and suggestions. Striking the balance of educating without lecturing is very challenging, and I suspect that mastering this balance is a lifelong endeavor. The strategy I have found most useful is simply to ask for permission. Patients will most often respond positively, and they typically appear genuinely moved by an otherwise small gesture. The information is then presented on their terms, which may increase their collaboration. In the rare event that a patient refuses, it does not preclude gathering information on their beliefs and understandings. Respecting the boundaries each patient establishes will also help him or her to feel more comfortable and increase the likelihood of his or her success in maintaining health and being fully engaged with the trainee at future encounters.

SELF-ASSESSMENT QUIZ

True or False?

1. MI is well suited to addressing many of the functional and clinical outcomes outlined in the chronic care model (CCM).
2. The amount and quality of an individual's training in MI is more predictive of outcome than his or her level of education and number of university degrees.
3. Focusing on the dangers and negative consequences of not changing a behavior is more effective than emphasizing the potential to prevent illness.
4. When presenting a menu of options to a patient, offering a limited, concise list of options is more effective than a lengthy list of choices.
5. An inpatient hospital stay should be viewed as an opportunity for an abbreviated, intensive MI-based intervention.

Answers

1. *True.* By establishing a sound therapeutic alliance that may be continued over a long period of time, MI complements the CCM, particularly with regard to the CCM's goal of producing "informed and activated patients." The CCM model is defined by six key components: self-management support, decision support, delivery system design, clinical information systems, health system, and community resources and policies.
2. *True.* Research demonstrates that the degree of MI training is a key indicator of outcome rather than a trainee's educational background, whether nursing, social work, psychology, or medicine, at the bachelor's, master's, or doctoral level.
3. *False.* Trainees should focus on positive outcomes, such as preventing illness or predictable consequences. Most people prefer to move toward healthy, positive goals rather than away from negative health repercussions.
4. *True.* Eliciting or providing a menu of three or four options promotes patient success by supporting patient autonomy and encouraging patients to choose their

own course of action. A clear, concise list is better; extensive menus may overwhelm patients, reduce confidence in their ability to choose wisely, and result in lower levels of motivation. Remember to begin this process by asking patients for their ideas regarding what elements/actions will promote success.

5. *True.* Applying MI within hospital settings is best achieved with short, intensive treatments. Through a graduated series of short interactions, patients are approached once or twice each day. The first step is to identify a behavior of concern that trainees might explore with patients in terms of the benefits that could result from implementing change. Discussing a patient's previous experiences with change plays an important role in building confidence and momentum. As patients prepare for discharge, a series of realistic, achievable interim goals are identified and discussed, as well as potential barriers to change, and the outpatient or community resources that could provide additional support.

11 Motivational Interviewing in Pediatric Settings

The spirit of motivational interviewing (MI) shapes every aspect of how we collaborate with our patients, and it is as important in our interactions with pediatric and adolescent populations and their families as it is when working with adult patients. In our encounters with younger patients, the traditional patient–physician dyad expands to a triad of patient–parent–physician, and our use of MI must be adapted to this change in circumstances. Our approach will also vary according to each child's developmental capabilities and maturity levels, the family's dynamics, and the nature of the presenting complaint. The clinical exchanges we discuss here demonstrate a variety of strategies that will facilitate your use of MI with children and adolescents.

WHY MOTIVATIONAL INTERVIEWING WITH PEDIATRIC POPULATIONS?

As discussed in Chapters 1 and 2, MI helps us establish therapeutic relationships with our patients through which they discover and enhance their own personal motivations for behavior change. A unique feature of pediatric settings is that a patient's interest, motivation, and ability to change may differ widely from that of his or her parent or caregiver, and MI has the potential to be especially useful in resolving these conflicts. The skilled use of empathy, respect for autonomy, and reflective listening often provides younger patients with the emotional space they need to express their views and perspectives. Recall that MI does not assume that patients agree with us concerning the objectives or goals of treatment, or even that a need for treatment exists. In using MI, our encounters become opportunities to elicit patients' perspectives as to what led them to be evaluated or treated, and it is this collaborative process that forms the basis of a therapeutic relationship.

GENERAL CONSIDERATIONS IN PEDIATRIC SETTINGS

Decision-making in pediatric settings is founded upon the belief that most, if not all, parents want what is best for their children. By extension, the paradigm of the "family as patient" must be kept in mind as we engage *both patient and parents* to promote healthy behaviors. Each family's dynamics and the developmental maturity of the patient will profoundly affect our interactions; sometimes we work more with parents, and at other times, primarily with the patient. As with other populations, common concerns include strengthening motivation to take medications as prescribed, improving attendance at appointments, and greater adherence to lifestyle changes such as diet, physical activity, and self-monitoring of blood pressure or blood sugar.

Navigating these interactions may prove more difficult than many physician–patient relationships, because discord between any two of the three parties is likely to reduce the chances of positive outcomes. Establishing rapport and building a therapeutic alliance is essential in these situations, and adhering to the core tenets of MI throughout interactions with both patient and caregiver will help minimize discord. Remember to ask open-ended questions; affirm patient choices; reflect what patients and parents *express*, in addition to what they *feel* and *mean*; and use summary statements to confirm your understanding and demonstrate that you are actively listening.

> ### KEY POINT
> ***Family as patient*** – Both patient and family can be engaged to promote healthy behaviors.

Children are highly sensitive to nonverbal communication such as eye contact, facial expression, head nodding, and—where appropriate—physical contact, and we must attend to the importance of these subtle signals, even as we communicate empathy and a sincere desire to understand the child's perspective. A helpful strategy is to begin by addressing the patient with open-ended questions; should he or she have difficulty expressing why medical help has been sought, closed-ended questions may prove useful in providing a sense of structure and security. Continue with open-ended questions to the parents or caregivers to help round out the story.

It is *paramount* to establish an alliance with both child *and* parent; this may be achieved by using reflective listening and affirmations to build positive rapport. Remember that while it takes time and patience to clarify the meaning of our patients' and their families' statements, and to identify the important differences between thoughts and behaviors, these actions are essential to the therapeutic dialogue. The process is often complicated when both patients and their parents/caregivers want us to support their points of view; consequently, it is crucial to find some element on which both parents and child agree.

DEVELOPMENTAL CONSIDERATIONS

One way to discuss a child's development is to consider three broad areas of maturation and growth: gross and fine motor abilities, language acquisition, and psychosocial skills. In this discussion, our primary focus is on how children's psychosocial development affects the use of MI and, in particular, the opportunities we have to engage with patients and their families. Naturally, a child's motor and language skills also influence how therapeutic relationships develop.

We begin by reviewing psychosocial development stages and how these pertain to MI (Fig. 11.1). Subsequently, we discuss strategies that are particularly well suited to each individual stage.

Very Young Children

- Before their first birthday, most children begin to exhibit a growing sense of autonomy and independence, combined with increasing cognitive and problem-solving abilities. Some of the changes parents describe in their children include the following:
  - expressing anxiety around strangers, often as early as 8–9 months
  - readily expressing pleasure/displeasure with specific toys, activities, people, and places

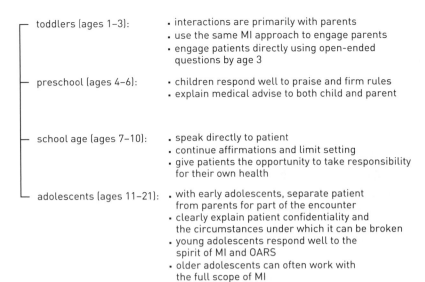

toddlers (ages 1–3):	• interactions are primarily with parents • use the same MI approach to engage parents • engage patients directly using open-ended questions by age 3
preschool (ages 4–6):	• children respond well to praise and firm rules • explain medical advise to both child and parent
school age (ages 7–10):	• speak directly to patient • continue affirmations and limit setting • give patients the opportunity to take responsibility for their own health
adolescents (ages 11–21):	• with early adolescents, separate patient from parents for part of the encounter • clearly explain patient confidentiality and the circumstances under which it can be broken • young adolescents respond well to the spirit of MI and OARS • older adolescents can often work with the full scope of MI

FIGURE 11.1 Engaging patients across developmental stages.

- actively responding to positive interactive behaviors such as holding, cuddling, and praising, in addition to verbal prohibitions against biting, hitting, and kicking
- demonstrating familiarity with daily routines
- recognizing and responding to pleasure/disapproval from their caregivers
- energetically exploring the world around them, both indoors and out
- frequent vocalizations, babbling, and acquiring simple words to indicate desires and intentions
- By 18 months, children devote more energy to social interactions, such as the following:
  - learning the concepts of choice and preference, and becoming assertive about their wishes
  - saying "No!" as a way of asserting autonomy
  - expressing frustration with the tension between insisting on independence versus physical and emotional dependence
  - increased mobility, which allows the child to actively pursue people, objects, and activities of interest

Toddlers

- Between 2 and 3 years of age, most children engage in parallel play in which:
  - groups of two or more children play alongside one another without interacting or exchanging toys; a child may observe other children and modify his or her behavior in response
  - they often wish to assert a choice yet have difficulty choosing
- 3-year-olds engage in trial-and-error learning and:
  - look forward to pleasurable activities and fear less desirable events
  - enjoy mastering new skills, whether gross/fine motor or language

- benefit from being included in family discussions
- need frequent reminding about safety hazards such as cars and hot stoves

A key point when engaging with young children is to approach the encounter in a relaxed, nonthreatening manner. Avoid using closed questions that invite "Yes" or "No" answers; instead, offer choices wherever possible: "Which ear would you like me to look into first?"

Preschoolers: 4–6 Years

- Beginning around age 4, children start to play collaboratively with others, and:
  - are driven by curiosity and a desire to explore
  - respond well to praise and clearly stated rules
  - are narcissistic but are beginning to be aware of how those around them feel
- The major transition in this age group is starting school:
  - they are expected to obey rules, play well with peers, avoid disruptive behavior, and tolerate negative consequences when rules are broken
  - team sports allow children the chance to learn sportsman-like conduct, improve physical competencies and coordination, and build friendships
  - language skills of comprehension and self-expression continue to expand
  - the ability to assume responsibility for simple tasks such as tidying up toys enhances autonomy and feelings of both competence and independence

Children in this age group typically possess an ability to talk about their family, friends, and experiences. Similarly, they are capable of understanding basic explanations concerning what is happening and why, and they are more likely to cooperate if they are addressed directly. Remember that a child's vocabulary sometimes exceeds his or her comprehension: therefore, use clear, simple words and expressions.

School Aged: 7–12 Years

- 7–8-year-olds: ongoing cognitive and emotional development, combined with improving communication skills, leads to more mature independence:
  - newly formed conscience allows greater comprehension of rules, relationships, and morals
  - problem-solving abilities improve as children demonstrate greater attentiveness, cooperation, and a capacity to focus on most aspects of a problem
  - the growing influence of peers may produce internal conflict as children discover differences between competing value systems, and family conflict as parents/caregivers adapt to new expressions of independence
- By age 9–12 years, a child's independence from family becomes increasingly evident:
  - parents acknowledge independence by providing youngsters opportunities to earn privileges in return for doing various household chores
  - many children are susceptible to negative peer pressure; this may be minimized by supporting the child's self-esteem and confidence
  - vulnerable children begin to engage in risk-taking behaviors as a result of peer pressure such as drug/alcohol use, smoking, or gang involvement

- some children begin to mature sexually and become aware of sexual themes and images in popular culture; it is important that they have access to accurate age- and culturally appropriate information from multiple sources

While parents of school-aged children maintain a key role in our therapeutic relationships, as trainees, we are now able to engage directly with our younger patients. As before, remember that a child's vocabulary and demeanor may not accurately reflect his or her comprehension of a given situation.

Adolescents: 13–21 Years

- In early adolescence (ages 13–14 years), children have a strong need to be part of a peer group, even as they pursue independence:
  - emboldened by a close group of friends, adolescents may disregard caution to satisfy their curiosity—occasionally this may be misinterpreted as overconfidence
  - the temptation to explore new experiences, especially those considered "cool" or likely to increase one's social status, is difficult to resist for adolescents unable to appreciate potentially negative consequences of their actions, or for those with low self-esteem who fear being ostracized by the group
  - a profound desire for independence combined with mood swings may cause conflict with family members and rebellion against household rules
- During middle adolescence (15–17 years), teens often become heavily involved with school and school-related activities such as sport, drama, band, and so on
  - these activities present important and enjoyable opportunities for building positive self-esteem through physical, intellectual, and emotional challenges
  - physical appearance is especially important at this time
  - friends become a primary source of both correct and incorrect health information:
    - many experiment with risk-taking behaviors such as tobacco, alcohol, and other drug use, and unsafe sexual practices
    - adolescents with chronic medical conditions often begin to question the necessity of long-term medications
  - interest in dating and physical intimacy/curiosity increases
- By age 18–21 years, physical development finishes, whereas cognitive development continues:
  - most older teens have established a self-identity and have begun to refine their moral, religious, and sexual values
    - they have a rational conscience and are able to compromise and make wise decisions
    - typically, autonomy increases as parental guidance decreases; however, life stressors and one's access to drugs and alcohol increase
  - young people now begin to look ahead to adulthood, especially with regard to career choices

Given the extremely wide variations in maturational level over the course of adolescence, chances are high that you will encounter an equally broad continuum of individual patients, ranging from those who resemble fragile schoolchildren to those who appear to function as adults. Attune yourself to subtle nuances of facial and verbal expression in your interactions with young people; often, these are as important, if not more so, than the actual words they use.

The marked differences in psychosocial development between young children and late adolescents illustrate why some elements of MI are more important than others, depending on a patient's age and maturity level. The following case studies help demonstrate how MI strategies may be tailored to suit different children's needs.

NEONATES, INFANTS, AND TODDLERS

When caring for either very young or nonverbal patients, parents/guardians are a prime focus in our interactions. A patient-centered approach is essential in your therapeutic conversations.

Exchange 1: Using Importance and Confidence Rulers in a Transplant Evaluation

A patient's candidacy for transplant depends, in part, on a family's ability to comprehend a complex medical condition, to maintain a high level compliance with medication regimes, and to attend frequent follow-up visits. Joey is a 7-month-old boy with hypoplastic left heart disease being evaluated for orthotopic heart transplant following continued and progressive heart failure after Glenn surgery.

TRAINEE: Earlier today, we discussed that even if Joey receives a transplant, he will not be cured. Instead, he'll be trading one disease for another. He will need to take immunosuppressant medications for the rest of his life. We also spoke about how he will need to stay in the hospital for a number of weeks following the surgery, that he'll need close follow-up in the weeks following discharge, and that, over time, we'll begin to increase the length of time between our visits. This is a lot of information to digest. What are your thoughts at this point? (Giving information followed by an open-ended question)

JOEY'S PARENT: There's definitely a lot to think about. We realize that this is a difficult process, especially at the beginning, with all the appointments he'll have and all the different medications he'll be taking ... but we're prepared to do whatever Joey needs us to do.

TRAINEE: You've told me that ensuring Joey gets his medications and attending all of his appointments is very important to you. If you had to rate the importance on a scale of 0 to 10, with 10 being the most important and 0 being the least important, where would you say you are right now? (Complex reflection followed by a closed question)

JOEY'S PARENT: Joey's health is the most important thing for us; we know he'll need his medications and that we'll have to be sure he attends all his appointments in order to ensure that he's doing as well as possible. It's the number-one priority for us, so 10 of 10.

TRAINEE: And using the same scale, 0 not confident at all and 10 extremely confident, how *confident* are you that you'll be able to give Joey all his medications and attend all those appointments? (Open-ended question)

JOEY'S PARENT: We'd like to say 10 again, but there's still so much we don't know. I guess I'd have to say an 8.

TRAINEE: I appreciate your honesty. Why do you say your confidence is an 8 and not a lower number like a 5? (Affirmation followed by an open-ended question)

JOEY'S PARENT: We still don't know if Joey is going to receive a heart, but just the same, it comes back to the fact that if he doesn't take his medications, he'll get very sick, and we need to come back for regular checkups and biopsies just to make sure he is doing OK. We don't want to have to deal with organ rejection, but it's not something we'd be able to see happening simply by looking at him.

TRAINEE: You really care about Joey and want to do everything you can to make sure he has the best result possible. What else makes your confidence an 8 instead of a 5? (Complex reflection followed by open-ended question)

JOEY'S PARENT: Well ... we've already gone through a lot together, and we know that as a family, we have the support and love we need to help us get through this experience.

TRAINEE: You get a lot of strength from your family, so you know you can make it through this really challenging situation. What else makes your confidence an 8 instead of a 5? (Complex reflection followed by an open-ended question)

JOEY'S PARENT: We stay optimistic, we try to look toward the future, and we talk about how to provide the best we can so Joey can be a healthy, normal little boy. That's really it.

TRAINEE: Being optimistic, supporting each other, and having the support of your family helps you be as confident as an 8. What do you think it would take for your confidence to move up to be a 9 or 10? (Summary followed by an open-ended question)

JOEY'S PARENT: We would need answers to several questions. We need to know how we're going to pay for all the hospital bills, and we also need to know how this is going to affect our jobs. We need to know what will happen if and when this heart transplant fails.

TRAINEE: With your permission, I can share with you some resources that might help you answer those questions, and you might also want to meet with our social worker, who can help with the financial issues. What else would need to happen to raise your confidence up to a 10? (Asking permission followed by an open-ended question)

JOEY'S PARENT: That's really about it.

A key strategy in this encounter is to ask the parents to describe why they do not assign themselves a *lower* number on the scale. This helps facilitate brainstorming about motivations for change by articulating the origins for the confidence that already exists. Once parents have a clear sense of where they *are*, they'll have a better chance of imagining where they'd like to *be*. Now the stage is set to identify potential barriers to achieving higher levels of confidence and to begin to find solutions to these issues.

SCHOOL-AGED CHILDREN

The school-aged child's rapid increase in language facility and vocabulary often obscures the child's emotional, intellectual, and social dependence on parents/guardians and family. We need to attend to this dichotomy and remember to use clear, simple language appropriate to each child's level of understanding, especially when we deal with them directly.

School-aged children are often highly interested in physician's visits, and although they may be reluctant to initiate contact, given half a chance, they are ready to engage and respond to questions. Children of this age are extremely sensitive to positive and negative feedback, and they tend to respond well to both affirmations and clearly stated expectations regarding what we expect of them.

Exchange 2: The E-P-E Sandwich in a Patient With Exacerbation of Cystic Fibrosis

Cystic fibrosis (CF) treatment includes the use of bronchodilators, antibiotics, pancreatic enzyme replacement, and mucous disruption. Alice is an 8-year-old girl with CF, admitted to the hospital for the third time this year with a serious bacterial infection.

TRAINEE: Help me understand what you know about cystic fibrosis so far. (Open-ended question)

ALICE: All I know is that I have a hard time breathing. I have to wear this big black vest that shakes me really, really fast, but then I end up coughing more, and I have to take lots of pills so I don't get sick, but sometimes I don't take all of them.

TRAINEE: OK, that is a pretty clear description, and thank you for being honest about how you take your medications. It's really important that we share all this information so we can work together to decide how best to take care of you. Would it be OK if I shared a little more information with you? (Affirmation followed by asking permission)

ALICE: Sure.

TRAINEE: As you already know, CF definitely affects your breathing. It makes your mucous really thick and that vest helps loosen it up so you're able to cough it out. If it stays there, you can get a really bad infection like you did a few days ago. One of the pills you take every day is an antibiotic, which we hope will kill the germs in your chest that make it especially hard to breathe. You also have breathing treatments, and the puffer to help you breathe more easily if you're finding it hard. CF also affects your tummy. It makes poop really thick and sticky, so you have a hard time going to the bathroom. One of the other pills you take is to help loosen the mucous in your tummy to help you go to the bathroom more easily. What else have you noticed lately? (Open-ended question)

ALICE: Well … now that you mention it, I've had a hard time going to the bathroom for a while and I haven't gone at all in the last couple of days. I do remember using my puffer when I first got sick, but it didn't help much, so we had to come to the hospital.

TRAINEE: (To the parents) I'd like to talk a little more about Alice's medications. How often would you estimate that she misses a dose, and what barriers do you think get in the way of Alice taking her medications each day? (Open-ended questions)

Beginning a therapeutic conversation with an open-ended question, asking permission to provide more information, and following up with another open-ended question helps us maintain the spirit of MI, while providing a smooth transition into a discussion about how to optimize healthy behaviors.

Young school-aged children may find open-ended questions confusing; generally, they wish to please, but they're not quite sure what we're looking for. One approach is to reduce the number of open-ended questions and to increase the number of affirmations; this will also help young patients engage with us. Another option is to adapt open-ended questions to an open-closed-open sandwich of questions, such as "How do you think you could increase your exercise? Could you join your soccer team ... or perhaps ride your bike with your friends and family every week ... or go to the park after school each day? Do you have other ideas? What do you think *you* would enjoy most?"

A third strategy is to ask either an open-ended question or a question with a restricted range of answers, make an autonomy statement, and then ask another open-ended question. This sounds complicated, but in practice, it may open up a productive brainstorming session. For instance: "What time of day works best for you to take your medication? First thing in the morning ... after school ... or before bed? Could there be another time that would work better? You're the best judge of what would work for you. What do you think?" Remember that context is key: Avoid peppering your patient with rapid-fire questions; rather, keep your tone friendly, open, and curious.

In our encounters with school-aged children on the cusp of adolescence, our approach needs to change yet again. While younger and mid-school-aged children tend to respond very positively to affirmations, adolescents often view these statements as patronizing, even demeaning. Similarly, while younger children like to know the "rules" of engagement, adolescents may perceive these guidelines as infringements on their independence, more of a punishment than a protective measure. Assess your patient's maturity level carefully, paying close attention to subtle cues of body language, facial expression, level of eye contact, and paralinguistic signals such as tone of voice, volume, inflections, and pitch, and tailor your approach to each individual.

ADOLESCENTS

As young patients approach adolescence, it is increasingly important to separate parents and children for a portion of the encounter to speak to each party regarding possible risk-taking behaviors. Parents and children alike need opportunities to express concerns and ask questions, secure in the knowledge that their confidentiality will be respected. In some instances, you will be unable to guarantee complete confidentiality, as when the intention to harm oneself or others is expressed, or in situations of sexual or physical abuse. Remember that in most instances, confidentiality is absolutely essential to young people, and it plays a key role in building therapeutic relationships with this age group.

The HEADSS template is a useful means of organizing a patient's social history according to the categories of Home, Education/Employment/Eating, Activities, Drugs/Depression, Sexuality, and Suicide/Safety/Spirituality. Moreover, HEADSS is comprehensive enough that by progressing through each area, you will discover a wealth of opportunity to establish rapport and explore how a teen's health is integral to the quality of his or her life. By accommodating both the spirit of MI and the OARS strategies, this instrument helps maintain a patient-centered approach to our conversations, identify a focus for behavior change, evoke our patient's motivations for change, and facilitate his or her plans for implementing long-term behavior changes.

Open-ended questions play a critical role in our interactions with adolescents, especially in our efforts to support a patient's autonomy while minimizing discord and status quo talk. Note how the following examples subtly acknowledge each patient's independence while prompting him or her to engage: "What is *your* understanding of what might happen if you stop taking your medications?" "How do *you* feel about your decision?" "What are you like when you drink/smoke pot/etc.?" When inviting your patient to articulate his or her thoughts and feelings in response to open-ended questions and statements, remember that maintaining a safe emotional environment is essential to an open, honest discussion.

Acknowledging teenagers' values and beliefs also reinforces our support for their right to make their own decisions. For example, statements such as "Only you can decide whether to use or stop using drugs" or "It's up to you to decide if, when, and how to make any changes" can defuse situations in which teenaged patients feel pressured to comply with parental or medical demands, whether real or imagined. Adolescents frequently disagree with adults, often because their respective value systems differ from one another. Recall, too, that young people may be highly influenced by their peers and consequently less concerned with either their parents' opinions or the long-term repercussions of their actions.

One strategy is to recognize and use "teachable moments," those brief, but exhilarating, occasions in which adolescent patients are truly ready to accept new information. Unfortunately, such instances cannot be scripted or even anticipated; all the same, they present an unparalleled opportunity for sharing knowledge in a timely and meaningful context. One of the great strengths of MI is that it maximizes the potential of teachable moments as catalysts for behavior change.

By contrast, direct confrontation or attempts to scare adolescents into compliant behavior serve only to create anxiety, increase defensiveness, and potentially destroy whatever rapport has been established. The adversarial approach also allows patients to avoid acknowledging that risk-taking behavior may result in devastating consequences, and it reduces the likelihood of sustained change in behavior.

Exchange 3: A "Teachable Moment" Related to Asthma Medication Adherence

George is a 14-year-old boy in ninth grade, admitted for a few hours following an acute asthma exacerbation.

GEORGE: Right … I want to go home! I'm feeling better now and I'm missing my field day for the last day of school.

TRAINEE: It's wonderful that you're feeling better and I can tell it's important to you to get back to your friends at school. Help me understand how you decided to come to the hospital in the first place. (Reflection, open-ended statement)

GEORGE: It's my asthma. I had trouble breathing outside and the school nurse couldn't control it with my inhaler, so I had to come here.

TRAINEE: So your asthma was so bad this time that your inhaler didn't help you breathe more easily. Do you have different kinds of inhalers, or just one? (Complex reflection, closed question)

GEORGE: Yeah, I've got the albuterol that I have at school and there's another one I use with a steroid. I can't remember the name of it.

TRAINEE: What's your understanding of how the steroid inhaler works? (Open-ended question)

GEORGE: I think I'm supposed to take that one every day, right? It never seems to do anything. It doesn't help me breathe any easier like the albuterol does, so I stopped taking it a while back. I mean, what's the point?

TRAINEE: You're correct, steroid inhalers should be taken every day and you might not notice a drastic difference in your breathing either before or after you take it. It's what we call a "controller" medication, and it works to keep down the inflammation in your lungs. When you use it daily, this medication prevents wheezing situations like you had this morning. You prevent the breathing problem before it occurs, and if, or when, it does occur, the problem is often less severe ... so you've got a better chance of being able to help yourself with the albuterol inhaler. What do you think about this information? (Giving information, open-ended question)

GEORGE: So if I take the Pulmicort®, I won't get sick with my asthma as often, and I won't keep missing stuff? Hmmm, maybe I'll go back to using it every day.

Acute hospital admissions often provide opportunities for adolescent patients to make connections between the lack of control of their illness and the negative consequences that result. This is especially true when teens have to miss enjoyable events because of poor health.

Another setting in which teachable moments can be particularly meaningful is the emergency department (ED). For many adolescents, the ED is the first place in which the all-too-real fallout from their actions is clear. Like most people, adolescents tend to respond more positively when they believe they are being helped rather than criticized or punished; under some circumstances, children and adolescents will withhold essential health information in order to avoid even a possibility of critique. Thus, establishing rapport with nonadult patients must take precedence on a first visit, rather than reviewing a long list of reasons why a particular behavior should have been avoided.

We cannot overemphasize the importance of confidentiality and the need to be as direct and truthful as possible, especially with regard to what information will be relayed to parents and others. A good place to start is by discussing your patient's perspective regarding how drug/alcohol use—or other behaviors—led him or her to be treated at an ED. Ultimately, adolescent patients themselves will decide whether we are trustworthy enough to earn the right to a frank and open discussion.

Exchange 4: The "Window of Opportunity" in an Alcohol-Intoxicated Adolescent

As a complement to the concept of teachable moments, the notion of a "window of opportunity" refers to the timeframe in which adolescents are ready and able to appreciate the profound connections between risk-taking behaviors and adverse consequences. This opportunity often presents in the aftermath of some sort of crisis that involves admission to the hospital, invasive procedures, and missing out on fun activities.

Jesse is a 19-year-old male sophomore in college who arrives in the ED after falling down a flight of stairs while in a state of acute alcohol intoxication.

JESSE: I've got to leave, *now*. You've already done more than I wanted, sticking that tube down my throat and giving me this "intravenous infusion" (IV).

TRAINEE: You feel as though these interventions were unnecessary and now we're holding you against your will. (Complex reflection)

JESSE: Yeah. I feel perfectly fine and I'm missing the after-party to my spring formal.

TRAINEE: You're feeling better now, and I understand that you have places you'd rather be right now. Would it be OK if I explain why we decided to start the IV infusion and pump your stomach? (Complex reflection followed by asking permission)

JESSE: I guess so, especially if it gets me out of here sooner.

TRAINEE: Your blood work when you arrived showed that you were very intoxicated, almost two times the legal limit for adults 21 and over. Your friends brought you in, after you'd fallen down a flight of stairs and banged your head. It would have been unsafe and irresponsible for us to send you out of the ED without checking anything. We needed to get you medically stable, obtain a CAT scan of your head to make sure you weren't bleeding, give you some fluids, and make sure your blood alcohol level wasn't still rising because of all the alcohol that was still in your stomach. What's your understanding about how alcohol affects you? (Giving information followed by open-ended question)

JESSE: Well, I never drink too much. I get a bit tipsy at times, but nothing bad will come of that. Sometimes I stumble and lose my balance and once in a while, I mumble when I'm talking. Mostly I just think a little slower when I'm drinking; it's like my brain doesn't work as fast as usual.

TRAINEE: You're quite correct that drinking alcohol decreases the speed of brain processing and that the more you drink, the worse your coordination becomes. May I explain a little more about what happens when you drink alcohol? (Giving information followed by asking permission)

JESSE: Sure, go ahead.

TRAINEE: By the time you're slurring your speech, you're already over the legal limit. What do you make of that? (Giving information followed by open-ended question)

JESSE: Wow ... Really? Are you sure? I had no idea.

TRAINEE: Yes. The limit is a blood alcohol concentration, or BAC, of 0.08, and in order to have slurred speech and slowed thinking, the BAC is typically around 0.1. And at a blood alcohol level of 0.15, people have much less muscle control and balance than normal. Our judgment is severely impaired when drinking alcohol, even at the limit of 0.08. Many people do things while drinking that they wouldn't normally do, such as having unprotected sex with someone they just met or driving while drunk because their judgment is impaired. These behaviors can lead to unwanted pregnancies, getting sexually transmitted infections, or losing your driver's license, sometimes even jail time. What are your thoughts about this information? (Information exchange followed by open-ended question)

JESSE: I know I feel less inhibited and that being with people is more fun when drinking, but I never imagined it could go that far. And now that I think about it, one of my sorority sisters slept with some guy she just met at a bar one time and ended up with gonorrhea. I always thought she just wasn't concerned enough to care about using a condom, but she's really smart, and I can't imagine she wouldn't know better. Maybe it was the alcohol.

TRAINEE: You've seen your close friends experience the consequences of poor judgment when intoxicated, and you don't want to experience that yourself. (Complex reflection)

JESSE: Yeah, and I definitely don't want that to happen to me.

This encounter engaged Jesse in a discussion about the consequences of his behavior using the "window of opportunity" and the E-P-E framework.

CHALLENGING SITUATIONS IN PEDIATRIC POPULATIONS

There are a number of concerns unique to pediatric settings that may restrict the use of MI. First among these is evidence of imminent harm to our patient, as in cases of childhood abuse, nonaccidental trauma, neglect, and expressions of either suicidal or homicidal intent. By law, we must report these events to the appropriate authorities in order that they may be investigated. Unfortunately, mandatory reporting may well damage the therapeutic alliance we have worked so hard to achieve; however, we cannot forget that the safety of the child or adolescent takes precedence over all other concerns. Informing adolescents of their rights to confidentiality includes the responsibility to clearly outline the limits of that confidentiality, and to do so at the outset of our interview. Adolescents have a right to know that some of the details they communicate to healthcare practitioners cannot be held in confidence, and why this is so. An honest discussion of these limitations has the potential to enhance an adolescent's trust in our judgments, and it may limit future damage to our therapeutic relationship.

Despite these challenges, the spirit and skills of MI that include sincere expressions of empathy, affirmations, reflective listening, and sensitively providing objective feedback is often a welcome element in challenging scenarios that support our explanations as to why mandatory reporting is necessary under particular circumstances, and it improves collaboration as the reporting process unfolds. As appropriate, inviting minors to participate in the reporting process allows them a modicum of control over the precise details they choose to share. Including young victims in this way may also mitigate some patients' anger and unhappiness that their confidentiality has been breached.

Other situations in which MI may not be appropriate include those that require emergency treatment or involve altered consciousness, such as acute asthmatic attacks requiring intubation or severe intoxication. Later, when the patient is stable, MI may prove advantageous in improving medication adherence or in changing risk-taking behaviors in order to avoid recurrences.

PERSONAL REFLECTION

While training as a medical student, I began to realize that *behavior* is what drives health outcomes. Antihypertensive medications are useless if they are not taken. Diabetes can often be avoided with lifestyle modifications. Suicide is the number-two cause of death among teenagers in the U.S. The examples are endless.

Unfortunately, I rarely witnessed my clinical teachers attempting to explore why people behave in ways detrimental to their health. Instead, patients were simply told what to do, or even worse, they were handed a prescription without any explanation whatsoever. This was true until my adolescent medicine preceptor introduced me to MI. Witnessing her use of MI skills during brief health interventions with adolescents and young adults allowed me to see the importance of learning MI should I hope to facilitate behavior change in my patients.

My first few MI sessions felt like disasters. Suddenly, my skill in establishing "excellent patient rapport" that had been commented on so frequently in my clinical evaluations seemed to vanish. I expressed my thoughts awkwardly, trying to phrase everything I said in an "MI way." Keenly aware of my own discomfort, in addition to that of my patient and observers, I asked rapid-fire questions, which are not only the antithesis of MI but something that I had never done before! I realized then that MI is not a script I had to memorize in place of my own techniques. Instead, it is a method to be used in conjunction with, and in addition to, the communication skills I already have.

Once I began to relax and engage my patients as I would in any other interview, I found it easier to practice MI skills because I was no longer trying to deviate from my natural style. I realized I could focus on a few MI skills at a time, such as increasing my reflection-to-question ratio. I no longer felt that I needed to start from scratch. As I became comfortable with the basics, I set goals for my interviews that were in line with the spirit and processes of MI, and I gradually became more comfortable adapting to the inevitable turns in my conversations with patients.

Since the inpatient psychiatric rotation where I first began to practice MI, I've had opportunities to continue to refine my skills during rotations in pediatrics and adolescent medicine. MI has fundamentally changed my approach to patient care; I no longer see myself as a "provider" of care, but as a collaborator. While I have not yet had the chance to follow patients long term, I've already noticed a difference in my interactions with acute, short-stay hospital patients. I see that individuals with a sense of autonomy, and who know their options, are more invested in their own care. Having experienced so many positive changes, I'm looking forward to incorporating MI into my training in child and adolescent psychiatry.

SELF-ASSESSMENT QUIZ

True or False?

1. MI's ability to clarify a caregiver's perspective with regard to seeking treatment for a child (the patient) makes it an ideal complement to caring for pediatric populations.
2. Open-ended questions are often confusing for school-aged children and other styles of questioning may be more appropriate.
3. Utilizing "teachable moments" is particularly important with adolescents as they are often less concerned about the long-term consequences of their actions.
4. Adolescents are particularly concerned about being punished or criticized and, consequently, may withhold potentially helpful information from healthcare professionals.
5. In its purest form, MI is an excellent approach in situations that involve imminent harm to patients, as in cases of abuse, non-accidental trauma, and neglect.

Answers

1. *False.* MI is an appropriate choice for use among pediatric/adolescent populations because of its effectiveness in (1) clarifying potential differences in motivations for treatment between younger patients and their caregivers, and (2) building a therapeutic relationship with all parties that facilitates open and honest discussion of these issues.

2. *True.* School-aged children may be confused by open-ended questions and uncertain about what information trainees seek. A more age-appropriate approach is to reduce the number of open-ended question and increase the number of affirmations. Other strategies include using an open-closed-open sequence of questions, and questions with a restricted range of answers, for example, three closed-ended questions in a row, followed by an open-ended question.

3. *True.* Teachable moments occur when patients demonstrate unexpected readiness to accept new information, thus allowing trainees to capitalize on so-called windows of opportunity. These occasions often occur in emergency settings, such as in the aftermath of a young person's threats of suicide while under the influence of drugs and alcohol, or during a discussion concerning contraception following a pregnancy scare. During such episodes, with adverse effects fresh in their minds, adolescents are more likely to connect risky behaviors with negative outcomes.

4. *True.* Adolescents tend to respond more openly when they perceive that they are respected, listened to, and understood; they may not report significant details should they fear censure or other negative consequences. As always, establishing rapport with patients is an essential preliminary to obtaining a thorough history and exploring the circumstances regarding why treatment was sought.

5. *False.* MI may be contraindicated in situations that present imminent or preexisting harm. Physicians are legally required to report such events, and contacting relevant authorities may damage a previously established therapeutic alliance. Nevertheless, the spirit of MI may be maintained under these conditions, particularly in terms of helping patients understand why mandatory reporting is necessary. Tactfully including minors in the reporting process has the potential to offer them a degree of control in extremely difficult circumstances.

12 Motivational Interviewing in Family Settings

Motivational interviewing (MI) enriches our encounters with families. Unfortunately, however, these contributions tend to be overlooked in medical education, as are most family-centered models of care. Instead, medical trainees focus on the conventional doctor–patient relationship centered around a state of ill health or disease, which both the trainee and the patient agree must be eradicated in order to best serve the interests of the patient. According to this paradigm, the focus of treatment is neither on the trainee–patient relationship nor upon the ambivalence many patients experience when an appropriate treatment regimen is begun. Rather, this model assumes that treatment begins and ends with a focus on eliminating a medical condition or injury, and in these situations, both the trainee and the patient are engaged in fighting that illness. This component of medical tradition focuses on the definition of a "patient as host to a defect or disease"; in effect, it is a closed system in which an error or deficit has been identified that requires treatment. This approach prioritizes physician knowledge and skill over patient perspective and life experience, and it derives from the assumption that physically-based conditions can be treated solely by physical interventions such as medication, surgery, or other treatments that involve manipulation of the body.

Despite its limitations, this model of healthcare is adequate for many uncomplicated physical illnesses. Nevertheless, we must remember that for psychiatric disorders and behavioral conditions, physical illness often serves to mask some type of psychological ill health that is commonly linked to one's interpersonal relationships. These difficulties may be challenging to discern and comprehend, and inevitably, inter- and intrapersonal conflicts arise when these symptoms begin to be treated. Recall, for instance, that effective treatments for many physically-based illnesses such as eating disorders demand that psychosocial factors be taken into account.

Few of our patients live completely solitary lives. Most have ties to family, friends, and colleagues; thus, the many psychosocial and interpersonal components of suboptimal health must also be understood according to how they help or hinder treatment and the healing process. These aspects play an especially important role in disorders of childhood and adolescence where the unique bonds between parent and child shape how illness is perceived and understood. Similarly, the nature and strength of marital ties also affect how illness in one spouse is comprehended by a partner.

Research demonstrates that emotional support plays a key role in the healing process, and trainees are well placed to encourage patients to make use of whatever emotional assistance is available. Our focus is generally directed toward the single individual we designate as the "patient." But in many circumstances, the problems facing our patients have profound effects on those to whom they are close. The healing process must be extended to include these individuals, particularly in terms of reducing the anxiety they experience in response to their loved one's illness. A trainee's ability to engage a patient's supports in a motivational way allows for powerful and evocative moments that can facilitate the process of change.

COMMON THEMES FOR FAMILY INVOLVEMENT IN PATIENT CARE

One group of patients seeks treatment because on their own, they lack sufficient resolve and confidence to make the behavior changes required for improved health and quality of life. As important sources of information concerning a given patient's struggles, family members can enhance medical treatment by offering support and reinforcing treatment goals. A second group of patients have been coerced into coming for treatment, either on the basis of family concerns or as a result of potentially negative consequences arising from persistent behavioral problems: loss of child custody, for instance, or other legal penalties. While family members may be more than ready for a patient to demonstrate significant behavior change, the patient may not express similar levels of readiness, motivation, and determination. The dissonance created between the conflicting desires of patients and their families can often work against the change process by increasing a patient's reluctance to engage in new behaviors while consolidating arguments in favor of maintaining the status quo.

WORKING WITH FAMILIES

The most important element of medical interventions that include families is to engage a patient's support system such that it becomes part of the process of change. Attending to complex and sensitive family dynamics may be both anxiety provoking and challenging for trainees; it sometimes seems as though there are simply too many elements to consider. However, by using MI skills to guide our interactions and by maintaining the spirit of MI in every patient encounter, we may begin to deconstruct, comprehend, and ultimately utilize an intricate web of relationships and interactions.

The core MI skills of OARS (see Chapter 4) are essential components of encounters with both individual patients and families (see Fig. 12.1). In practice, the two primary objectives of family interventions, improving communication and restructuring relationships, cannot be achieved if a trainee is unable to accurately hear, reframe, and reflect each person's expectations as family members attempt to resolve their differences. Trainees can encourage and facilitate accurate and genuine communication between family members, but this can occur only when each person feels understood.

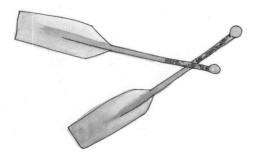

FIGURE 12.1   Using OARS to engage families.

For understanding to take place, trainees must be able to maintain a therapeutic alliance with the group as a whole and to elicit change talk. Sometimes trainees need to offer support for each family member's position; at other times, they must be able to tactfully suggest that a particular family member consider the perspectives of other individuals. By remaining empathic and using MI skills consistently, you will discover that providing support at one time and withdrawing it at another can be negotiated without damaging the therapeutic relationship. Other key elements include maintaining objectivity and offering timely affirmations, accurate reflections, and expressions of concern for the good of the family unit.

As always, you must be mindful to avoid arguments in favor of change that have the opposite effect of pushing patients away from behavior change. As delicate issues arise from members of a patient's family, these must be addressed with tact and sensitivity. There is no fixed set of principles related to using MI in family settings, but a number of common situations demonstrate how MI processes, its spirit, and its skills may be tweaked to fit particular circumstances.

KEY STRATEGIES FOR USING MOTIVATIONAL INTERVIEWING WITH FAMILIES

Stay Balanced Between the Patient's Perspective and the Family's Perspective

> KEY POINT
>
> Stay balanced in family interactions. It is crucial to maintain equipoise between patient and family.

We can easily find ourselves allied with family members who seem to be asking for reasonable change in the patient's behavior. For instance, a young man living in his parents' home and using drugs not only jeopardizes his own health but that of other family members as well. Accordingly, we might view his parents' demand that he stop using drugs as quite reasonable. While this response may appear both rational and objective, such a position opens a number of unnecessary and counterproductive issues. Should we be unable to explore and accept the young person's point of view, we will also be unable to establish a therapeutic alliance with him and little will be accomplished. Remember that we do not need to agree with a patient's position in order to elicit and accept that point of view. Rightness or wrongness about a behavioral problem is also unimportant. The critical issue is to elicit and listen attentively to all perspectives, find common ground between opposing views, and recognize the potential value and worth of every family member's opinion in resolving differences.

Recall that a key aspect of MI spirit is *acceptance*. Commonly, members of a family have different roles and positions of authority, and it is essential to give time to each person's point of view. Similarly, each individual who is part of the engagement process has the potential to help, assuming it is properly evoked. Remember that you are enlisting *the family* to become a part of the change process for your patient.

When family members feel their opinions have not been heard, discord is often manifested by undue focus on a particular "agenda," which in turn reflects a high level of frustration concerning the patient's current behavior. When this occurs in a session, patients frequently become defensive and express their own anger as rationalizations for why they behave as they do. In turn, family members may begin to argue that the patient's conduct in the session illustrates how out of control he or she is, and that these behaviors cannot be tolerated. These interactions revolve around the status quo and offer little prospect of change; furthermore, they can undermine a patient's interest or attempt to implement behavior change. By validating each person's perspective using the MI spirit, trainees avoid the risk of eliciting discord from those who may provide meaningful support to the patient.

Stay Patient-Centered

> **KEY POINT**
>
> If the divide between patient and family is too wide, you may need to favor remaining patient-centered.

Just as we can find ourselves siding with a family, so too we may be biased toward our patient in the mistaken belief that a family is either too demanding, or that they unfairly blame our patient for the maladaptive behaviors. Family therapists have long identified various roles that people play in dysfunctional families, one of the most well known being that of the scapegoat, the person other people view as "the problem." When we recognize that we are having difficulty maintaining our objectivity, we give ourselves a philosophical reminder that we must side with the patient's struggle. This realization helps guide our interventions and keeps us focused on what really matters.

Ambivalence in this setting commonly involves the identified patient experiencing a high degree of anger that he or she has been unjustifiably maligned. These feelings must be explored in individual sessions in order to articulate them and understand them. Similar explorations may then take place in the presence of family members in order to help everyone involved recognize and discuss how ambivalence might be resolved. This principle requires that we remain focused on brainstorming, instead of allowing family members to engage in personal attacks and accusations. When a family personalizes a problem, the risk for defensiveness and discord increases, patients are likely to maintain the status quo, and open conflict may arise between patient, family, and trainee.

The following examples demonstrate how trainees might communicate acceptance and inclusion to family members:

a) "Your brother asked you to come today because he believes that your perspective is very important as he takes his first steps toward not using drugs. Since your point of view is so meaningful, the best place to start is for me to ask you to share your perspective on your brother's struggle. . ."

b) "You've seen more clearly than anyone your father's struggle with drinking and how different he can be from the person you feel so much closer to when he's sober. That's why providing your perspective here today is so important. Would you be willing to share your views with us?"

> KEY POINT
>
> If family conversation devolves into blaming, redirect the session toward a specific problem behavior all can agree to work on.

A session in which we engage with patients and families about problematic behaviors can be emotionally laden. Frustrated and angry family members may express sentiments that are undermining and destructive. Individuals who are hurting commonly veer away from problem behaviors and instead list patient character flaws and personal failings. While emotional sharing is often a key part of the process, an interview may degenerate into accusations and recriminations as old wounds are reopened.

Patients and families can agree to constructively discuss problematic behavior, but we cannot permit name calling, or talking about personal flaws or failings, to thwart the process of change. Setting ground rules at the beginning of each session helps everyone to remember to treat one another's perspective in a nonjudgmental way. That said, it is crucial that we intervene quickly and effectively to refocus attention back to the problem whenever a discussion turns personal. One method to transition away from hurtful comments is to discuss how challenging it may be for the patient to implement the changes that are being considered. Note that this intervention may occur without invalidating an angry family member. But by refocusing attention away from anger toward the struggle and vulnerability shared by all, a new basis for empathy and understanding may emerge. A primary technique is to reframe what has been said into a statement that reflects what might be considered "normal" or "usual" under similar circumstances.

MOTHER [TO YOUNG ADULT SON]: I know you're depressed, but using drugs can't be helping you. I know the doctor has told you this many times. We've been dealing with this for 5 years now. You were doing better just last year when you had that job. I know you weren't using drugs when you were working. Why did you start again and why did you stop working? Sometimes it seems like you do these things on purpose. You say you're depressed but sometimes I think you're just lazy. I want to keep helping you, but I am coming to the end of my rope here.

SON: Yeah, yeah, I've heard it all before. You don't know what I am going through. [To the trainee] See? I told you, all she does is criticize me. I want to stop using and I've made some progress. She's right, I was better last year, but I get stressed and I get cravings. And when she hammers me about being lazy, I just feel like going out and using more drugs!

TRAINEE [TO MOTHER]: You're frustrated with your son's drug use and the long course of his illness. We see this with other families and it's common for parents to feel the way you're feeling. I can tell that your frustration isn't just with the burden it places on you. It comes from your concern for your son and what will happen to him if he doesn't get this under control.

MOTHER (CRYING): Yes, I am so worried about him. I want him to be more independent because I won't be around forever. I want to be able to think he can take care of himself.

TRAINEE: Yes, that's what I'm hearing. You know, there is a support group I know of for families of people who are abusing substances. There are at least 150 families in this support network. They have much in common and meet monthly at the local hospital. They have other activities, too. How do you feel about considering to join?

MOTHER: Yes, I would like that.

TRAINEE: When families experience illness, it places a burden on the family that is not normal. When one or more of the members is ill, everyone must be even more supportive than they usually are. [To mother] When we first met, you told me how hard it was when your husband was ill, before he passed. That was 3 years ago, right?

MOTHER: Yes, I had to work during the day and take care of him at night. [To son] That's one time when you helped me a great deal. I remember telling people I didn't know what I would have done without you being there.

SON: I remember. I was into drugs then but not as much as now. I was 17 and angry a lot because I couldn't go out as much as I wanted to, but I wanted to help him and you, too.

TRAINEE: How much different is this situation now? The two of you had your own frustrations 3 years ago, but you found a way to work together. It's reasonable that family members become frustrated with the process of helping each other, especially during times of family crisis. It's more than is normally expected, and when we get upset, it's because of that extra burden that is no one's fault but rather, part of the current circumstances the family is going through. [To mother] "I think you'll find that many others go through something similar when you speak with people at the support meetings we talked about. What's important now is to see that one thing everyone in the family has in common is the need to deal with the problems. One strategy that can be helpful is to realize that each time you get frustrated, it's more effective to think through it, just as we've done here."

Then focus on the behavior or situation you want to change, not on the emotion that accompanies your frustration:

"The two of you have just expressed your feelings in a highly emotional manner about how drug use is affecting you individually. But you each noted some common ground when you indicated in your own way that stopping the drug use is key to starting the recovery process. If we start there and look at what might be helpful in reducing drug use, we can make the most of your individual strengths. [To son] In what ways might your mother help you stop using drugs?"

In this scenario the trainee does not respond to the heated exchange between the mother and her son. Rather, he or she uses selective reflection in showing empathy for the mother and her position and offers to help her find emotional support that may prove helpful in restoring her depleted emotional reserves. The trainee also reviews a previous situation similar to that of the present time. In the past, mother and son worked together to help one another and reviewing this experience reinforces a sense of mutual self-efficacy. Finally, the trainee emphasizes that what they are going through is "normal," and he or she focuses on how de-emotionalizing the situation will help them cope with the son's drug abuse.

Validate and Affirm Family Members Who Assert Their Concern and Facilitate Family Engagement

> **KEY POINT**
> OARS works just as well to engage families as it does to engage a single patient.

Use OARS skills to uncover and explore avenues for engagement and, at the same time, affirm and validate each family member's concerns within the family setting. Pay attention to the content of each comment and remember to attribute valuable insights or suggestions to the appropriate individual. For instance:

- "You make a valid point."
- "You've offered an important insight into the situation."
- "You've pointed out an important perspective."

By consistently expressing feedback in this way, you are crediting people for their help and creativity, and you reinforce that individuals who may be at odds most of the time can also work together. In family sessions, even a single statement may be modified in a number of different ways. When we highlight different ideas and insights, we tacitly invite others to offer their opinions as to how problems may be resolved.

Use language that helps family members express themselves in a way that improves how a patient understands their concerns. When we use other vocabulary to reframe a particular reflection or statement, we encourage a family member to begin to talk about the problem using new terms and new expressions. Hearing new language in use is a reassuring sign that progress is under way and suggests a new understanding of the patient and the problematic behaviors.

As family members exchange perspectives, make use of spontaneous opportunities to discuss the pros versus the cons of changing. This is a part of the directive nature of MI. At times, attentive silence is the most appropriate response; use these moments to observe nonverbal communication in addition to other behaviors that warrant feedback. When an especially raw or emotional perspective is shared, intervene to clarify what was said and reflect the emotion to facilitate further discussion. Family encounters can abound with unpredictable moments and, while sessions may be loaded with painful or negative emotions, they may also present moments of exhilaration as powerful insights concerning problem behaviors are spontaneously expressed. When such moments occur, remember to pause and reflect upon what has happened and note their significance as a sign of improved communication.

- "As a daughter, you've shared a compelling summary of the effect of your father's drug use. I get the impression that this type of sharing has not happened very often in the past. [Turning to address the father who is the patient] What's your take on the perspective your daughter has just expressed?"
- "You've shared how hurt you were when your brother chose not to take his diabetes medications and suffer from a stroke, and now he is seeking your support in helping him focus on taking care of his diabetes and his overall health. [Turning to the brother who is the patient] What's it like for you to hear your brother share his experience of the effects of your not taking care of your diabetes had on him?"

Another technique is to use an intervention designed to facilitate more constructive communication among family members. For example, reframing personal criticism as a complaint can help defuse the defensiveness prompted by personal attacks. Moreover, a clearly articulated complaint has the potential to become a point of discussion around which family members can exchange perspectives and resolve problems.

a)

A PATIENT'S DAUGHTER: You always cared more about doing drugs with your friends than making time for me. You've always been so selfish!

TRAINEE: You've been hurt by past events. But your father has made it a priority to get treatment, and it is important that you've taken time to come and share your perspective. I think one reason your father wanted you here today is to acknowledge the low confidence he feels about facing these obstacles without your support.

TRAINEE TO FATHER (THE PATIENT): What are your feelings about your relationship with your daughter? How do you think your daughter might help you deal with the challenging process of staying in recovery?

b)

A PATIENT'S HUSBAND: Not long after we got married, your drinking spiked. Most days, I feel like I married someone else. I don't know if it's because of work or because of me. This just isn't what I agreed to, I feel betrayed, and I am really angry.

TRAINEE: Your wife's drinking hurt you in many ways. You've struggled ever since she increased her drinking, and now it affects your relationship in very significant ways. You mentioned not knowing whether it is work or other things. So it is clear that you are committed to trying to change, if you can understand what needs to be worked on. [To wife, the patient] What comes to your mind as some reasons that cause you to want to drink?

Even when a family has steadfastly taken sides about problematic behavior, it is crucial that we remain neutral about the behavior itself. Recall the basics of MI techniques used in an individual encounter. Rather than allowing yourself to be drawn to one side or other of the ambivalence, remember to take your time and use open-ended questions and reflections to explore and understand the issues that contribute to emotional conflicts. Similarly, remaining objective and nonjudgmental with family members allows us to consider and value each person's perspective. Just as internal ambivalence may be resolved by an ongoing exploration of pros and cons, so too an ongoing review of family members' opinions may help evoke change talk. For example:

A PATIENT'S SISTER: You have to quit drinking! Can't you see all you have lost because of it? You'd think this would be enough to make you stop!

TRAINEE [TO SISTER]: It's been a struggle for you. And the decision about continuing to drink continues to be a struggle for your brother as well. Yet your brother has asked that you come here today to support him in his struggle to be sober. People often ask others to help them in different ways. [To brother] It may be best to begin by asking you to share how your relationship with your sister is important to you and what she, as a particular person in your life, might do to show her support and help you to work on recovery.

Share (and Model) the Motivational Interviewing Spirit With All Who Are Involved in the Engagement Process

While patients are the center of concern in any family setting, MI spirit has the capacity to enrich everyone engaged in the present encounter. The spirit of MI is founded upon a patient-centered approach, characterized by the key concepts of collaboration, evocation, compassion, and acceptance. To establish a collaborative environment, an essential first step is to value and accept each person's perspective. In doing so, we model a collective approach to problem solving based on the belief that each family member has a role to play in a *partnership* that is central to the process of change.

Evocation is the one aspect of the MI spirit that is uniquely augmented within family settings. An underlying premise of MI is that a patient's strengths already exist within that particular individual, and that change occurs as these strengths are awakened, reinforced, and used effectively. Similarly, including MI as part of family interventions assumes that struggling families already possess the competencies and strengths required to resolve problematic patterns of behavior. Eliciting family members' perspectives on the strengths of the patient they care about can be a powerful reminder for patients who have lost track of their inner strengths. These reminders become an impetus for change that, in turn, has the potential to strengthen engagement among the family as a whole in ways that would not have been possible in individual encounters.

Within a family context, compassion implies that we understand what the problematic behavior has meant to each family member; recall that this information takes time to uncover and is often exceedingly painful to articulate. By reframing each perspective in such a way that our patient understands precisely how his or her behavior has affected others, we can then help patients resolve ambivalence and move toward behavior change.

By accepting the intrinsic value and worth of each person in a family, we encourage honest expression of what the problematic behavior has meant for that individual. A second part of acceptance is to affirm each family member's struggle, in addition to highlighting how that person might best assist the patient to bring about, and maintain, behavior change. Use accurate empathy to demonstrate your understanding of each family member's perspective and acknowledge the autonomy of each family member and of the family as a whole.

During a one-on-one MI session, patients may express little reason for change. However, facilitating engagement between patient and family can play a key role in helping a patient move through the stages of change. One's readiness can significantly increase when a family member shares an experience that a patient had not previously known of or considered. In this instance, a trainee's role is to facilitate evocation from within the family, in order to evoke reasons for change from within the patient.

PATIENT: I just didn't think my drinking was that big a deal. I mean, sometimes I have a hangover the next day and feel kind of lousy, but I've kept my job, earned income for the family. I've held it together.

TRAINEE: Sometimes you've seen how your drinking has been affecting you, and today your family has shared their concerns about your drinking. What questions do you have about their experience with your decision to drink?

PATIENT: I just haven't really thought about it that way. [Turns to daughter] What has this been like for you?

DAUGHTER: Well … one thing is that I feel like I'm the only kid on Saturday mornings whose dad isn't there when my soccer game starts. I mean, I know why you aren't there. What makes me nervous is what I should say if someone else asks me where you are. I don't want to tell them that you drink a lot.

PATIENT: You think I am late because I've been drinking?

DAUGHTER: Dad, it's like that every weekend.

PATIENT: I just never thought about what not being there on Saturday mornings meant for you. I didn't even think you'd miss me.

PERSONAL REFLECTION

I have discovered that using MI in family settings does not mean learning a new mode of MI; rather, it means adapting the spirit, processes, and skills to a wider context in order to evoke the power of a family's perspective and to elicit new sources of support for patients in the process of change. Working with families also opens up opportunities for much personal satisfaction as we share the spirit of MI with others. One such moment occurred when I observed a colleague concluding an interview with a family in which a mother and daughter had recently confronted the daughter's serious issue with self-injury. Through sharing what the impact of self-injury had been for each party, and the significance of the daughter's ability to change this behavior, they were able to communicate long standing painful feelings which resulted from a divorce and family move, and which had been either shut down completely or expressed in self-destructive behaviors.

At the end of this family's work, they told my colleague, "We're quirky, crazy, and a load to deal with, but you've never judged, you've always listened, and you've always focused on us and our struggles. We can tell you anything. You get us. You accept us. Thank you, thank you." The significance of sharing the spirit of MI is evident. This is the kind of gratification we receive only when using family-centered interventions to help patients and families find themselves again. Through MI, the humanity our patients search to retrieve is found.

SELF-ASSESSMENT QUIZ

True or False?

1. The traditional understanding of patients as "host to defect or disease" is limited to treating and managing chronic medical conditions.
2. The two primary objectives of family sessions are to allow family members to express their concerns and to provide an environment in which patients see how their illness or behaviors affect their family.
3. Focusing on the patient's perspective is an essential element in using MI during family encounters.
4. Remaining patient-centered when using MI in family encounters is critical.
5. Exploring a patient's character flaws and personal failings during an initial family encounter is a useful technique for prompting engagement.
6. Validating patients' experiences over those of family members is key to successfully using MI in family encounters.

Answers

1. *True.* No patient should ever be viewed as a mere "host," and trainees must always remember that patients live and work within a social context. While it is true that some patients lead relatively isolated lives, most have a network of relationships with family, friends, and colleagues, all of whom are important sources of information regarding patients' struggles, and potential sources of support as patients approach the goals of treatment. The healing process is maximized only when the psychosocial and interpersonal components of suboptimal health are acknowledged.

2. *False.* The objectives of family interventions include improving communication patterns between patients and family members, and restructuring family relationships. To facilitate this process, trainees must maintain a therapeutic alliance with the group as a whole, by listening, reframing, and reflecting each individual's experiences and expectations.

3. *False.* When using MI in family encounters, trainees must assume a balanced position between a patient's perspectives and those of family members. Aligning with one perspective over another is tempting, but failing to maintain an equitable therapeutic alliance between all will likely have little effect.

4. *True.* During MI family encounters, trainees must remain focused on brainstorming and working through a patient's ambivalence. Trainees cannot allow family members to personalize a problem or engage in personal attacks and accusations; these will result in patient defensiveness and discord. Family sessions cannot be allowed to degenerate into arguments.

5. *False.* Family members who are suffering and struggling to confront unhealthy behaviors commonly revert to listing a patient's character flaws and other deficiencies. Patients and family members must not be allowed to use personal attacks or name calling in a family session; instead, everyone present must remain confident that constructive comments and observations are welcome.

6. *False.* It is important to validate both patients and family members during clinical encounters; doing so helps trainees maintain a therapeutic alliance with everyone present. By affirming family members, trainees acknowledge the contributions that others make in the interest of bringing about positive change, despite perhaps being at odds with a patient.

13 Special Populations and Settings

This chapter explores how motivational interviewing (MI) enriches the care we provide for patients with particular health concerns in a variety of settings: screening interviews for unhealthy/risky behaviors, sexual health, chronic pain, eating disorders, substance use during pregnancy, palliative care, psychiatric disorders, and substance use disorders. Evidence demonstrating the value of MI in these groups varies, but research is ongoing.

What is known is that MI helps patients bring about behavior changes that have the potential to mitigate, even avert, catastrophic medical consequences. The first step is to assist each patient to identify unhealthy behaviors so that the appropriate, MI-related interventions may be planned and implemented. Unfortunately, we often contribute to a systemic failure to help patients recognize and acknowledge problematic behaviors. Sometimes we lack familiarity with appropriate screening tools and strategies, while in other instances, we lack sufficient confidence or expertise to address the unhealthy behaviors we do identify. MI provides a sound foundation for screening, identifying, and exploring a wide range of harmful behaviors, we must acquire these skills in order to serve our patients to the best of our abilities.

You'll notice that many of the dialogues presented in this chapter are longer than those in previous chapters. This is a deliberate choice; our goal in doing so is to highlight, in an extended fashion, the pacing of the encounters with patients regarding particularly sensitive issues.

SCREENING

As obvious as it may seem, it's worth remembering that one cannot tell whether a patient is struggling with certain behaviors simply by observing him or her. Earlier chapters have reviewed a plethora of nonverbal cues that we should attend to in our patient interactions; let these signals guide how the interviews unfold. Even within a relatively short screening interview, establishing a therapeutic alliance with the patient is essential; a safe and secure atmosphere encourages patients to share their perspectives regarding specific health concerns, and it increases their readiness to request, listen to, and learn from the information we share in return. Screening interviews call for a unique combination of medical knowledge concerning specific illnesses blended with an ability to use empathic, reflective listening in the pursuit of an open, trusting relationship with each patient.

Medical screening refers to the process of integrating data gathered through observation, written self-reports, patient interviews, laboratory tests, and physical examinations to determine whether patients are (1) engaging in behaviors that increase their risk of contracting an illness or worsening an existing condition, or (2) experiencing clinical manifestations of a secondary problem. The patients we interview in the clinical exchanges often experience feelings of shame or guilt about themselves or their behaviors, and they may be reluctant to share intimate information. Fear of disapproval or an acute sense of the social stigma that accompanies various signs and symptoms is another deterrent. In some situations, patients will acknowledge symptoms and/or behaviors but minimize their frequency, significance, and possible sequelae.

By improving the likelihood of honest, open reporting and emphasizing a spirit of collaboration and support for a patient's autonomy, MI helps us engage with patients who might otherwise fall between the cracks in our healthcare system. Important skills include expressing empathy, using reflective listening with an egalitarian approach, maintaining a nonjudgmental tone, and providing objective feedback regarding high-risk behaviors, diagnoses, treatment options, and prognoses.

The Screening Process

Screening for a particular condition should be prefaced by a short discussion outlining what will be explored in the encounter. Do not overlook this element; it plays a key role in reducing the potential for discord that may arise when patients feel ambushed, surprised, or offended at the content of your questions. In the following interview, MI skills are incorporated from the outset:

TRAINEE: Hi, I'm Doctor Jones, you're here for a routine physical exam, is that right? (Closed-ended question)

PATIENT: Yes, that's why I'm here.

TRAINEE: It's nice to meet you. Part of our interview will include talking about your lifestyle, which includes topics like drug use and sexual activity. Are you OK with us having a discussion about this? (Providing information followed by asking permission)

PATIENT: I'm a little bit uncomfortable talking about some of this stuff, but I understand that's important. Overall, I'm pretty happy with my life and my choices right now.

TRAINEE: It's up to you to decide what, if any, changes you'd like to make, and it's important that you know this won't affect our working relationship. I may make recommendations, but these are not meant to be judgmental. (Autonomy statement)

PATIENT: Phew! I'm relieved that you're not going to tell me what to do.

TRAINEE: You've had some experiences in the past in which doctors haven't seemed to listen or understand you. You don't have any specific health concerns right now, and at the same time, by coming here today, you demonstrate that you value your health. (Complex reflection)

From the moment of introduction, this trainee demonstrates a transparent approach to the interview that emphasizes collaboration. On a more subtle level, the trainee reinforces respect for patient autonomy and self-determination and a genuine interest in promoting patient health.

Screening for Unhealthy Alcohol Use

The US Preventive Services Task Force (USPSTF) ranks screening and counseling for unhealthy alcohol use as third among the top five health-related prevention priorities for American adults. Given the strong contribution overconsumption of alcohol

FIGURE 13.1   Brief interventions using FRAMES.

has on morbidity and mortality rates, this type of screening is widely recognized as a highly cost-effective measure, and virtually any patient interview that includes reference to alcohol use will be enriched by integrating the MI approach. Attitudes and approaches to alcohol range from abstinence, infrequent or low-risk use, to higher risk behaviors, including problem drinking, alcohol abuse, and the less common, but more severe, alcohol dependence.

Brief interventions for unhealthy alcohol use typically last from several minutes to an entire visit and may occur within a single session or multiple sessions. These patient-centered, motivational conversations focus on increasing insight and awareness regarding alcohol use and supporting patients' motivation for behavioral change; they are suitable as stand-alone interventions for at-risk individuals, as well as for those who need more extensive care.

The acronym FRAMES summarizes the six key points of brief interventions:

- **F**eedback regarding personal risk or impairment is offered to patients following assessment of alcohol use patterns and consequences.
- **R**esponsibility for the decision to change, and to bring about change, belongs solely to our patients.
- **A**dvice concerning how to modify substance use is shared in a nonthreatening, nonjudgmental manner.
- **M**enu of options regarding strategies to modify behavior and/or possible treatments support autonomy and encourage patients to participate in their own care.
- **E**mpathic approach assumes that we demonstrate warmth, respect, and understanding at all times.
- **S**elf-efficacy and a patient's belief that he or she is capable of behavior change are supported when we elicit and reinforce change statements.

Following is a sample of statements during a brief intervention using the FRAMES model (Fig. 13.1):

Feedback (Summarize current assessment): What I understand you saying is that, on average, you have five or six drinks in a single day, two or three times each week. Earlier today, we discussed why monitoring your blood pressure and taking your antihypertensive medication as prescribed is so important to your health. These two behaviors are connected in that the amount of alcohol you consume is in the range of what is called "high risk," partly because of how it might affect your blood pressure. What are your thoughts about this relationship? (Elicit patient's reaction and listen)

Responsibility: It's up to you to decide when, or if, you're ready to reduce your alcohol consumption or to stop drinking altogether. Whatever you decide will not affect our working relationship or your treatment with us. (Emphasize patient responsibility)

Advice: Would it be okay if I shared with you which actions you might take to improve your health and, in particular, your blood pressure? (Wait for permission: proceed if permission is granted) My suggestion would be to limit your drinking to seven drinks or fewer per week, and no more than three drinks on a single occasion; sometimes don't drink at all when you're out. What are your thoughts about this advice? How do you feel about reducing your drinking? (Recommend changes with patient's permission)

Menu of Alternatives: I realize that reducing or giving up drinking might be really challenging, and I'm wondering if we could brainstorm strategies that could help lessen your exposure to situations that prompt you to drink. I could also make some suggestions about programs and community support. (Present alternative options)

Empathy: Sorting out what you need and want to do about your drinking is not an easy decision. (Respectful, nonjudgmental approach)

Self-Efficacy: Could we spend a few minutes reviewing what you've done in the past to manage your drinking? These experiences, regardless of how successful they were, provide important clues as to what works or doesn't work for you. (Wait for permission, and then proceed) I believe that, together, we can come up with a strategy that will work for you when you decide you want to change your drinking. (Eliciting and reinforcing hope and optimism)

Sexual Behaviors

In the area of HIV/AIDS prevention, MI helps to target patients' ambivalence about acknowledging and reducing high-risk sexual behaviors. For example, the randomized clinical trial of the EXPLORE study investigating behavioral interventions in a large sample of men who had sex with men demonstrated a significant reduction in the rate of HIV infection among those who received MI, compared with those who were given standard counseling sessions regarding risk reduction. One reason for this finding may be that MI's effectiveness is closely related to the strength of the therapeutic alliance practitioners establish with their patients over an extended period of time. Another possibility is that MI allows practitioners to address substance use and risky sexual behaviors simultaneously.

Although little research has been conducted on MI's effectiveness in screening for sexually transmitted diseases (STDs), MI is more effective when compared to standard care, among patients being rescreened for these diseases.

Primary care settings and sexual health clinics provide a wealth of opportunities to engage patients in therapeutic conversations about risk-taking behaviors, and the skillful use of MI techniques, even in brief interventions, has tremendous potential to affect behavior change. Prefacing your conversations with an emphasis on confidentiality, supporting autonomy with empathic statements, and providing personalized feedback regarding the health risks associated with particular sexual activities will help patients feel more comfortable discussing their behaviors. Remember that the content of your discussions will include highly personal and private details; a sensitive, tactful approach is a must.

The OARS skills, informed by the spirit of MI, are well suited to the process of screening for, and discussing, high-risk sexual behaviors:

1. **O**pen-ended questions:
   - "What made you decide to come to the clinic today?"
   - "What would you like to address during this visit?"
   - "How did you decide to come for HIV/STDs testing?"
   - "What are your thoughts about using condoms?"
   - "What makes you think you may be at risk for HIV/STDs?"
   - "What do you think are the riskiest behaviors you've engaged in prior to our meeting today?"
   - "How do you see your alcohol or drug use fitting in with your behaviors prior to and during sex?"
2. **A**ffirmations:
   - "I appreciate your willingness to speak openly with me."
   - "You've taken the first step to seek treatment."
   - "You see that it's important for you to be tested and begin to sort out what your thoughts are about your sexual behaviors."
   - "You really care about your health and want to take action to stay as healthy as you can."
3. **R**eflections:
   - "On one hand, you like the spontaneity of sex without condoms; on the other hand, you worry about not knowing the sexual history of your partner."
   - "You sometimes get caught up in the nightlife scene and decide to have unprotected sex. At the same time, you've been thinking about being more careful in your choice of sexual partners."
   - "You got angry at your boyfriend and had unprotected sex with someone you met at a party; now you regret doing things that may have put you at risk for HIV."
   - "You've been thinking about reducing your risk of HIV and you've already started practicing safer sex by not getting drunk during sex."
4. **S**ummaries are synopses of the most salient points made by a patient in response to open-ended questions. Here is a sample summary based on a patient's description as to why she came to the clinic that day:

TRAINEE: "So ... let me check to see if I understand you correctly. About 3 months ago, you broke up with your boyfriend; since then, you've been drinking alcohol several times a week and hitting the bar scene more. Your drinking interferes with your ability to stay safe during sex; you've had unprotected sex with six different people in the past 2 months. You're concerned that you may be at risk for contracting HIV. What have I missed?"

A helpful approach for exchanging information and providing feedback to patients regarding their behaviors is to use the framework of E-P-E. We continue the previous exchange next:

TRAINEE: We've discussed a number of concerns, including that you feel angry, possibly depressed, over the loss of your boyfriend, that you're drinking more than you think you should, and you've engaged in high-risk sexual practices. You see these behaviors as being linked together; if you were to change one of them, which one would you choose first and why? (Elicit)

PATIENT: I'm not sure. They seem all connected but I've been feeling pretty down and drinking a lot, and that seems to lead me to making bad judgments about the people I sleep with.

TRAINEE: You're saying that it starts with your feelings. Would you like to hear about what we offer in the clinic that might help you cope with your feelings about breaking up with your boyfriend? (Provide then elicit)

PATIENT: Yes, I guess. I've talked to my friends about it, but it hasn't helped. As a matter of fact, we're usually at the bar, or we talk while I'm drinking at home … so I guess that's not good.

TRAINEE: We have a counselor here at the clinic who could speak with you about working on how to break the cycle of anger, depression, drinking, and risky sexual behaviors. How do you feel about setting up an evaluation by our counselor? (Provide then elicit)

PATIENT: Yes, I think I need to do it and discuss some treatment options.

Many trainees feel uncomfortable asking patients about their sexual practices. In these situations, remember that your role is not to judge or evaluate your patients' behaviors, but to explore how best to support their desire to behave in ways consistent with their aspirations and values.

CHRONIC PAIN

Chronic pain management poses significant challenges in all healthcare settings and benefits from a interdisciplinary approach. As patients struggle with significant pain, they often become aware of the variables that affect their perceptions of discomfort, such as anxiety, fatigue, support of friends/family, and one's intrinsic coping style; these insights often prompt an interest in exploring how to proactively self-manage pain.

Self-management describes the ongoing process which encourages patients to assume a greater role in the management of long-term conditions through (1) learning about the condition, (2) gaining confidence in their knowledge base and ability to make informed decisions, (3) changing unhealthy behaviors in favor of more positive options, and (4) acquiring technical skills, such as monitoring blood glucose levels, using exercises to decrease pain or learning how to make effective use of the Internet. A patient's degree of motivation is a key factor in determining his or her level of engagement in the self-management process, which in turn, influences the likelihood of following recommended strategies, functional improvement, and overall treatment outcomes.

The Motivational Model of Pain Self-Management suggests that patients' motivation, or readiness, to engage in pain management behaviors is the crucial element in their ability to adapt to pain. One's degree of motivation is influenced by two primary variables: (1) beliefs regarding the *importance* of engaging in pain self-management, and (2) beliefs concerning one's *ability* to engage in these behaviors, that is, one's sense of self-efficacy. Given this emphasis on motivation and self-efficacy, MI is an ideal complement to this model of pain management.

Chronic pain is both physically debilitating and emotionally demoralizing, and it should come as no surprise that nonadherence and high dropout rates are common in pain rehabilitation. MI has been shown to improve patient adherence to recommended treatments and strategies, either as a stand-alone intervention or in combination with physical therapy/exercise programs. This may be a result of MI's attention to a sound, well-established trainee–patient relationship that provides strong support for a patient's sense of self-efficacy.

As in many areas of medicine, we've often been tempted to "lecture" or "push" our patients into adopting behaviors that we believe will improve pain management; in effect, we behave as though *we* know best. Alas, such is not the case, and inevitably, our efforts to cajole or coerce are doomed to failure. Forcing unreceptive patients to listen to unwelcome advice creates discord in the relationship and lessens the possibility of behavior change.

Consider the following encounters:

Scenario 1

PATIENT: I'm having so much pain! I feel as though I can't bear it! I can't take a step without wincing ... it's just so awful.

TRAINEE: Hmmm ... well, I see that you're supposed to be taking the medications we prescribed last time we saw you. Aren't you taking them? (Directing, closed-ended question)

PATIENT: Yes, I'm taking them, but they just don't seem to be working anymore.

TRAINEE: Are you going to physical therapy? (Closed-ended question)

PATIENT: Not all the time. I'm in so much pain that it's been hard to drive myself there. What else am I supposed to do?

TRAINEE: You need to have physical therapy and you need to do the exercises we discussed; these should help reduce your pain. (Ordering)

PATIENT: (Sighs) Okay ... I'll try but I'm not sure it's going to work. I just can't see things getting better.

TRAINEE: You know, if you don't try, we can't tell whether these things will work or not. (Directing, blaming)

PATIENT: I know you're right ... but I feel too discouraged to keep trying. I think I'm a little depressed and that makes it so much harder to deal with the pain.

Scenario 2

PATIENT: I'm having so much pain! I feel as though I can't bear it! I can't take a step without wincing ... it's just so awful.

TRAINEE: You are really upset with what you are going through. You're struggling more to cope with the pain and it's affecting your ability to function. (Complex reflection)

PATIENT: Yes! The medications you gave me aren't working anymore, and I don't know what else to do to get some relief. I just want to take a few pain-free steps.

TRAINEE: Your sense is that the meds aren't controlling your pain very well. You want to feel better and you're not sure what other options are available that you can rely on. (Complex reflection)

PATIENT: Well, the physical therapy hasn't been helping either ... I just don't feel like driving myself there.

TRAINEE: You're feeling stuck. And you are overwhelmed by the amount of pain you're experiencing. Would it be OK for us to discuss some of our options, such as reviewing your medications and exploring other treatment choices? (Complex reflection followed by an open-ended question)

PATIENT: Yes, thank you, thank you. I would really appreciate it. I'll do whatever it takes to help me feel better. I hate living like this; I feel so dependent on everyone else.

In the first encounter, there is no attempt to engage with this patient's struggles with pain management; instead, a rigid plan of action is dictated without consultation or collaboration. In response, the patient expresses sustain talk concerning her inability to manage the high levels of pain she is experiencing. The second encounter demonstrates how to engage the patient in a discussion about her pain: how she is managing it, what works, and what doesn't work. This empathic exchange allows the patient to share openly and honestly, uses reflective listening to elicit change talk, and nurtures a sense of patient-directed decision making; in other words, this trainee actively supports the goals of self-management.

One of MI's strengths is to nurture a patient's sense of self-efficacy, which in those who suffer chronic pain is closely tied to perceptions of pain intensity and tolerance, level of day-to-day functioning, and the use of analgesics. Each patient's readiness to self-manage pain should be assessed along a continuum designed for each of the different self-management strategies. For instance, while patients may be eager to engage in light exercise to alleviate pain, they may not be ready to explore how coexisting depression affects their willingness to go out for a walk. MI helps to guide how we assess a patient's readiness for change, and making use of tools such as the importance and the confidence rulers helps to determine which behaviors patients are most likely to engage in. By eliciting change talk and evoking a patient's motivation for adaptive behavior change, MI introduces the possibility of hopefulness and optimism. An open discussion of the advantages/disadvantages of modifying self-care behaviors, and the creation of a pain management agenda will reinforce patient autonomy and empowerment.

EATING DISORDERS

The category of eating disorders includes anorexia nervosa, bulimia nervosa, binge-eating disorder, and eating disorders not otherwise specified; together, they are highly prevalent mental illnesses associated with a range of physical and psychosocial consequences. Often, these disorders are further complicated by patients' reluctance to disclose their behaviors and symptoms on account of feelings of guilt or shame and/or the belief that they will be judged or punished. An additional obstacle to successful treatment is the low motivation for change that many patients with eating disorders express.

Family dynamics influence the clinical manifestations of eating disorders; thus, any treatment plan must include working with family members and/or other supportive individuals. Clinical evidence points to an association between one's readiness for change and both short- and long-term outcomes of improved health status. Patients with eating disorders often experience marked fluctuations in their motivation to address the signs and symptoms of illness; thus, a crucial element in their care is that trainees avoid a "mismatch" between treatment goals and patient readiness for change.

Effectively treating eating disorders takes time, and establishing a sound therapeutic relationship is crucial to building trust. From the first moment of contact with a patient with an eating disorder, MI skills guide accurate assessment of your patient's readiness for change and complement other treatment modalities such as food diaries and cognitive-behavioral therapies. MI may also be beneficial for reducing the anxiety and emotional distress family members experience when caring for someone with an eating disorder.

Consider screening most, if not all, patients for eating disorders, particularly girls and women between 10 and 30 years of age; recall that overall, women are three times more likely to develop anorexia or bulimia nervosa than their male counterparts. In the spirit of MI, use the OARS skills to assess your patient's present behaviors; from here, begin to formulate a personalized approach to your care, remembering that reinforcing each patient's autonomy is critical, not solely to long-term behavior change, but for recovery itself.

Open-ended questions/statements:

- "How do you feel about your weight? Do you think you're too thin, too fat, or just right? How do you see yourself?" (Open-closed-open sandwich)
- "Describe for me what would happen if you gained weight."
- "What might you feel if you were to gain/lose 5 pounds?"
- "What is it like for you to eat around other people?"
- "Which part of your body would you change if you could?"
- "What are your exercise goals?"
- "What is it like for you when you feel you can't stop eating or control what you're eating?"
- "What is it like when you weigh yourself and how does this make you feel?"
- "In what circumstances do you take laxatives or diuretics to control your weight and how does this make you feel?"
- "What are your thoughts about your eating habits/restricting?"
- "Help me understand the downside of your eating habits."
- "What is it like when you gain/lose weight?"
- "Tell me how your eating habits differ from those of your friends."
- "How do your eating habits differ from those of your friends?"
- "Tell me about your expectations regarding your appearance and weight."
- "What needs to happen in order for you to change your eating habits?"

Affirmations:

- "You are a very resilient person to have dealt with these feelings for so long and not fallen apart."
- "You've worked hard to increase the protein in your diet and exercise more often, despite how challenging this has been."
- "You're courageous in your decision to seek treatment, knowing that it's hard for you to discuss your struggles with your eating habits."
- "You've been feeling more confident about following an exercise program and you feel good about that accomplishment."

Reflections:

- "Restricting what you eat helps you feel more in control of your life."
- "You worry what other people will think if you're overweight."
- "Your eating behaviors never cause any difficulties for you."
- "You feel that your family doesn't understand and just wants to see you eat the way they think is right."
- "You're afraid of the effect intensive treatment might have on your social life."

- "You feel more beautiful when you're losing weight, and at the same time, it makes it impossible for you to enjoy activities with your friends that include food."
- "On one hand, eating comforts you when you're upset, and on the other hand, you often feel more upset after overeating."
- "You feel uncertain that you can overcome your illness, and at the same time you realize that you've already made many positive changes."

Summaries:

- "Before we begin looking at your ideas about incorporating exercise on a regular basis, would it be ok for me to review my understanding of what we've discussed so far today?" (Requesting permission to summarize)
- "You know that you're a strong person. You've decided to follow a routine exercise program and you feel confident that you can stick to it while watching your diet. Your ultimate goal is to maintain your weight, feel healthier, and be more active with your grandchildren. You've also decided to discuss your smoking with your primary care physician and you're willing to review options that would help you quit, permanently. What else are you thinking about changing?"
- "You feel satisfied about having gained some weight and being able to think more clearly. You see a connection between your depression and your struggles with your weight. Now, you've decided to work on your depression and continue to stay on track with gaining weight to reach a normal BMI."

Many patients with eating disorders present in pediatric or adolescent medicine settings, where being attentive to an age-appropriate communication style is essential. This includes drawing attention to the importance of confidentiality, particularly under circumstances in which parents/family members are asked to leave the exam room, as with older adolescents. Another challenge is the need to collect additional data from family members even as you build a therapeutic alliance with your patient. We suggest interviewing parents/family members in the patient's presence; this promotes trust, while reducing any implication of secrecy.

If time does not permit a joint interview at your first meeting, plan to meet with both parties as soon as possible. Addressing maladaptive patterns of communication within families is an indispensable part of treating eating disorders, and helping family members acquire some MI skills may well be included in your treatment plan. Patients should be encouraged to discuss their illness with trusted family members, especially those whose support will be required in the weeks and months ahead.

The following dialogue illustrates how the spirit of MI informs all aspects of this clinical encounter, including OARS skills and other strategies:

TRAINEE: You're concerned about gaining weight, and you've been making yourself throw up once a day. You exercise on a daily basis, running about three miles. You're 5 feet, 8 inches tall, and you weigh 125 pounds. What else is important for you to tell me so I can better understand your situation? (Collecting summary followed by open-ended question)

PATIENT: Well, I'd like to weigh 110 pounds; I think that would be a good weight for me. I'm trying hard to lose another 15 pounds.

TRAINEE: You believe you need to lose more weight; you're not satisfied with where your weight is now. (Complex reflection)

PATIENT: Yes, I thought I'd be OK at 125 pounds, but when I look in the mirror I still look fat, especially my legs, so I think I just need to lose a bit more.

TRAINEE: When you lost weight in order to meet a previous goal, it didn't feel satisfying. What do your parents think about your weight and weight-related behaviors? (Complex reflection followed by open-ended question)

PATIENT: My father thinks I look nice and always says it's good to stay in shape. But he doesn't know what I'm doing, and I really don't want him to find out. You won't tell him, will you?

TRAINEE: Our conversations are confidential—unless you ask me to share certain details with your parents or I become concerned that some of your behaviors may put your life in danger. I don't think that's happening right now. What are your thoughts about discussing your weight with your parents? (Emphasizing autonomy and confidentiality, followed by open-ended question)

PATIENT: My mother doesn't care. She always pays more attention to my younger sister and doesn't say much to me. And, really, most of my friends think I look good. A couple of them tell me they think I have an eating disorder ... but they're girls who don't care about how they look, so I don't really pay attention to what they think.

TRAINEE: You feel strongly that your mother isn't there for you. On one hand, some of your friends have expressed concern about your eating habits, and on the other hand, you don't see any problems with your eating. (Summary)

PATIENT: Well, I know I do some things that are like an eating disorder, but I'm not out of control. I mean, I don't binge on food for hours, so I don't have to make myself throw up too much—usually just after dinner because that's when I eat the most. And I think it's good to exercise. All the doctors on TV are always saying we need more exercise.

TRAINEE: You feel you're able to control your behaviors and you believe that what you're doing is the right thing to stay healthy. (Complex reflection emphasizing autonomy)

PATIENT: Yeah, that's right. I still don't think I should stop exercising. I feel OK and I think if I stop throwing up or exercising I'll gain weight, and I sure don't want to get fat!

TRAINEE: You don't see any reason at this time to make changes in your eating behaviors or exercising. I'm wondering how you would feel about asking your parents to join us for a session to discuss your relationship with them and your expectations from them? (Complex reflection, followed by open-ended question with a suggestion)

PATIENT: I guess it won't hurt to talk to them.

TRAINEE: I appreciate your willingness to have the family meeting, and I'll set it up very soon. (Affirmation)

Notice the gentle pacing of this encounter and the care with which the trainee clarifies her understanding of the patient's statements. A spirit of nonjudgmental collaboration and support for patient autonomy underpin the beginnings of a therapeutic relationship; establishing a safe, nonthreatening environment is a key element that fosters open, honest communication. The patient is relatively (but not completely) content with her approach to eating and clearly states that she has no interest in changing any of her behaviors. The patient's agreeing to attend a joint session with her parents should not be understood as a signal to rush headlong into an aggressive treatment plan; to do so would be to succumb to the righting reflex and its temptation to "fix too much too soon." Remember that creating discord, particularly in the early stages of a patient–trainee relationship, will likely promote ongoing sustain talk and lessen the possibility of behavior change.

SUBSTANCE USE IN PREGNANCY

As in all clinical settings, MI has the potential to improve relationships between pregnant women and their physicians regardless of context. On its own, MI has not been successful in significantly reducing either smoking or drug use during pregnancy, as compared to standard treatments; however, MI may increase a pregnant woman's readiness to stop smoking and thus improve smoking cessation efforts. With regard to alcohol use, MI has been shown to reduce heavy alcohol consumption among pregnant women, in addition to helping women who drink and who do not wish to become pregnant to use contraception more effectively.

The following clinical encounter demonstrates how MI might be used to help a pregnant woman struggling to quit smoking:

TRAINEE: You've said that you want to be a good mother and that you know it's bad for your baby when you smoke. (Summary)

PATIENT: Yes, I've read about how smoking affects my baby's development, reduces birth weight, and sometimes, babies of moms who smoke aren't as healthy as other babies. But I can't stop! I've tried, but I really need to smoke. (Crying) I can't take all this stress … I don't know what to do.

TRAINEE: You've shared a lot about wanting to do the best for your baby and you've made many efforts to quit. You would try again if you thought you could quit successfully. Right now, you're terribly frustrated that you haven't been able to stop smoking. (Affirmations, complex reflections)

PATIENT: Absolutely, I feel so angry about it; I just don't know how to do it.

TRAINEE: Tell me what you like about smoking. (Open-ended question)

PATIENT: It makes me feel good. It relaxes me. When I haven't smoked for a while, I get a weird sensation in the back of my throat and then the thought comes to me that I just need a feeling of smoke to stop feeling worried or stressed out.

TRAINEE: Smoking makes you feel more relaxed and takes away an uncomfortable feeling. What else? (Complex reflection followed by an open-ended question)

PATIENT: Well, I usually smoke with a latté; it just seems to taste better with a cigarette. I really like that.

TRAINEE: You like the taste of coffee when you smoke and the two go hand in hand. It's hard to imagine having coffee or a latté without a cigarette. What else do you like? (Summary and complex reflection followed by open-ended question)

PATIENT: Well, I seem to smoke more when I'm sitting around with friends. I like doing it when we're chatting, catching up on news, all that stuff.

TRAINEE: You enjoy socializing more when you smoke. What else can you think of? (Complex reflection followed by open-ended question)

PATIENT: Well, I used to think it looked cool when I smoked. I think a lot of girls get into that as teenagers, you know those glamorous images from the movies. But that really isn't important to me anymore.

TRAINEE: So ... the way you looked or felt was important when you were younger, but this doesn't mean as much to you anymore, especially when you think about how smoking could hurt both you and your baby; and now, you feel it's time to quit. (Complex reflection)

PATIENT: Yes, I know that I've got to do it. I don't think I could stand what might happen to my baby because of my smoking.

TRAINEE: Your concern about the impact of smoking on your baby's health is your main reason to quit. (Complex reflection)

PATIENT: Well, right now, like I said, I don't want it to hurt my baby. I'm really worried about it.

TRAINEE: The problems you and your baby might have because of smoking outweigh the pleasure you get out of smoking. What other reasons do you have for quitting? (Complex reflection followed by open-ended question)

PATIENT: Well, it sure costs a lot of money, even when I buy the cheapest ones I can find. It's really beginning to add up.

TRAINEE: You spend more on cigarettes than you want to, and you can think of plenty of other things to spend that money on. About how much would you say you spend on cigarettes every month? (Complex reflection followed by an open-ended question)

PATIENT: Oh God, it's scary ... I try not to think about it. I smoke ... say, 15–20 cigarettes a day and they cost $7.00 a pack, so ... probably at least $200 a month. Wow ... that's a lot of money. That would certainly help when the baby comes along.

TRAINEE: You've thought about the amount of money you spend on cigarettes, and it doesn't make sense to you to spend that much, especially when you consider the costs to your baby's health. What else concerns you? (Complex reflection followed by open-ended question)

PATIENT: I know it's hurting me, too. I mean, besides the risk of cancer, I have a bad cough most of the time, especially first thing in the morning. It's gross. And it seems I can't walk very far without needing to rest. Last week, I went shopping with my mom and I had to stop every few minutes just walking through the mall, simply to catch my breath.

TRAINEE: So, you cough up a lot of phlegm most mornings and you've noticed some physical limitations because of shortness of breath. What other concerns do you have? (Complex reflection followed by open-ended question)

PATIENT: Well, I hate the way my house smells. It doesn't bother me quite so much anymore, but you know, I don't seem to have much of a sense of smell. But someone told me it's from smoking. Is that really true?

TRAINEE: It's not uncommon for smokers to have a reduced sense of smell; it happens very gradually and many people don't notice. What else are you worried about? (Giving information, open-ended question)

PATIENT: Well ... I argue with people who tell me I should stop. Not everyone gets on my case, but I have only three friends who smoke—they're the ones I visit with—and we drink coffee and talk and smoke together. But my mother—she's the one who tells me that my house stinks, my hair and clothes stink, and that I should stop, at least for the baby. Another friend in the neighborhood won't even come to my house anymore because of "secondhand smoke." She says she's fine going out together, but when I light up a cigarette, she goes somewhere else until I finish it—she doesn't want to be around it. She and I used to be really close . . . but not so much anymore. I miss not seeing her as much as I used to, before she decided to stay away because of my smoking.

TRAINEE: Let me see if I've understood everything you've shared with me: you have a few reasons why you like smoking—it helps you relax, it tastes good with coffee, and it's part of socializing with three of your friends. At the same time, you have a number of reasons why you believe you should quit: the health of your baby, the money it would save you, the smell that pervades your house, the support of your close friend whose company you miss, the support and approval of your mom, and perhaps most important, your idea of what it means to be a good mother. (Summary as a double-sided reflection, ending on the side of change)

PATIENT: Yes, I guess that's right. I never thought about it like that before. And the things we just talked about are really important for both me and my baby. I really need to stop.

TRAINEE: You value being a good mother, and you're concerned about the effects smoking could have on your baby. In the past, you've tried hard to quit. Tell me what it's been like for you when you've tried to give up cigarettes. (Summary followed by open-ended question)

PATIENT: I tried both the patch and the gum, but I didn't stay with them.

TRAINEE: You struggled with taking them as prescribed. How do you feel about considering counseling and perhaps medication to help you quit? You're the best judge of what will work for you. (Complex reflection followed by open-ended question and autonomy statement)

PATIENT: That would be great. I'm willing to do whatever it takes to quit. The nurse told me I might not be able to use the gum or patch since I'm pregnant. Is that true?

TRAINEE: Not necessarily. Studies show that people who want to quit smoking and who attend counseling, in combination with using either the patch or the gum, are twice as likely to quit, compared with people who try only one method or the other; this is quite a significant improvement. Since you're pregnant, you might want to start with a counseling program and should you decide to explore further, you could discuss nicotine replacement therapy, or possibly a medication option, with your obstetrician. Recent studies show that, depending on the stage of pregnancy, it's safer to take medication than to smoke. How does this information fit into your desire to stop smoking? (Providing information followed by open-ended question)

PATIENT: Right now, smoking prevents me from being as good a mother as I'd like to be. I feel that smoking has begun to control my life, and I want to be free of it.

TRAINEE: We have a smoking cessation program in our clinic. Many of my patients have benefitted from it: They felt more confident about quitting, once and for all. How do you feel about considering being involved in the program? (Providing information followed by open-ended question)

PATIENT: Good, why not. Could you give me some of the details?

In this scenario, the patient expresses considerable ambivalence about smoking cigarettes, describes past failures to quit, hints at a low sense of confidence in her ability to stop smoking, and describes some of the stigma experienced by pregnant women who smoke. Instead of emphasizing the many adverse effects cigarettes impose on both mother and child, the trainee takes time to elicit the high value this patient places on being a good parent; this is followed up by using a decisional balance technique of reviewing the pros and cons of smoking in order to help the patient resolve her ambivalence about trying, again, to quit. The desire to quit is affirmed, and it is linked to the desire to be as good a mother as is possible.

Note how the decisional balance technique is introduced by asking the patient what she likes about smoking, before moving on to consider the negative aspects of the behavior. This order is important; typically, patients are more likely to remember, and be motivated by, whatever is discussed *last* in the balance exercise. This strategy also allows the trainee to frame the adverse effects of smoking as potentially motivating factors to quit. The difference is subtle, but contrasting the positive aspects of smoking—as something one likes but does not *have* to do—against various factors representing the benefits of quitting, shifts one's focus onto the significance of the reasons to stop smoking.

This movement elicits change talk from the patient; the trainee responds by summarizing and introducing possible options to help this patient stop smoking. With permission, information concerning the effectiveness of smoking cessation programs is offered and the positive experiences of previous patients are used to illustrate the benefits of these programs. In this scenario, the patient welcomes these recommendations; often, however, patients need more time to resolve ambivalence. Remember that the decision to commit to changing one's behavior always rests with the patient; our role is to support and guide the patient along the way.

PALLIATIVE CARE

MI's emphasis on active, empathic listening complements care to both patients and families in palliative settings. Empathy helps us accurately reflect the full range of what patients express, whether it be ambivalence, fear, hope, or any other human experience. The major challenge with implementing MI into palliative care is that the ambivalence at the core of the intervention is associated with decision-making related to the end of one's life, just as most patients are grappling with the concept of self-determination in an unfamiliar and difficult way.

Among other populations, the therapeutic conversations of MI focus on identifying and resolving issues of ambivalence regarding changes in behavior that contribute to positive health outcomes. Patients have the choice whether to implement change, and our place is to guide, not to judge. In a palliative setting, however, patients know that the end of life is approaching and this unavoidable reality sheds new light on the context in which change is considered and brought about.

Patients in the process of dying may be reluctant to discuss any aspect of choice with regard to the end-of-life care they receive, but wherever possible, they should be invited to express their thoughts and concerns. As with all patients, those approaching death must be allowed time to consider whatever changes, large or small, they would like to implement. Given the circumstances, this may seem counterintuitive; recall that the *process* of deciding to bring about change is more important than the decision itself. We sometimes feel the need to hasten the decision-making process, either by confronting our patients and/or their families or by assuming responsibility for decisions that are not ours to make. As one might expect, these actions create discord in therapeutic relationships, which in turn, affects the quality of care we provide.

Another potential source of conflict occurs when we disagree with a patient's or family's decision(s) regarding end-of-life care. In these situations, we must strive to counsel from a position of neutrality. Fundamental differences of opinion regarding value systems, moral judgments, and locus of control are bound to occur, and we are obliged to control any sense of disappointment, disapproval, or frustration. Miller and Rollnick (2013) uses the term "equipoise" (see Chapter 7) to describe counseling sessions in which we consciously and deliberately explore both the pros and cons of a given behavior, taking care to balance the attention we devote to both sides of the discussion, and to avoid steering our patient toward one choice over another. In these instances, making use of the decisional balance tool discussed earlier is a helpful strategy that places responsibility for decision-making right where it belongs: with our patient.

MI enhances palliative care in a variety of ways, such as helping patients decide which treatments to accept, resolving ambivalence regarding amount and type of pain relief, making the decision to move into a hospice or remain at home, or articulating what an individual wishes to experience or accomplish prior to death.

Following are two versions of a clinical consultation with a patient experiencing end-stage lung cancer who is ambivalent about modifying pain regimens. Although he has severe bone pain, he is concerned that increasing narcotic use will affect his ability to remain alert during family visits, particularly those with his grandchildren.

First Scenario

TRAINEE: I see you're in a lot of discomfort; you feel the medications you're on are not helping. We really need to adjust the doses or perhaps add some new ones. (Appears attentive to patient's experience but takes a directing approach.)

PATIENT: Yes, I'm in a lot of pain, but I don't want to feel like a zombie. I'm not sure I want to take bigger doses and more meds.

TRAINEE: But you're suffering, and we have to do something about it. The only way to help your pain is to increase your dose of painkillers. (Directing, advising without permission)

PATIENT: I know if I take a bigger dose, I'm going to feel groggy; I won't be able to enjoy my grandkids and that would kill me.

TRAINEE: Well, I don't think there's any other way to relieve your pain other than to increase the medication. (Subtly argumentative, also directing)

PATIENT: I'd rather put up with the pain and deal with it for the time being without taking a bigger dose of medication. I want to enjoy the grandchildren for as long as I can.

Second Scenario

TRAINEE: I see you're in a lot of discomfort; it looks like the medications you're on are not helping. How do you feel about brainstorming some options to address your pain? (Summary followed by open-ended question)

PATIENT: Yes, I'd like to talk about it … I'm in a lot of pain, but I don't want to feel like a zombie. I'm not sure I want to take bigger doses and more meds.

TRAINEE: You're concerned about possible medication changes, and you want to make sure you're alert and able to function as normally as possible. (Complex reflection)

PATIENT: You bet! I want to make sure that when my grandchildren come to visit, I'm fully awake and able to enjoy them; they're great kids and I really don't want them to see me zoned out.

TRAINEE: Being able to interact with your grandchildren brings a lot of joy into your life, and you're worried that a change in medication might interfere with it. (Complex reflection)

PATIENT: Well, if we could work together on finding a good medication plan that would help ease the pain without making me groggy, I'd consider it.

TRAINEE: I appreciate your willingness to discuss possible options. Are you OK with us taking some time to review all your meds, with the goal of finding out how you could be more comfortable without becoming too drowsy? (Affirmation followed by a request for permission)

PATIENT: That sounds great. Thanks a lot.

In the first scenario, the trainee is unable (or unwilling) to either collaborate with the patient or listen to the patient's concerns; instead, he or she barges ahead with plans to change the medication orders. When confronted with an unreasonable either/or decision, the patient declines any change, and in effect, chooses to experience unnecessarily high levels of pain rather than risk not enjoying visits with beloved grandchildren.

In the second scenario, MI skills abound in a collaborative, patient-centered interaction. The patient's concerns about overmedication are acknowledged and validated, as is patient autonomy. By responding tactfully and sensitively, the trainee nurtures patient engagement and encourages a trusting, therapeutic relationship. This does not mean that the patient's pain will be controlled as precisely as one would hope; but it does mean that this patient is participating in his care to the fullest extent possible.

PSYCHIATRIC DISORDERS

The use of MI in mental health settings is becoming more common, as either a preamble or an adjunct to the treatment of a wide range of psychiatric disorders, including anxiety disorders, eating disorders, suicidal behaviors, depression, psychotic disorders, and co-occurring psychiatric and substance use disorders. A major problem in this field of care is the ambivalence many patients feel about seeking help, complying with treatment programs, and changing unhealthy behaviors. As we know, resolving ambivalence is a primary goal of MI, which makes it particularly well suited for this group of patients.

To date, most studies concerning MI recommend that it be incorporated into existing therapies in order to promote patient engagement with treatment and thus improve clinical outcomes. One of the major challenges in applying MI within psychiatric settings is the complex presentation of target behaviors, which in many cases, are observed in a variety of psychiatric disorders. For example, among depressed patients, the goals of treatment concern not only behavioral changes, such as reducing social withdrawal or disruptions in sleep/eating habits, but also less well-defined targets such as feelings of guilt and shame, obsessive thinking patterns, and a profound sense of worthlessness. This scenario is further complicated by the dynamic nature of these targets, which may require modification over the course of therapy.

MI may have a synergistic effect when combined with other treatment modalities such as cognitive-behavioral therapy (CBT). In the case of depression, MI personalizes what is referred to as manualized CBT—that is, direct, short-term treatment interventions—by promoting the therapeutic alliance, enhancing patients' engagement with treatment, reducing discord, and effecting specific changes in the behaviors associated with depression. The MI/CBT combination also facilitates adherence to therapeutic tasks, such as homework assignments, among patients struggling with significant anxiety.

Patients with generalized anxiety disorder (GAD) report that MI creates a safe and supportive atmosphere, increases mindfulness and awareness of themselves, improves motivation for treatment, and reduces symptoms specific to GAD. Similarly, integrating MI into the care of patients with obsessive-compulsive disorder (OCD) has the potential to increase and sustain patient engagement with a treatment regimen. Typically, this consists of what is known as "exposure and ritual prevention therapy," which is designed to help patients confront their fears and reduce/eliminate maladaptive responses.

Another potential application of MI is as a brief intervention for suicidal ideation, followed by CBT. Making use of a decisional balance strategy by eliciting reasons for suicide and reasons to live may promote the exploration and development of a personalized plan to make life worth living; even a brief, single session has the capacity to enhance a patient's engagement in treatment. MI adaptations have also been developed to better suit patients with cognitive deficits, such as speed of processing, ability to reason and problem solve, and diminished verbal comprehension, that often accompany psychotic disorders. These adaptations include increased flexibility in the structure and duration of MI sessions.

KEY POINT

MI and CBT are synergistic modalities that can be used in conjunction.

The following excerpt occurred during an initial interview with a depressed patient who presented to the emergency department reporting suicidal thoughts:

TRAINEE: What made you decide to seek treatment now? (Open-ended question)

PATIENT: I can't keep going anymore … I know I'm severely depressed.

TRAINEE: What does this feel like for you? (Open-ended question)

PATIENT: I've just about had it; everything is too much for me. Even getting here took way more energy than I've got. I'm exhausted.

TRAINEE: You feel overwhelmed, and very, very tired, even with things that you used to be able to manage. (Complex reflection)

PATIENT: Totally overwhelmed. First I lost my job, then my wife left me. Now she won't let me see the kids unless I get treatment for my depression.

TRAINEE: You've suffered a lot because of your depression. I'm wondering if you've been feeling depressed to the point of having thoughts of suicide. (Complex reflection followed by an invitation to share)

PATIENT: Sure, I think about ending it, all the time … but I'm not sure whether I want to follow through with it. It would really hurt my kids … maybe even ruin them.

TRAINEE: You care very much about your children. You realize that if you followed through with your suicidal thoughts, it might destroy them. (Complex reflections)

PATIENT: Yeah, but my life feels so out of control. I'm hurting so much … I miss my kids a lot … I need to be there for them, but I can't.

TRAINEE: You feel so horrible that sometimes you want to end your life. At the same time, you think about your kids and you want to be part of their lives, to support them as they grow up. They're really important to you, as you are to them. (Complex reflection)

PATIENT: My gut feeling is that killing myself is a cop-out. I need to get back into treatment, back on my medications. I stopped taking them a year ago after I started feeling good.

TRAINEE: You're willing to take responsibility for your life. You're willing to start the process by resuming treatment for your depression. (Summary)

PATIENT: I don't really want to get back on medications, but I know that if I do, and if I get back into therapy, I'll start getting my depression under control … and maybe start rebuilding my life. I've done it before.

TRAINEE: You've lived through similar experiences in the past, and you've learned about what helps and what doesn't help. Would it be OK if we talk about some of the resources that are available for you? (Complex reflection, support for autonomy, request for permission to share information)

PATIENT: Sure, go ahead. I guess the least I can do is listen.

The spirit of MI is evident throughout this encounter, particularly in the care taken to gently encourage the patient to openly discuss his depression, sense of hopelessness, suicidal thoughts, and the adverse effect these experiences are having on his quality of life. Notice how the trainee elicits and validates the high value this patient places on his children and their relationship. Secondly, note how the patient's ambivalence about following through with suicide is acknowledged and explored. We sometimes feel apprehensive about addressing suicidal ideation, as though talking about it openly may make it a reality. Most trainees have experienced similar feelings. Observe how trusted colleagues and consultants deal with the issue of suicidal statements and ask for guidance. Finally, note how the trainee elicits this patient's personal motivations for change and supports both his autonomy and his ability to bring about meaningful behavior change in his pursuit of improved mental health.

SUBSTANCE USE DISORDERS

MI is at least as effective as more intensive treatments for a number of substance use disorders. Among patients with these problems, MI is typically included as part of brief interventions, over a course of one to four sessions, with a considerably higher cost-effectiveness than alternative treatments. Not surprisingly, greater changes in behavior have been observed with four sessions, as compared to one. MI appears to be particularly effective when practitioners and patients are not matched on the basis of racial, ethnic, or cultural characteristics, and it has demonstrated positive results in diverse clinical settings, regardless of patients' age, gender, or severity of the substance use disorder.

MI is especially effective with challenging patients, such as those who are angry or withdrawn. One adaptation of MI is known as motivational enhancement therapy (MET), which includes specific evaluation of a patient's substance use and personalized risk feedback; treatment is designed to occur over four sessions. Adding or integrating MI in the treatment of patients with co-occurring psychosis and substance use disorders has the potential to enhance engagement in treatment, reduce substance use, and increase medication adherence.

KEY POINT

Motivational Enhancement Therapy (MET) – a four-session adaptation of MI with normative, personalized feedback

---

The following excerpt comes from a clinical encounter with a young adult who presented intoxicated with alcohol. Accompanied by the police, he was aggressive and uncooperative, and was admitted on an involuntary commitment order; after sleeping for lengthy periods, he was awakened for the session that follows. After initially refusing to attend, he agreed to join our team for a session.

TRAINEE: Thank you for coming to meet with us. What's your understanding of why you're in the hospital? (Open-ended question)

PATIENT: I'm here because I got to a break point, I called 911, and they brought me here.

TRAINEE: You got to a breaking point when you felt you needed help. What was going on for you? (Complex reflection followed by an open-ended question)

PATIENT: I was angry, man! Really angry.

TRAINEE: You were angry, and you felt so angry it got to a breaking point. What was that like for you? (Simple reflection and open-ended statement)

PATIENT: Yeah ... I thought I was going to do something violent.

TRAINEE: You felt so angry that you were out of control. You thought you might do something you would regret if you didn't get help. What were you angry about? (Complex reflection followed by open-ended question)

PATIENT: My situation. I'm homeless.

TRAINEE: You were feeling angry about being homeless. How did you become homeless? (Complex reflection followed by open-ended question)

PATIENT: I lost my job in February and couldn't pay my rent. By April, they kicked me out and I've been on the streets ever since.

TRAINEE: You've been dealing with being homeless for a while, and it makes you angry. You were afraid you'd become violent and do something you would regret. (Summary)

PATIENT: Well, not really afraid. Probably nothing would've happened, and I could have just gone to a friend's.

TRAINEE: You're not sure you would have gotten violent, and at the same time, you were feeling so angry that it was overwhelming and you felt out of control. So you decided to call 911. (Complex reflections)

PATIENT: Yup.

TRAINEE: Then what happened? (Open-ended question)

PATIENT: I came here ... with a bit of help.

TRAINEE: How do you feel about being here now? (Open-ended question)

PATIENT: I think I made a mistake. I have to go to court Thursday and Friday for my hearings and if I don't make it I'll have to go back to jail. I don't want to go jail, and that's what will happen if I miss the hearings.

TRAINEE: You feel like it was a mistake to come here because you're concerned you'll miss your hearings. (Simple reflection)

PATIENT: Yeah, and I can't go back to jail.

TRAINEE: And it's really important for you to go to court because you don't want to end up in jail again. (Complex reflection)

PATIENT: Well, would you want to?

TRAINEE: That's a big consequence for you, or anyone, and it's really important that it doesn't happen. (Complex reflection)

PATIENT: Right.

TRAINEE: And you're wondering if you made the right decision coming here and at the same time, last night you felt so angry that it became overwhelming and out of control, and you felt you needed to call for help. (Summary)

PATIENT: Yeah, well, I never would have called if I wasn't drinking. I would have gone to a friend's house and probably nothing would have happened.

TRAINEE: You were drinking and you think that made you lose control and prompted your call. How long had you been drinking? (Complex reflection followed by close-ended question)

PATIENT: A few hours.

TRAINEE: What else was going on yesterday? (Open-ended question)

PATIENT: Nothing, I spent some time with some friends.

TRAINEE: You've been homeless since April ... what happened that made your anger reach a breaking point last night? (Complex reflection followed by an open-ended question)

PATIENT: I was just getting angry about my situation.

TRAINEE: Your situation. (Simple reflection)

PATIENT: I just keep getting turned out of places and don't have so many options.

TRAINEE: And you've been angry ... at your situation, at the people who have been turning you out. (Complex reflection)

PATIENT: Yeah, and that I got into this situation.

TRAINEE: And a little angry at yourself, for getting into this situation. (Complex reflection)

PATIENT: Yeah.

TRAINEE: What happened that made you homeless most recently? (Open-ended question)

PATIENT: Some so-called friends said I could stay with them, and then they changed their minds and kicked me out.

TRAINEE: You had some friends offer to help you out, and they betrayed your trust. (Complex reflection)

PATIENT: Yeah, betrayed ... they just kicked me out.

TRAINEE: How did you initially become homeless? (Open-ended question)

PATIENT: I was renting a place, and I asked a friend to give my rent money to my landlord for me one time, and she just pocketed it instead.

TRAINEE: So you trusted your friend to help you, and instead she betrayed you. How did that make you feel? (Complex reflection followed by open-ended question)

PATIENT: Angry! And hurt.

TRAINEE: You felt angry at your friend, at your situation, at yourself for trusting her because she hurt you. (Summary)

PATIENT: Wouldn't you be?

TRAINEE: Well, it hurt that she violated your trust … I think anyone would be hurt and angry about that. (Complex reflection)

PATIENT: Yeah, for sure. That's why I can't trust anyone.

TRAINEE: You feel you can't trust anyone because you've had that trust violated so many times before. (Complex reflection)

PATIENT: Yeah.

TRAINEE: You were also feeling angry about what happened … how do you usually handle things when you're feeling that angry? (Complex reflection followed by open-ended question)

PATIENT: It just rolls off.

TRAINEE: Sometimes it just rolls off. And at the same time, from what you're saying, sometimes it builds up until it gets overwhelming, like last night. What's the difference between anger that rolls off and anger that gets overwhelming? (Complex reflections followed by an open-ended question)

PATIENT: Well, a lot of times it's something little and it'll just roll off. But the big things that don't go away kind of build up.

TRAINEE: So more recently, the big things—being homeless, and feeling like you can't trust anyone—didn't go away, and your anger kept building up. I know you said you wouldn't have called for help last night if you hadn't been drinking. (Summary)

PATIENT: Yeah.

TRAINEE: And at the same time all this anger was building up. How do you think the alcohol played a role in your calling for help? (Complex reflection followed by open-ended question)

PATIENT: Alcohol makes me think about my situation, and my anger more … it makes me focus on it.

TRAINEE: When you're drinking, you focus more on how you're feeling. (Complex reflection)

PATIENT: After I'm done drinking I do.

TRAINEE: After you stop drinking you start to focus on your feelings, and that makes them more intense, more overwhelming. (Complex reflection)

PATIENT: Yeah.

TRAINEE: What's it like when you're drinking? (Open-ended question)

PATIENT: While I'm drinking, I feel happy, feel good. Then when I lay down for the night and I'm still drunk, I start thinking about my situation.

TRAINEE: And then you feel worse. So when you're drinking, it's like an escape from how you feel about being homeless, and then after you're done you feel even worse than when you started. (Complex reflections)

PATIENT: Yeah.

TRAINEE: So you've been struggling with being homeless, feeling like you can't trust anyone who offers help, feeling hurt by others, and feeling angry about your situation and at yourself for being in the situation. And that makes you want to drink to get away from it. And when you drink, you end up feeling even more angry and sad afterward. (Summary)

PATIENT: Yeah, when I focus on it, I feel worse.

TRAINEE: I understand that you wish you hadn't come here—what do you think would happen if you left now? (Complex reflection followed by open-ended question)

PATIENT: I'll be fine if I don't drink.

TRAINEE: If you don't drink, you feel you could manage. How does drinking get in the way? (Complex reflection followed by an open-ended question)

PATIENT: Well, it makes me end up here, and then I miss my hearings … and go back to jail.

TRAINEE: Drinking makes your emotions feel out of control and then you need to get help, which gets in the way of the rest of your life. How else? (Complex reflection followed by open-ended question)

PATIENT: I run out of money, and then it's hard to get an apartment and get to meetings and everything.

TRAINEE: Drinking keeps you from getting to meetings and making steps that would help you get housing, which is a major goal for you. How confident are you that you can stop drinking? (Complex reflection followed by open-ended question)

PATIENT: I'm confident.

TRAINEE: What makes you confident? (Open-ended question)

PATIENT: I know myself, and when I set my mind to something, I do it.

TRAINEE: You're the kind of person that follows through when you set your mind to something. (Affirmation)

PATIENT: Yeah, and especially when there's something important motivating me, like I need to get to those hearings. I can't go back to jail.

TRAINEE: When you have important things in mind that you know drinking interferes with, you feel more able to keep from drinking. Like making it to your court date, getting money, and getting to appointments for housing. (Complex reflection)

PATIENT: Right.

TRAINEE: What can we work on together while you're here to help you be able to reach those goals? (Open-ended question reflecting collaboration)

PATIENT: I just need to do it.

TRAINEE: Okay, we'll be working with you during your stay in the hospital to help you get some resources in place so you can be able to stay sober and get more stable housing.

This therapeutic encounter emphasized the importance of meeting the patient where he is and engaging him to better understand his perspective on his use of alcohol and its connection to his struggles. The spirit of MI was maintained consistently throughout the session and the use of OARS skills facilitated the patient's ability to open up and to start engaging in treatment.

CULTURAL FACTORS AND MOTIVATIONAL INTERVIEWING

In our increasingly diverse societies, we inevitably encounter people whose backgrounds differ from our own, and cross-cultural miscommunications are a fact of life for many trainees. Our own experiences have taught us the need to recognize that each party within a therapeutic relationship—patient, family member, trainee—identifies with at least one cultural group. As we know, one's culture may be defined in a number of ways: nationality, language spoken in the home, gender, marital status, age, income level, profession, special interests and hobbies, and so forth. Keeping this short list of cultures and subcultures in mind before we begin our interviews helps us avoid pigeonholing patients within one group or another, instead of seeing them as the individuals that they are.

Avoid making assumptions about your patients' beliefs and behaviors. Stereotyping, that is, attributing preconceived and oversimplified qualities or characteristics to a patient, serves only to limit our ability to approach him or her with openness and honesty. The spirit of MI encourages us to understand each patient's frame of reference and to appreciate that all behavior occurs within a cultural context.

Language barriers pose a number of important challenges between patient and trainee, especially in terms of incorporating MI. One suggestion is to avoid using family members as interpreters, particularly when the content of a conversation involves sensitive material. In any event, address your comments to the patient him- or herself, rather than the interpreter; doing so helps maintain a patient-focused approach. Remember that nonverbal cues are culturally dependent and that what you consider to be "encouraging and supportive" eye contact may be understood as aggressive or offensive behavior.

For many first-generation, low-income immigrants, the notion of a private hospital room is unsettling, perhaps even lonely or threatening; oftentimes, the hustle and bustle of other patients and staff provides welcome distraction. For others, the thought of sharing a room with a stranger is to be avoided at all costs. Our best suggestion is to ask patients directly about their preferences.

Another cultural challenge is the clash that occurs between medical culture and our patients' views of themselves as dependent/independent individuals. Some patients are discomfited when trainees assume the collaborative approach MI advocates; this makes sense when one recalls that in some cultures, an authoritative, direct approach is understood not as paternalistic, but as confident, knowledgeable, and professional. In these situations, be especially attentive to the nuances of interpersonal communication, and wherever possible, confirm what you intuit with a patient's family and friends.

Remember that the concept of patients as "experts" regarding which health-related choices and behaviors are best for them is new and unfamiliar to many of the people we treat. Just as it takes time for us to gain competence in learning MI, so too patients, and sometimes their families, need time to recognize and accept the role they play in the therapeutic process.

PERSONAL REFLECTION

In my first year of osteopathic medical school, my classmates and I had a short human sexuality course at the beginning of our second semester. One of our assignments entailed watching a brief video clip of a patient telling a physician that she did not want to have a pelvic exam and pap smear performed. Our "job" was to be the physician and document how we would respond to that patient. We were told to discuss the scenario in small groups to brainstorm ideas.

Having received no training in MI thus far in medical school, most of my classmates immediately responded by saying they would explain the benefits of having a pelvic exam and pap smear to the patient in an attempt to persuade her to have the exam done. In our History and Physical course, we were instructed to "educate" the patient without being taught to first ask for her permission to give advice, an explicit nonadherent MI behavior. In addition, we were never trained to follow up by asking the patient what she thought of the information or how she might incorporate it into her decision-making. Despite being taught to ask open-ended questions in the History and Physical course, many of my classmates said they would ask questions such as "Have you ever had this procedure done before?" and, if so, "Did it go well in the past?" These are clearly close-ended questions that do not elicit much response from the patient. We were also instructed to listen closely to what our patients had to say; however, the concept of reflections was never mentioned. A simple reflection may be equated with "listening closely," but a complex reflection goes beyond this—a complex reflection conveys a deeper understanding of what the patient means or feels. It shows that the physician is engaging the patient in a balanced, meaningful conversation rather than passively listening in an authoritarian role.

Despite the holistic approach to the patient that is encompassed in the osteopathic principles, we were not taught the specific skills of MI that enhance the patient–physician relationship.

Having had the opportunity to learn MI before beginning medical school, my response to the assignment is as follows:

Before giving the patient any advice, I would explore the reasons as to why she does not want a pap smear and pelvic exam by asking an open-ended question such as "Help me understand your reasons for not wanting a pelvic exam and pap smear." This will allow the patient to respond in her own words and is more likely to elicit an explanation rather than prompting her with a set of closed-ended questions or trying to persuade her to agree to the exam by giving her more information about it. The patient may respond by voicing concerns related to recent sexual activity and a fear of STDs, sexual abuse, or discomfort during a prior pelvic exam. As an active listener, I would reflect on what I heard from the patient to gain a fuller understanding of her reasoning. I would then further explore the patient's reluctance by asking her to tell me more about her previous experiences (pertaining to her specific reasons). I would acknowledge any concerns, fears, or discomfort the patient may be feeling and assure her that this conversation is confidential and that she can decide whether any of this information goes into her chart. If the patient is reluctant to respond to the open-ended question, I would then proceed with more specific questions exploring her history of sexual activity, possible fear of STDs, sexual abuse, or discomfort during a prior pelvic exam as potential contributors to her refusal to have the pelvic exam.

Before giving any information, I would explore what the patient knows about the purposes and benefits of having the exam and ask the patient's permission to provide her with that information, if her knowledge about it is inaccurate or missing. If she agrees, I would then explain to her the benefits of a pelvic exam and pap smear for both preventive measures and as an early diagnostic tool. After giving the information, I would ask the patient a question such as "What are your thoughts about the information I gave you?" If the patient's reluctance was partially due to lack of knowledge, the information provided may change her decision about having the pelvic exam. If the patient still refuses, I would acknowledge her autonomy with a statement such as "You know what's best for your health." It is always the patient's choice to decide what she wants to do, and continuing to pressure her into changing her decision can evoke resistance and stifle any change talk that may have been present. Furthermore, leaving the discussion in this manner makes it likely that she will be more open and flexible during future contacts with her.

SELF-ASSESSMENT QUIZ

True or False?

1. Screening for unhealthy alcohol use is less important than screening for colorectal cancer, breast cancer, cervical cancer, and cholesterol screening.
2. According to the acronym FRAMES, "R" represents the Reasons individuals have to address or change particular behavior(s).
3. The EXPLORE study, which looked at the use of MI in screening for HIV/AIDS, demonstrated that MI is as effective as other interventions.
4. Early evidence now suggests that the use of MI among patients with chronic pain may be beneficial.
5. In general, MI is not recommended for use within palliative care settings, especially as patients confront end-of-life decisions.
6. When combined with CBT and other therapeutic interventions, MI is particularly helpful in treating depression.
7. Motivational enhancement therapy (MET) is an adaptation of MI that has been shown to be successful in treating patients with substance use disorders.

Answers

1. *False.* Unhealthy alcohol use is ranked third among the top five prevention priorities for US adults, according to recommendations by the US Preventative Services Task Force (USPSTF).
2. *False.* FRAMES is a mnemonic that guides brief interventions using MI. The elements of FRAMES are as follows: Feedback regarding personal risk or impairment; Responsibility for change rests with patients; Advice, not insistence, is offered in regard to change; Menu of options encourages patient involvement in key decisions; Empathetic approach; and encouraging and developing patient's Self-efficacy.
3. *False.* The EXPLORE study found that MI interventions reduced acquisition of HIV infection during an 18-month follow-up among a large sample of men who have sex with men, as compared to standard, twice-yearly counseling on risk reduction.
4. *True.* The Motivational Model of Pain Self-Management is a recently proposed model that suggests that the motivation to manage pain is influenced by two key factors: beliefs about the importance of engaging in pain self-management, and beliefs about one's own ability to engage in these behaviors. MI has been shown to enhance these two factors, in addition to having demonstrated improvement in patients' pain self-efficacy.
5. *False.* MI is effective in palliative care settings, particularly with regard to the usefulness of counseling with neutrality. With this goal in mind, trainees may help guide patients toward making difficult decisions, while not advocating for any particular decision.
6. *True.* The combination of MI and CBT facilitates patients' engagement with therapy, adherence to treatment plans, and the ability to follow through with homework assignments, among those with depression and anxiety disorders. Research also suggests that MI, followed by traditional CBT, is effective when applied as brief interventions among patients with suicidal ideation.
7. *True.* MET, a very successful adaptation of MI, is a four-session therapeutic intervention that includes addressing patients' substance use and strengthening motivation for change.

14 Integrating Motivational Interviewing Into Using an Electronic Medical Record and Electronic Communication

Are electronic medical records (EMRs) a necessary evil and potential pitfall—or a tool to enhance communication?

Background on Electronic Medical Records

A rudimentary electronic medical record was described in the 1960s by Lawrence Weed, MD, who saw it as an opportunity to organize problem lists, reduce medical error, and clarify medical decision making. It was not until the 1990s, however, that health systems and physicians began to use EMRs more consistently. In 1991, the Institute of Medicine published a report recommending that every physician use an EMR by 2000; however, only 18% of physicians were using an EMR at that time. As of 2011, 54% of US physicians had office-based EMR (CDC). Medicare is deploying financial incentives to healthcare practitioners who have "meaningful use" of EMR, which is accelerating EMR use. Universal EMR use is now considered inevitable. Given that we are moving toward computers in each exam room, how do we not only preserve but also enhance the patient–trainee relationship? By viewing the computer as a tool, rather than an obstacle, we can enhance our therapeutic alliance with our patients.

The advantages of EMR are many: simplified billing, improved documentation, and reduction in medical errors; additionally, it is a useful tool for implementing practice guidelines and sharing medical information between practitioners. Frequently cited disadvantages are cost, time, and the human resources needed to implement and use the EMR. We will focus here on an entirely different (potential) disadvantage—the negative impact the EMR can have on the patient–trainee relationship. Understanding how the EMR alters this relationship is crucial; as you have seen elsewhere in this book, better outcomes are strongly correlated with a positive therapeutic alliance between patient and trainee.

Electronic Medical Records and Motivational Interviewing

Numerous interpersonal pitfalls of EMRs have been described in research literature: physicians working with EMRs have been observed to focus more on detail-oriented tasks and less on exploring the psychosocial issues, including how an illness affects a patient's life. Practitioners who use EMRs in the exam room have been found to have decreased eye contact and less awareness of patients' nonverbal cues. EMR use can also disrupt a patient's narrative of illness, yielding a less nuanced and detailed history. From an MI-specific perspective, we are concerned about placing the trainee in the expert role; encouraging the question-answer trap; and turning the interaction into a trainee-, rather than patient-centered interaction.

Before discussing optimal use of EMRs in an MI-centered practice, it is worth noting that the EMR has several clear advantages in practicing MI:

1. Trainees can collect data from the EMR and use time during the visit for discussion and review as well as enhancing motivation rather than data collection with many open- and closed-ended questions in a row.
2. Easy access to data provides the ability to provide personalized feedback by sharing and graphing test results (BMI, HbA1C, blood pressure, weight, etc.)—visual/printout helps information to stick.
3. Patient and trainee can search for and discuss appropriate patient education materials (including from the Internet).
4. EMR use can facilitate shared decision-making when plans are completed in a collaborative manner.
5. EMR use can increase a patient's ownership of treatment by seeing his or her own suggestions printed out in the treatment plan.
6. EMR use can increase self-efficacy by connecting patient to online resources with the assistance of the trainee.
7. Practitioners and trainees are more likely to share charting when using EMR.
8. EMR and using a shared health portal can enhance patient–trainee relationship (depending on each patient's computer literacy/access).
9. EMR can use prompts for eliciting values related to healthcare.

Incorporating a patient health portal into an EMR has been shown to give patients a greater sense of control over their health as well as improving communication with practitioners. While there is scant research into the use of MI using electronic media, it is known that brief interventions and personalized feedback delivered via e-mail can be helpful. As individuals become increasingly reliant on electronic communication, adapting to patients' preferred methods of communication is another method for increased patient-centeredness.

Strategies for Using Electronic Medical Records in a Motivational Interviewing–Consistent Way

Several strategies can enhance the use of an EMR in an MI-consistent way. Situating the room such that the patient and medical trainee are able to see each other and the computer screen as well as participate in nonverbal communication is key. Similarly, allowing the patient to see the computer screen enhances the patient's sense of collaboration. Turning away from your patient to face the keyboard and screen while typing or looking past or over your computer screen to a patient does not facilitate rapport building. EMRs are particularly useful when patients can enter their medical history or acute health concerns and review of systems in advance of a visit (even if this is in the waiting or examining room prior to the trainee's arrival). This allows the trainee to spend more time reviewing together with the patient the data that he or she entered, using open-ended questions and reflections to delve deeper into patient's problems, as well as opportunities to give affirmations regarding patient's knowledge about his or her own history, diagnosis, and treatment options and for the past efforts in self-management.

As in all interactions, introductions set the stage for optimizing a patient's experience with the encounter. Coming into the room, making introductions, and asking patients for their preferred name and gender emphasizes that the patient is the expert on himself or herself and builds rapport. The preferred name as well as preferred gender can be added to the EMR so on all future visits the trainee and ancillary medical staff are prompted to use the preferred name as well as preferred gender; this is particularly important when providing transgender care and ensures that patients are addressed properly in a respectful way that is tailored to their identity.

When introducing the use of the EMR, it can be helpful to explain that the computer is there for more than just charting the visit; it is a tool to facilitate sharing of patient and trainee viewpoints and understanding more about the patient's concerns and to assist in forming a collaborative plan together to optimize the patient's health.

When assessing the reason for a visit, it is helpful to start with open-ended questions such as "What is the reason you are here today?" or "What made you decide to seek treatment today?" and reflect the reason(s) (especially when different from the Chief Complaint documented in the online schedule or nurse's notes). It can be helpful to reflect back any triage notes and ask for more detail with open-ended questions such as "Help me understand what happened after the last visit on November 2 when you met with Dr. Jones about your headaches." EMRs allow seamless transition between today's record, past visits, lab tests, vitals, medications, and other critical information with a single click, all of which can be looked at by the trainee and the patient together.

When the patient has already entered the history and review of systems into the EMR, the trainee can then review the entered data and use open-ended questions, as well as simple and complex reflections to further explore issues and any ambivalence regarding behavior change. Trainees can identify and give affirmations about patients knowing their own history, medications and reasons for use, family history, treatment options, and so on, as well as affirmations about self-management, focusing on one's own health, knowing one's own body, and about learning from past experiences to help figure out what will work best for oneself in the future.

When using an EMR, there are ample opportunities to integrate the E-P-E framework (see Chapter 4). Starting off by saying, "What do you know about different options for treating your symptoms?" or "What do you know about how your medication works to control your symptoms?" This can elicit a wealth of information regarding patient knowledge as well as tailor offerings of medical information so they are most salient and useful to the patient. When patients verbalize misinformation or lack information, the trainee can ask the patient, "Would it be okay if I told you more about that or about some options I know about and you can tell me what you think of that?" As long as the patient gives permission to be given information or advice, the trainee can do so and then end by asking, "So what do you think of that or how does that information or those suggestions help you?" The EMR provides a unique opportunity to ask the patient if it would be okay to look at information together online, for example, to review an up-to-date article on how to diagnose and treat lichen sclerosis or insomnia. After reviewing the information together, the trainee can elicit from the patient what he or she makes of the information and then transition to a treatment plan elicited from the patient based on the new information that the trainee and the patient found together. This interaction is extremely collaborative and embodies the true spirit of MI.

There is also a role for using the EMR to convey the trainee's findings from the physical examination portion of the visit. As the examination is conducted, the trainee can share with the patient his or her clinical findings and these can be recited aloud a second time if the trainee chooses to type the results of the examination into the EMR while the patient is in the room.

Another way to integrate MI into using an EMR is to collaborate on the treatment plan. The plan should include decisions about treatments as well as when the patient will follow up with the trainee and how (e.g., in person, by phone, or e-mail). The E-P-E framework is a natural fit when working together on composing a treatment plan with the patient. Once the collaborative plan is written, the trainee can offer to print out the plan if a printout of the plan is desired. The same is true for using the EMR as an aid to offering educational handouts and referrals, but the trainee should only print these out and give them to the patient if the patient requests them. Finally, the EMR can be used to order medications electronically so that prescriptions are waiting for the patient when they arrive at the pharmacy. However, it is important to always ask permission to send an electronic prescription versus a written one because the patient may wish to determine which pharmacy to use.

Many EMRs also have e-mail portals for confidential communications with patients via e-mail about follow-up on health issues, lab results, or answering patients' questions. E-mail messages can be composed in an MI-adherent way by using open-ended questions, reflections, and affirmations.

In conclusion, EMRs are here to stay and they are changing the way medical care is provided. They have many advantages but also have the potential to interfere with rapport and collaborative care. When EMRs are used in an MI-consistent manner, they have the potential to greatly enhance patients' care experience and facilitate health behavior change.

SELF-ASSESSMENT QUIZ

True or False?

1. The advantages of EMR include the following: simplified billing, reduction in medical errors, and improved documentation.
2. EMR provides easy access to clinical data that facilitates the use of the E-P-E framework and personalized feedback.
3. When EMRs are used in an MI-consistent manner, they have the potential to strengthen the alliance with the patient and facilitate health behavior change.
4. EMR doesn't have a role in discussing with the patient the trainee's clinical findings from the History and Physical Examination (H&P).
5. EMR does not have the capacity to facilitate the process of self-management of chronic medical conditions and shared-decision making process using MI spirit.

Answers

1. *True.* EMR has many advantages including simplified billing, improved communication, reduction in medical errors, and facilitating the implementation of practice guidelines and sharing medical information between practitioners.
2. *True.* When using an EMR, there are ample opportunities to integrate E-P-E framework. For example, E-P-E is a natural fit when working collaboratively with a patient on a treatment plan.
3. *True.* When data in EMRs are utilized to facilitate a dialogue with the patient about clinical findings, it has the potential to improve the patient-trainee relationship and initiate a conversation about change.
4. *False.* EMRs can play a significant role in conveying in an MI-consistent manner the trainee's findings from the H&P.
5. *False.* EMR can positively influence the process of behavior change and patient empowerment to self-manage medical conditions and also strengthen the process of decision-making using the MI approach.

15 Learning and Experiencing Motivational Interviewing

Learning motivational interviewing (MI) is as much about being attuned to avoiding behaviors that might present roadblocks to communication as it is about learning and strengthening new approaches to behavior change. Focusing too much on new skill acquisition can often derail the process of self-reflection on one's ability to communicate effectively. Carefully reflecting upon how we approach patients—that is, our "bedside manner"—is an essential component in evaluating our knowledge, skills, and attitudes toward MI. In this regard, it is imperative that we recognize the value of the foundational skills of MI, particularly reflective listening, open-ended questions, affirmations, and an emphasis on promoting self-efficacy, which are critical to establishing rapport with patients and to gaining a fundamental understanding of each patient's experiences and motivations.

PERSONAL REFLECTION

What Motivational Interviewing Means to Me

To me, MI is a "game changer." Before learning MI and reading *Motivational Interviewing: Helping People Change* (Miller & Rollnick, 2013), I relied heavily on simply being a "nice person" and obtaining information for diagnostic purposes. I felt I could build great rapport but that I did not provide the solutions I assumed patients were seeking. I now realize that the solution is within them. It lifts a great burden off my shoulders to find out that I don't have to come up with solutions. I now understand that the patient knows best, and I am acquiring the skills to assist patients in searching for their solution and to evoke it from them. I feel more competent as a physician. I have been able to see change before my eyes in a matter of hours or days, and the experience is both enlightening and empowering. I have gained confidence in myself, in my field, and in my ability to help my patients help themselves. It motivates me to seek and perfect other skills. This approach is not only critical in my professional life, but it has shown me more effective ways to interact with people in general. I have a better understanding of the dynamics of certain conversations, particularly those involving ambivalence. This is an essential skill that can be used in all clinical encounters and can be helpful throughout training in medical school.

CHALLENGES OF LEARNING MOTIVATIONAL INTERVIEWING

One of the most challenging, yet rewarding, aspects of learning MI is to ensure that you find and receive regular supervision and coaching. Key to the process of learning is finding a mentor who can guide you in learning the process of MI and who can guide your learning through videos, observed patient therapeutic encounters, readings, and Web-based materials. Making audio and video recordings of selected sessions can facilitate the learning process. Furthermore, a proper mentorship fit provides pause to the hurried accumulation of skills that derails so many trainees. Our mentors have been instrumental in helping us slow down the process and avoid being too ready to falsely reassure ourselves that we have successfully gained competence in a newly learned skill. We often have found ourselves attempting to quickly move to the next set of skills—as is common in learning most medical procedural skills acquisition—without going through guided self-reflection on that skill to assure that we have learned and practiced it thoroughly. A mentor is extremely helpful in pointing out challenging areas that could be improved and guiding the process of change. This is why it is important to have close mentorship while learning MI, particularly since so much of learning MI is experiential. No matter what metric or evaluation tool is used, there are subtleties of language and behavior for any trainee that can only be addressed through observation and in-vivo coaching by a skilled supervisor.

KEY POINT

Finding a mentor who can guide you through the process of learning MI is fundamental.

Learning MI is also a collaborative process that is enriched by shared learning. As you progress through your learning, it is important to share your learning experiences and enthusiasm with your colleagues. Collaboration with your fellow trainees invites candid sharing with the end goal of expanding your practice repertoire and developing confidence in counseling patients on behavior change. This is exemplified in role plays and practice group exercises that allow trainees to assume the role of the patient, practitioner, and feedback provider.

We have had the opportunity to share our knowledge and experiences with colleagues in an academic pediatric residency training program. Guided by a multidisciplinary team of Motivational Interviewing Network of Trainers (MINT), we created a longitudinal MI curriculum for pediatric residents. Key to this was assembling a diverse group of trainers to guide the process of developing the curriculum. The curriculum is based on current, evidence-based MI interventions and is trainee-driven, such that multiple surveys and self-assessments have led to targeted revisions to ensure that the learning process is adapted to trainees' (pediatric residents and fellows) focus and professional needs.

As trainees in psychiatry and pediatrics, we understand the time demands and needs of our colleagues. We customized the MI curriculum to best fit these needs, and we supported each other through personal reflections and experiences to allay anxiety related to the initial process of learning MI. We developed a yearly workshop that provides an intensive training and accommodates the needs of busy pediatric residents.

We embedded regular booster discussions and practice sessions during the adolescent medicine rotation, with dedicated supervision and coaching provided during that rotation. The intent is to create a culture that fosters learning and training in MI, such that it can be a part of everyday clinical practice. This is supported by an MI pocket guide we originally created for pediatric residents and modified to provide regular reminders throughout daily practice. Furthermore, we developed a modified evaluation tool to facilitate regular observation and feedback on the psychiatry resident's behavior change counseling and communication style with trained faculty in adolescent medicine.

The initial implementation has been challenging. Many preexisting notions about MI needed to be addressed. The perceived time constraint of using MI was the most noted barrier, followed by the idea that MI was "a type of psychotherapy" that would not be applicable to everyday practice. The interactive workshop helped tremendously in obviating these misconceptions. We found improved subjective and objective knowledge, skills, and attitudes following the MI workshop. Furthermore, we were able to personally refute these concerns and share the value we have found in routinely using MI in our practice.

As incorporation of our curriculum has gained footing, there has been an increasing adoption of MI into routine clinical practice at our institution. This is apparent both through observation in the Adolescent Medicine clinic, and also through objective data compiled using the Helpful Response Questionnaire (HRQ). MI has become part of regular discourse, not only on the adolescent medicine rotation but also on general pediatric and subspecialty rotations. Although we are still in the process of analyzing our work, to date the results appear to be very promising. In summary, the development of our MI curriculum has resulted in assembling a group of individuals with diverse backgrounds and perspectives, who have guided all who have participated in learning and training in MI. Most importantly, it has been a reminder of the importance of reflecting on our own training and practice of MI and being cognizant of our own strengths and limitations.

EIGHT STAGES IN LEARNING MOTIVATIONAL INTERVIEWING

First introduced by Miller and Moyers in a seminal paper in 2006, the underlying idea was to create a framework to customize training for trainees by defining eight discrete developmental stages (Fig. 15.1) that all trainees progress through to establish competence in the practice of MI.

Getting stuck is inevitable and a normal process of learning; we all go through this. The stages are points in training where trainees may get stuck. It is extremely important to know when you get stuck and to seek the guidance needed to help you get unstuck. Identifying the stage of learning and attending to these challenges can be useful in facilitating continued advancement as you go through training in MI.

Stage One: Understanding the Spirit of Motivational Interviewing

Understanding the spirit of MI is fundamental. The spirit originally included collaboration, evocation, and supporting patient autonomy. More recently, MI spirit

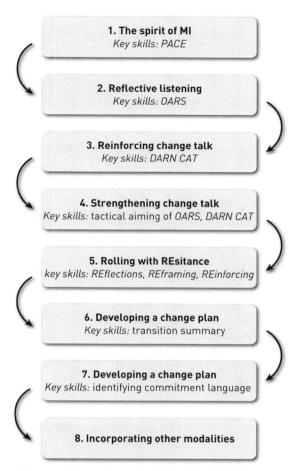

FIGURE 15.1 The eight stages of learning motivational interviewing.

was broadened to include two changes: (1) adding *Compassion*, defined as promoting the patient's own best interests rather than the practitioners' motivations for patient change, and (2) reframing support for autonomy as *Acceptance*, defined as creating a friendly atmosphere of autonomy support. A willingness to offer a patient-centered approach and elicit the patient's motivations for change is essential. In turn, this attitude fosters greater consistency in MI-adherent behaviors and the language we employ, resulting in improved patient receptiveness. Trainees get stuck when they are not open to the spirit of MI and have assumptions about patients or about their role in counseling. This can lead the trainee to become confrontational, overly directive, or overly advising. The early-stage trainee must understand the importance of being open to the spirit and how the spirit guides the MI approach. Accepting the spirit of MI is emphasized when teaching trainees, particularly as it allays anxiety related to the experience of learning. The spirit of MI provides a context and fits well with one's role as a medical trainee. It makes MI digestible and provides a foundation for the cumulative process of learning MI.

```
                            TOOLBOX
PACE

Patient autonomy
Acceptance
Collaboration
Compassion
Evocation
```

Stage Two: Patient-Centered Counseling Through Reflective Listening

Reflective listening can be a difficult skill to master and being able to consistently engage requires continuous development. We make an effort to spend twice as much time in reflective listening as we do in asking questions. We find that we listen better by using not just simple reflections of what the patient just stated but also by formulating accurate reflections that embody a summation of the patient's experience. Paying careful attention to the explicit and implicit information that is shared by the patient during clinical encounters is crucial.

You are interviewing a 22-year-old man who is slouched in his chair, head in hands, looking down, and who is not responding to your initial greeting. A reflection might be, "You look upset about being here today."

Reflections can express empathy, enhance patient confidence, reinforce collaboration, convey compassion, develop discrepancy, and increase expressed motivations for change (Miller & Moyers, 2006). They are subsumed in the acronym OARS (*O*pen-ended questions; *A*ffirmations; *R*eflections; *S*ummaries).

*O*pen-ended questions:

PATIENT: I have been in a weight management clinic for nearly 2 months.
TRAINEE: What has your experience in the weight management clinic been like?

*A*ffirmations

PATIENT: I hate taking my insulin, none of my friends have to, and I have so many things going on at school right now.
TRAINEE: Even though you would rather not take it, you take your insulin because staying healthy is really important to you.

*R*eflections

PATIENT: Marijuana just reduces my stress and allows me to chill and get things done. So many other things in my life are horrible; marijuana is the only thing that helps.
TRAINEE: You can't imagine your life without smoking marijuana.

*S*ummaries

PATIENT: I know I have COPD, but when I am not taking my medications, I'm fine. It's just every once in a while that my lungs start to act up. The medications are expensive, and it's hard to remember to take them. But my wife is concerned, and I guess I do feel healthier when I've taken my meds.

TRAINEE: Although COPD medications are costly and cumbersome to take regularly, others around you are concerned and have noticed the medications help you and, in fact, you feel better when you are taking your medications regularly.

OARS skills are tremendously useful. As these skills are strengthened, they can increase the likelihood of success in later stages of learning MI. It's not enough simply to know the components of the acronym; we must understand how best to use these elements over the course of a therapeutic encounter.

Stage Three: Reinforcing Change Talk

There should be a conscious effort to focus and guide the counseling session with a specific goal in mind. We are charged with helping the patient to resolve ambivalence and elicit motivations for change. It is important to key in to "change talk" (i.e., Desire, Ability, Need, Reasons [DARN]; Commitment, Activation, Taking steps [CAT] statements):

TOOLBOX
DARN CAT
Desire, Ability, Reasons, Need, Commitment, Activation, Taking steps

Desire
  "I really want to start exercising regularly, it's just so hard."

Ability
  "I could stop smoking if I wanted to."

Reason
  "My blood pressure is too high for me not to do something about my weight."

Need
  "I really need to start taking my medications."

Commitment
  "I am definitely going to stop drinking."

Activation language
  "I am thinking about going to some Alcoholics Anonymous (AA) meetings to help me stop drinking."

Taking steps
  "Last night I got rid of all my ash trays, threw out the remainder of my cigarette carton, and decided to use the patch that my physician gave me."

You respond to change talk by reinforcing change talk and minimizing sustain talk. Increasing change talk leads to increasing commitment language. In our experience, incorporating ways of ranking or measuring motivation for change is a useful strategy in helping generate change talk. Don't stop with one piece of change talk; keep probing for further change talk by using different techniques such as asking, "What else?" This open-ended question continues the process of eliciting more change talk:

TRAINEE: On a scale of 0 to 10, 0 not confident at all and 10 extremely confident, how confident are you that you can stop smoking?

PATIENT: Probably like a 6 or 7.

TRAINEE: A 6 or 7. What made you say this rather than a 2 or 3?

PATIENT: I don't know, I guess I know it's affecting my health and my wife would be happy.

TRAINEE: You know it will help improve your health and it will make the ones you love happy. What else?

Increasing commitment language and reducing sustain talk directly correlate to behavior change.

Stage Four: Building on and Strengthening Change Talk

The ability to actively elicit and reinforce change talk distinguishes MI from other modalities. Recognizing and facilitating change talk occurs through repeated reflections, affirmations, and open-ended questions, thereby continuously evoking reasons for change. We need to listen closely in order to pick up on change talk. Reflections can be essential to ensuring that you understand accurately what the patient means; however, our statements also reflect the change talk itself and can be used to strengthen it. Change talk must be supported by a clear intent and gentle guidance from the trainee. Frequent change talk expressed by the patient shows that the trainee is on the right track and is an accessible feedback mechanism for the trainee to guide the session. Hearing change talk provides a great feeling of confidence and it cues you in that you are on the right track. However, change talk does not guarantee commitment language, so it is important to not jump too quickly to eliciting commitment language.

Stage Five: Responding to Sustain Talk—Rolling With Resistance

Responding to sustain talk is different from confronting or opposing sustain talk (see Fig. 15.2). The proper technique is to not elicit sustain talk but also not to ignore it.

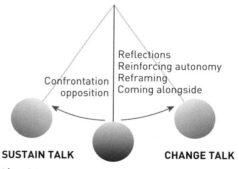

Reflections
Reinforcing autonomy
Reframing
Coming alongside

Confrontation
opposition

SUSTAIN TALK   CHANGE TALK

FIGURE 15.2   Rolling with resistance.

Rather allow and accept it. If you attempt to negate sustain talk by directly challenging it, it will come back stronger. You can reflect it and often you will get change talk as a result.

Imagine a swinging pendulum: Opposition to sustain talk will lead a patient to defend the status quo; instead, supporting patient autonomy reinforces patient-elicited reasons for making changes. As we discussed in previous chapters, strategies to use include selective reflections, reinforcing autonomy, reframing, and coming alongside the patient.

TOOLBOX

Rolling with **RE**sistance

REflections

REframing

REinforcing autonomy

Stage Six: Developing a Change Plan

The presence of sustain talk suggests the patient is not ready to enact a change plan. As change talk becomes more frequent, commitment language is more likely to emerge and grow. Transitioning from change talk to planning for change requires tact and timing. If you are unsure about whether a patient is ready to engage in commitment language, use a reflection to determine his or her readiness. "You have been talking a lot about wanting to make changes, at the same time I can't tell if you want to discuss what might work for you or how to get started. Help me understand where you are with that." Also, a transitional summary of change talk followed by an open-ended statement prompting patients to discuss plans for change can be an effective introduction to a new way of thinking. "You've mentioned how changing your eating habits would help you live long enough to travel and enjoy your grandchildren. And you want to have a good quality of life. Living longer and enjoying your life are great goals. What do you think about brainstorming with me now about two or three things you could introduce into your lifestyle to help you get there?"

Stage Seven: Consolidating Commitment Language

In general, once a change plan is discussed, it can be detrimental to revert back to eliciting motivation for change because the discussion can regress back to sustain talk. It is tempting to continue to identify reasons for change, but when you hear commitment language and the patient prepares for this, you should transition and support this momentum. The trainee has an important role in directing the plan and offering information, as long as the patient permits it. Furthermore, while we can assist by eliciting and consolidating commitment language, a common mistake for us is to miss the expression of commitment language or fail to solidify the patient's commitment to the plan. However, behavior change is unlikely when patients are not explicit in describing and verbally committing to a particular plan for change. It is important to remember (and to remind him or her) that it is the patient's change plan. The plan should be structured from what is elicited or approved by the patient. In this way the patient "owns" the plan.

Stage Eight: Incorporating Other Therapeutic Modalities

MI was never intended as a be-all, end-all therapeutic method or even as a long-term therapy. MI must be used first as a part of the engagement process. The MI style assumes nothing about the symptom, problem, or issue at hand. Rather, MI leaves it to the patient to define it. As this is accomplished and ambivalence is reduced, behavior change treatment works optimally when MI is integrated with other therapeutic modalities, such as cognitive behavioral therapy.

STRUCTURAL FRAMEWORK OF MOTIVATIONAL INTERVIEWING TRAINING

The most common forms of training are combinations of lectures and experiential exercises in a workshop setting. The workshop format has been shown to help trainees improve knowledge, attitudes, and confidence in using MI. However, without continued training and practice, results are rarely maintained over time. The lecture component should be succinct and relevant with an open invitation to comment or ask questions. The focus of trainings should be on small group exercises, observation of interviews, feedback, and coaching. Modeling is a significant component of training, predominantly through videos and live demonstrations. We have found that modeling is best approached by reviewing and periodically stopping to break down a video or interaction. From our experience, it is best to focus readings on shorter, succinct, and relevant research and practice articles. When you agree to provide training, make sure to become familiar with your audience and their particular needs. Doing so ensures that everyone is "on the same page" regarding expectations for the training, which enhances enthusiasm for learning.

METHODS OF TRAINING

Role Play and Use of Standardized Patients

Use of standardized patients for training medical trainees to improve communication skills is well established. However, role playing among colleagues has several advantages over the use of simulated patients. They include the ability to role-play a patient situation that has truly happened in practice, which is instrumental in understanding the patient's perspective. Furthermore, role plays engage trainees in discussing their own personal challenges and experiences in practicing MI. In our MI curriculum for pediatric residents, we use role plays and have found that it is fundamental to understanding the patient's experience. We often explore this after a role-play interaction and find that it works well.

Skill-Building Workshops

The most common approach for communication skills training, and particularly training in MI, are skill-building workshops. They consist of a variety of activities, including lectures, discussion, and skills practice sessions using audiotaped or videotaped interactions with a real or standardized patient. Training in MI is just as much about reducing old counterproductive habits as it is about learning new skills. Active experiential training, targeted feedback to the trainee, and sustained supervision are essential for skill development. It is very important to be aware of your communication and behavior in a given interaction. We emphasize audio-taping or videotaping yourselves. It can be a humbling experience to view or hear yourself because, we often inflate our skills and can exhibit MI non-adherent behaviors without even knowing it. It is critical to be continuously reflecting on your skills and ensuring that you receive objective feedback.

Feedback

I quickly became accustomed to receiving feedback, as well as offering it, though both were uncomfortable at first. Through this constructive environment, we pushed each other to excel, take risks, and be honest about our perceived struggles/successes. It was so much fun to watch each other's MI skills progress. The feedback during my 6 weeks of training was an essential part of learning MI and embracing its spirit. We had a supportive and keen team and pushed each other to work hard and do our best every day … A key concept that my mentor really helped me grasp was how to mobilize the process of change, once the patient is expressing change talk and commitment language. An incredibly effective strategy was to "go deeper" with my reflections, for example, take more risks with my hypotheses of the underlying meaning to a patient's words. This set the stage for using more powerful evocative questions, and many of my patients really embraced exploring their internal worlds and external interactions.

EVIDENCE-BASED TOOLS FOR PROVIDING FEEDBACK

Feedback and coaching in MI should focus on training practitioners in skills that can be reliably measured. This resulted in the development of several tools routinely used in the evaluation and feedback of trainees. Common to all these tools is attention to the spirit of MI and a focus on a particular target behavior in the trainee–patient interaction. It is beyond the scope of this chapter to provide extensive details of these tools (see References). The following is a brief overview of the most practical tools.

Motivational Interviewing Treatment Integrity Scale (MITI 3.1.1)

This behavioral coding system focuses on specific trainee behaviors and is aimed at assessing clinical skill in practicing MI (Moyers MITI 3.1.1). The initial intent was to provide a measure of treatment integrity for clinical trials of MI and a means of providing formal, structured feedback. It is the most commonly used tool for assessing MI adherence of a counseling session and for providing feedback for the trainee.

KEY POINT

MITI 3.1.1 is the most commonly used tool for assessing MI adherence of a counseling session.

Behavioral Change Counseling Index (BECCI)

Behavior change counseling (BCC) is an adaptation of MI that is a brief intervention primarily employed in healthcare settings. It is designed to help patients discuss the "how and why of change" and help them understand how their perceptions of current situations affect their behaviors and choices for behavior change. The difference between BCC and MI is that MI is focused on eliciting change talk and developing discrepancy, while BCC is focused on simply listening and understanding the patient's perspective to determine how best to guide the patient to behavior change. BCC focuses less on the psychotherapeutic elements of MI, particularly less of a focus on eliciting change talk. From this adaptation, the Behavioral Change Counseling Index or BECCI was developed as a 12-item scale that measures specific MI behaviors for the provision of feedback in both practical and research settings. It is the first instrument specifically developed to assess health behavior change, while incorporating measures of skills used in both MI and BCC.

The focus of the BECCI is on trainee's consulting behavior and attitude and not the behaviors of the patient. It is designed to be scored easily and quickly, given the time constraints of the healthcare setting.

We have found the MITI to be a great tool for review key areas in MI with supervisors and trainees. However, it is structured to provide great detail, and the inherent time constraints limit its practicality. Therefore, the BECCI may be a better evaluation tool for everyday use in a healthcare environment, with the MITI being available for observed clinical interactions in a more structured setting for coaching and feedback purposes. The BECCI has been our choice for our MI curriculum as it is brief and easily scored, with good interrater reliability and relevance to the healthcare setting. We have also added a qualitative piece to the BECCI to give our supervisors more flexibility in providing feedback.

Helpful Response Questionnaire

The HRQ is one of the older and more frequently used scales when evaluating MI skills and behavior. It was developed to assess the use of empathic language. HRQ is a brief, free-response questionnaire that can be administered to groups or individuals. It consists of six scenarios of simulated patient interactions that are likely to be seen in clinical settings. After each scenario, the trainee is instructed to play the role of the counselor and provide a helpful response. The average administration time is approximately 15 to 20 minutes.

COACHING AND MODELING

Watching my mentor was a fundamental part of how I learned MI. His compassion toward patients and passion for the art of MI was incredibly inspiring. In some of his sessions, I felt like I was in a concert hall, watching a conductor fervently evoke music from the orchestra. I also took in a lot through observation of body language and tone. In many interviews I would write down what I felt were particularly effective/evocative phrasings and review them later. I think one of the benefits of having an MI mentor is that like any apprenticeship, you observe the mentor's skills and techniques and incorporate/deliver these through your own personal style.

TRAINING OUTCOMES

The goals of training in MI are to demonstrate competency in the use of skills, the optimal use of skills in practice, and the long-term retention of skills. Primarily three areas define competence: knowledge, skills, and attitudes.

The effect of MI training on patient behaviors is mixed. In one study, after 1 year after MI training, patients of MI-trained trainees were more motivated to change and had a better understanding of factors that help prevent complications of disease, compared to controls (non-MI-trained trainees). In studies of patient behaviors, observed, audio-taped or videotaped assessments of skill are more reliable than self-assessments. Another study demonstrated the last point as it found that trainees' self-reports overestimated their skills and that there is a limited correlation between self-reported skill and outcomes.

Self-reported belief that one has learned a technique that has not been learned can be a detriment to both pursuing further training and improving MI-consistent skills. Inherent in using and evaluating MI skill and competence is the trainee's ability to continuously assess one's own communication and clinical practices, both subjectively and objectively.

> **KEY POINT**
> Belief that one has learned a technique that has not been learned can be detrimental to MI.

MOTIVATIONAL INTERVIEWING NETWORK OF TRAINERS

Given the rapidly expanding adoption, training, and research relating to MI, a centralized source for education and resources was needed. This resulted in the development of the Motivational Interviewing Network of Trainers (MINT). MINT held its first meeting in 1997 and has now grown to represent 35 countries and more than 20 different languages (MINT Web site). MINT is a group of individuals with specialized training and competency in both practicing and educating others in MI. MINT has become an international organization with a diverse group of trainers who apply MI in a variety of settings. The focus of the organization is to improve the quality and effectiveness of counseling as it relates to behavior change. MINT promotes the use of MI and advocates for MI practice through research, education, and training that it sponsors. Resources, communications, publications, and other shared practice opportunities are disseminated through their Website, www. motivationalinterviewing.org, including the e-journal: *Motivational Interviewing: Training, Research, Implementation, Practice* (www.mitrip.org). MINT has an annual meeting alternating with both a national (US) site and an international site with Train the Trainer (TNT) workshops. Admittance to workshops is competitive as it is based on merit and availability. The annual meeting also holds several didactic plenary sessions and small group workshops presenting new data on the practice of and training in MI.

FINAL THOUGHTS

MI places the responsibility of change on the patient, making the trainee a guide in the process, which prevents trainee's burnout and compassion fatigue in practice. In addition,

MI provides tools for both enacting behavior change and guiding communication with patients, which reduces trainee's anxiety in the process of counseling patients. The sense of collaboration espoused by MI allows trainees and patients to work together rather than be in conflict or struggle. It is important to keep the goals of a clinical encounter realistic and to remind yourself that you do not have to do everything during an encounter. You can select skills to use and help guide the patient together. A big hurdle for early trainees is to keep in check the idea that you need a quick fix for your patients. Change is the patient's responsibility; the trainee is there to offer guidance and skills in the process of change and to assess whether this offer is acceptable to the patient.

Training in MI has increasingly become more diverse and innovative, yet the staples of training continue to be predominantly workshop and experiential based. As we discussed earlier, the necessary ingredients to high-quality training in MI are instruction, practice, feedback, and coaching/modeling. Instruction is the book learning, which should be fluid. Deliberate practicing is practicing mindfully and should feel effortful. It requires focus and attunement toward rough areas and improvement. That means practicing skills that are beyond your ability. Real and straightforward feedback encourages a growth mindset, a construct developed by Carol Dweck. Growth mindset versus fixed mindset means that your abilities may be developed through education and hard work; you can make mistakes and fail because these are necessary for development; and you can take on difficult work and persevere because you know this is how you truly improve. If during our training we create a culture of showing our work and soliciting constructive feedback, we are acknowledging that looking at our flaws and errors is important to getting better. This is how we learn how to do a better job, and this is how we can do better for our patients. Keep in mind that, at first, it may be hard to accept the feedback and difficult to become accustomed to it. However, with time one becomes more comfortable. If you struggle, you succeed—that is the growth mindset. Complementary to the feedback, modeling from our mentors is incredibly helpful in learning MI.

We clearly need to develop an atmosphere of continual improvement. We need to try solutions that are on the cutting edge of best practice research because we want to master best practices approaches rather than continue the status quo. We should challenge ourselves and those around us to have the utmost respect for our patients, to drop judgmental attitudes and enhance our empathic skills, and understand where someone is and be able to help that person get where he or she wants to go. MI is particularly well suited as a framework for our type of work.

SELF-ASSESSMENT QUIZ

True or False?

1. MI is best learned and practiced with the supervision and coaching of a mentor who is experienced in MI.
2. The spirit of MI comes last, after a trainee has mastered other skills and techniques.
3. Reflections are only used to demonstrate to the patient that the trainee has been listening.
4. "I need to quit using heroin because I want to be around for my kids and even my grandkids" is an example of "desire" change talk.

5. When a trainee hears change talk, it is important to move quickly to commitment language, so as to not lose momentum.

6. Once a patient has begun to share commitment language, it can be detrimental to continue exploring motivation for change.

7. There is a strong, positive correlation between a trainee's self-reported skill and patient outcomes.

8. Motivational Interviewing Network of Trainers (MINT) is a source for education and training in MI.

Answers

1. *True.* A key process of learning MI is to find a mentor who can guide the learning process and can offer feedback on a trainee's sessions. A proper mentorship also offers a pause to the hurried accumulation of techniques that can derail trainees, as well as offer honest perspective on the progress of a trainee's skills.

2. *False.* Understanding the spirit of MI is a fundamental step as trainees begin their MI training. A solid grasp of the spirit makes MI digestible and provides a foundation for the cumulative process of learning it. Additionally, the spirit of MI offers a context and fits well with an individual's role as a medical trainee.

3. *False.* While reflections can demonstrate to a patient that a trainee has been actively listening, they also express empathy, enhance patient confidence, reinforce collaboration, convey compassion, develop discrepancy, and increase expressed emotions for change.

4. *False.* This statement is an example of "need" change talk. Recall the helpful acronym DARN CAT (Desire, Ability, Reason, Need, Commitment, Activation, Taking steps), to categorize types of preparatory and mobilizing change talk.

5. *False.* While change talk provides a great feeling of confidence and cues trainees that they are on the right track, it is important to remember that change talk does not equal commitment language. It can be hazardous to jump too quickly from early change talk to commitment language.

6. *True.* When a trainee hears commitment language, it is important to allow for a smooth transition and support the momentum. By revisiting motivation for change after a patient has clearly demonstrated commitment language, a trainee runs the risk of making the patient regress to expressing sustain talk.

7. *False.* In studies of patient behaviors, observed, audio-taped or videotaped assessments of skill are more reliable than self-assessments. Another study demonstrated that trainees' self-reports overestimated their skills and that there is a limited correlation between self-reported skill and outcomes.

8. *True.* MINT is an international organization of diverse trainers who specialize in the practice and training in MI. The focus of the organization is to improve the quality and effectiveness of counseling as it relates to behavior change. MINT promotes the use of MI and advocates for MI practice through research, education, and training.

16 Future Directions of Motivational Interviewing in Medical Training

I first heard the term "motivational interviewing," or MI, at the beginning of medical school. It was among the hundreds of new terms thrust upon us in those early days, and I must admit, it flew past me. I didn't understand what it meant and beyond one elusive reference, the following 2 years of training provided little, if any, insight regarding the spirit, processes and skills of MI. In fact, scant attention was paid to teaching us the importance of building rapport with patients during our encounters, whether for history taking or for those related to ongoing care or discharge planning. I felt a significant gap in my training: Something essential was missing, but I didn't know what it was. To my chagrin, I had a difficult time engaging with patients, regardless of the clinical setting. Despite good intentions, even my best efforts often left me feeling distant and disconnected from my patients. Although I tried diligently to listen actively to every patient I met and felt genuine empathy in even the most challenging situations, the feeling persisted.

Early in my third-year psychiatry rotation, I learned that my problems were common among both trainees and practitioners, and that they do not reflect a lack of compassion or concern for a patient's well-being. Rather, it is an inability to communicate empathically. I wasn't fully engaging my patients because I was unable to convey the acceptance and empathy I felt for them; consequently, I could not establish therapeutic relationships grounded in collaboration. The result: suboptimal outcomes for both my patients and for me.

I trained in MI while working with patients who have co-occurring psychiatric and substance use disorders, a field in which MI was first established as an effective, evidence-based therapeutic approach. Throughout this period, I saw firsthand how MI could improve every aspect of communication with patients and, consequently, promote the collaborative spirit that leads to improved outcomes. I practiced MI skills throughout the clinical rotations that followed, through an array of clinical settings with different patient populations, and I continued to see positive results. While MI is a potent tool for working with patients with substance use disorders, it has also enriched my clinical encounters among those who presented with both acute illnesses and the many challenges of chronic disease, such as cancer, chronic respiratory disease, diabetes, heart disease, obesity, and stroke.

Research confirms MI's value as an integral part of patient care within a variety of clinical settings, including family medicine, internal medicine, emergency medicine, pediatrics, and the surgical specialties. MI also lends itself to being adapted for use in highly specific contexts such as brief interventions. As Miller and Rollnick remind us, MI is, first and foremost, a particular style of a therapeutic conversation designed to help individuals change unhealthy behaviors. With today's increased focus on evidence-based interventions, MI may well become the standard of care for engaging patients in any setting, and perhaps even the norm against which all clinical interactions are measured.

Currently, MI training is emphasized primarily in the fields of psychiatry and behavioral medicine, and even in these settings, MI is usually reserved for those at the graduate level, that is, house officers, residents, registrars, and fellows. Here lays one of the major dilemmas confronting how best to incorporate MI skill into the junior levels of medical training: If, as the literature suggests, the use of MI is expanding to the point of becoming the basis for engaging patients in a variety of settings, training practitioners in these skills will need to expand as well.

At which point in medical education should MI be taught? In my experience, learning MI at the beginning of my training would have been extremely useful. I believe the early days of medical school are the ideal place for future practitioners to acquire this approach, which may then be carried into patients' encounters throughout undergraduate training and into specialty programs. Beginning the MI training process at the introductory level would ensure broader inclusion as a component of general medical education. In this way, MI could contribute to the sound foundation required for effective medical interviewing and be further refined for use in specific specialties.

Is it possible to teach MI to medical students as a fundamental approach in providing care? An expanding body of research regarding MI education suggests that individuals across a wide range of academic abilities and experience have the capacity to learn the MI approach. Indeed, it is not intelligence that limits one's capacity to learn and make effective use of MI. Rather, it is an inability to feel empathy and/or the lack of interpersonal skill. Many medical students appear to have chosen medicine in response to a strong sense of empathy for others, and from this perspective, it opens a window of opportunity to make the most of the empathy skills by working with trainees on how to foster those through learning and implementing MI in patient care.

It is unclear why MI teaching and practice remain primarily within the purview of psychiatry and behavioral medicine. A possible explanation is the lack of consistency in medical school training, particularly regarding communication skills. No standardized curriculum exists for basic medical interviewing skills, and interviewing is often viewed as more of an art than a science, something intrinsic to an individual that may, perhaps, be acquired, rather than taught. The research demonstrates, however, that just as MI may be taught, so too it may be practiced by individuals with diverse background, in almost every conceivable clinical setting. What makes it more challenging is how to incorporate practical and easy access to good supervision and coaching to guide the learning process in the training environment. It is our responsibility to be proactive in seeking supervision and promoting the importance of it.

Integrating MI across many fields of medicine will require transforming the culture of the medical profession. Practicing MI across various specialties will not only change the way practitioners communicate with their patients but will offer improved outcomes to patients with a wide range of maladies. There is no shortage of evidence in support of wider MI use, yet we are still waiting for it to be fully incorporated into clinical practice.

Over the centuries, an attitude of paternalism pervaded clinical practice, and although it sometimes seems that communication patterns are entrenched in outdated traditions, this aspect of our profession is, in fact, undergoing significant change.

A paradigm shift relating to the nature of the doctor–patient relationship is under way which presents all practitioners with the possibility of improved rapport with those who come to us seeking help. Better still, this change offers profound gains in the sense of satisfaction experienced by both physicians and patients.

The importance of recent advances in medical education is exceeded only by that of medical/scientific research, and we're on the front lines of far-reaching changes. The responsibility for consolidating innovations—such as MI—into physician–patient relationships rests with us. How will we respond?

Appendix 1
Motivational Interviewing Quick Guide

The following appendix outlines and summarizes key points covered in previous chapters. This guide will provide you with a quick reference to tools and strategies for utilizing MI in daily clinical practice.

DEFINITION OF MOTIVATIONAL INTERVIEWING
Collaborative, goal-oriented style of communication designed to strengthen personal motivation for, and commitment to, a specific goal by eliciting and exploring patients' own reasons for change within an atmosphere of acceptance and compassion.

Communication Continuum:

Directive → **Guiding** → Following

Instructive, Giving advice, ***Active Listening, Eliciting, Collaborating,*** *Seek to understand only*

Typical Medical Style **Motivational Interviewing** No advice

SPIRIT OF MOTIVATIONAL INTERVIEWING
The underlying spirit of MI adheres to the ethical concepts of beneficence, nonmaleficence, justice, and autonomy (not meant to be manipulative).

Four aspects of the spirit of MI:

1. Partnership: think dancing versus wrestling
2. Acceptance*: unconditional positive regard
3. Compassion: actively promote another's welfare
4. Evocation: people already have change inside of them; it simply needs to be called out.

---

* Acceptance is composed of absolute worth (prizing and respecting a patient's inherent worth/ potential for change), accurate empathy (communicating active interest in an effort to understand a patient's perspective), autonomy support (honoring and respecting a patient's autonomy, irrevocable right, and capacity for self-direction), and affirmation (acknowledging a patient's strengths and efforts).

CORE COMMUNICATION SKILLS—OARS

Open-Ended Questions: Questions that cannot be answered with yes/no response or a one-word response

Affirmations: Statements that accentuate the positive/highlight positive steps toward change

Reflections: Statements that verbalize meaning or feelings, sometimes hypothesizing what is not actually verbalized

Summarizing: Bringing together and juxtaposing information for the patient to see in a new light

COMMUNICATION SKILL	DO's	DON'T's	USES
Open-ended questions	– Begin questions with "what," "how," and "in what ways"; "tell me about"; "describe for me" – Intersperse questions with reflections in a 1:2-3 ratio on questions to reflections	– Barrage the patient with a myriad of questions in a row – Compound multiple questions together – Give yes/no or multiple-choice questions (not open)	– Assess motivation for change and perceived self efficacy – Facilitate patient's exploration of self – Develop rapport
Affirmations	– Highlight patient attributes, strengths, or acts that might aid change efforts – Include patient-specific references – Maintain positive regard – Best if started with "you"	– Become a cheerleader – Use language of personal judgment such as "good" or "great" as an affirmation – Make an "I" statement	– Acknowledge a patient's efforts – Bolster confidence and self-efficacy – Convey empathy – Shown to increase retention and decrease defensiveness
Reflections	– Be succinct; use clear language – Use 2–3 reflections for every question you ask – Use complex reflections to add meaning or emphasis – Continue the paragraph	– Use wordy/vague reflections – End reflections with an upward inflection, lest they be considered questions – Make prefaces ("I think," "it sounds like," "what I hear you saying is…")	– Convey understanding of patient viewpoint, emotions, or meaning – Confirm engagement – Keep person talking, exploring, and considering
Summaries	– Use three types: collecting, linking, or transitional – Take sufficient pauses after reflections to encourage dialogue	– Use wordy/vague statements – Summarize for summarizing sake—have a clear purpose in mind (such as collecting data or transition conversation)	– Convey understanding of patient viewpoint – Reiterate that practitioner is listening – Especially effective for summarizing ambivalence

Processes of Motivational Interviewing

Four processes may emerge in order, but they are recursive throughout sessions:

1. Engaging: Establishing trust and working relationship
2. Focusing: Collaboratively developing direction/agenda
3. Evoking: Eliciting patients' own motivations for change
4. Planning: Strengthening commitment and making plans

Engaging

Three aspects of engagement:

1. Establish mutually respectful relationships
2. Agree on treatment goals
3. Collaborate on negotiated tasks

Key points for engaging:

- Active and reflective listening
- Stay patient-centered
- Nonverbals actually say a lot (give undivided attention, good eye contact, mirror with facial expressions, etc.)
- Explore goals and values

Largest threat to active engagement: communication of nonmutuality (i.e., lack of positive regard)

Avoid these traps: Assessment, Expert, Premature Focus, Labeling, Blaming, and Chat Traps

Focusing

Focusing is the process of becoming clear about goals and directions
Somewhere between following where the patient happens to go and dictating where the patient should go
This is a *collaborative* process.

Agenda Mapping:

- Used when there are multiple behaviors to change
- Meta-conversation about direction and plan
- Involves structuring/set-up choices, considering options, then zooming in and agreeing/negotiating on a path

Evoking

Ambivalence = simultaneously conflicting emotions/arguments
Process of evoking helps people move through natural process of resolving ambivalence
Goal is to increase "change talk": ratio of change to sustain talk is a predictor of future change actually happening

Evoking Strategies:

1. Importance/Confidence ruler: scale 0–10 of how important/confident patient is; follow-up/explore (if 6, why not a 3?)
2. Querying extremes: explore both positive and negative
3. Looking back: consider time before problem
4. Looking forward: consider changed future

5. Exploring goals and strategies: look at discrepancies between these and current behaviors
6. Normalizing ambivalence: create safe atmosphere and promote engaging

Hope and Confidence: Important to elicit hope and evoke strengths. Strategies include menu of options (either elicited or offered with permission), confidence ruler (above), exploring past successes and highlighting the implied strengths, and reframing past failures as "tries" and learning from experiences

Change Talk: Any self-expressed language that is an argument for change

Preparatory Change Talk: "**DARN**" (These alone do not indicate change will happen):
Desire (I wish, I want)
Ability (I can, I am able)
Reasons (If I do x, then y)
Need (I need, I must)

Mobilizing Change Talk: "CAT" (Signals movements toward resolution of ambivalence):
Commitment (I will)
Activation (I intend to)
Taking steps (I have)

Responding to Change Talk: **REFLECT IT, Ask about it, Summarize**:
Continue to use OARS to build on it and evoke more change talk
When change talk appears vague, disingenuous, or naïve, take person at his or her word and become interested/try to focus on statistics.

Sustain Talk: Opposite of change talk; language that is argument against change

Responding to Sustain Talk:
1. Straight reflection
2. Amplified reflection
3. Double-sided reflection ("and at the same time")
4. Emphasizing autonomy
5. Reframing
6. Agreeing with a twist
7. Running head start
8. Coming alongside

Discord = Dissonance between patient and trainee; look for signs (defending, squaring off, interrupting, and disengaging). Function of relationship, not just of the patient.

Planning
Signs of Readiness:
1. Increased change talk: both frequency and strength
2. Diminished sustain talk
3. Taking steps: Important to affirm these
4. Expression of being resolved
5. Envisioning future
6. Questions about change

Implementation intention = Specific plan of action + interpersonal statement of intent to do it

Summarize Change Talk, then ask "key question": "(change talk) ... What's the next step?"
Step of planning: confirm goals → itemize options/develop plan → elicit preference for options → summarize plan → troubleshoot
When developing a new plan from scratch, *brainstorm* to generate possible options or steps

Exploring reluctance can actually aid in commitment by discussing possible pitfalls and potential solutions

EXCHANGING INFORMATION

Offering information and advice is a two-way exchange. It's easy to overestimate how much information and advice a patient needs:

E-P-E Approach:
Elicit: explore patient's prior knowledge and query re: what information is wanted or needed, ask permission to give information or advice
Provide: give personalized information or advice, prioritize what the patient most wants/needs to know, give information clearly and in small doses, and use autonomy-supportive language
Elicit: check back in re: person's understanding, interpretation, or response to provided information

For large load of information, divide up into manageable pieces → **Chunk-Check in-Chunk:**

Chunk of info provided (remember keep it personalized), **Check In** re: thoughts and understanding of info, **Chunk** of additional information.

EQUIPOISE

Equipoise = Neutrality. Conscious decision to NOT use one's professional skills/position to influence a specific choice or decision

BRIEF INTERVENTIONS

MI has been shown to be effective in brief encounters. Components of effective brief intervention: **"FRAMES"**:

Feedback of personal status relative to norms
Responsibility for personal change
Advice to change
Menu of options from which to choose in pursuing change
Empathic counselor style
Support for self-efficacy/autonomy

Always remember—**Do not focus on specific skills so much as to lose focus on truly listening to the patient and maintaining the spirit of MI**

Appendix 2
Video Clips of Clinical Encounters

You can access these videos at: http://oxfordmedicine.com/motivationalinterviewing

1. CLINICAL ENCOUNTER WITH AN ADOLESCENT

In this encounter, a young woman meets with the trainee in the primary care outpatient setting to discuss her concerns about possibly having a sexually transmitted infection. This clinical exchange demonstrates the effective use of motivational interviewing (MI) with an adolescent patient, illustrating the MI spirit, OARS skills, and the elicit-provide-elicit framework.

2. CLINICAL ENCOUNTER WITH AN ANGRY FAMILY MEMBER

In this encounter, a distraught father confronts the medical trainee about his seriously injured son. The trainee utilizes the motivational interviewing approach to minimize discord in the exchange, to help to engage the patient's father, and to gain a better understanding of his concerns. The trainee demonstrates the skillful use of reflective, careful listening, while minimizing the use of questions.

3. BRIEF INTERVENTION IN THE EMERGENCY DEPARTMENT

In this encounter, the trainee meets briefly with a patient prior to her discharge from the emergency department, where she was evaluated following a car accident related to alcohol use. The trainee uses this window of opportunity to do an motivational interviewing–based brief intervention (BI). By virtue of its brevity, this BI is focused on enhancing the patient's motivation and mobilizing her own resources for change.

4. CLINICAL ENCOUNTER WITH A PATIENT STRUGGLING WITH DEPRESSION AND COCAINE USE

In this encounter, the trainee meets with a man who is struggling with chronic depression and cocaine use. The patient was involuntary committed after he got into an altercation with police officers. Motivational interviewing is utilized to engage a withdrawn patient to help him open up about his feelings and experiences. In this encounter, the patient's autonomy is clearly supported.

5. CLINICAL ENCOUNTER WITH A PATIENT WITH CHRONIC OBSTRUCTIVE PULMONARY DISEASE (COPD)

In this encounter, an older man meets with the trainee in an outpatient clinic for a routine examination and prescription renewal. This clinical exchange illustrates the use of the evoking process of motivational interviewing (MI) in the context of helping the patient explore and resolve his ambivalence about quitting smoking. The trainee maintains the person-centered, nonauthoritarian, and collaborative style of MI throughout the encounter.

6. CLINICAL ENCOUNTER WITH A PATIENT STRUGGLING WITH DEPRESSION AND ALCOHOL USE

In this encounter, the trainee meets with a patient, in the inpatient psychiatric setting, who was admitted with depression and heavy alcohol use. The two meet shortly after the patient was involved in a physical altercation with another patient in the unit. The trainee uses the motivational interviewing spirit and skills to engage and guide the patient to help her to gain a better understanding of the connection between depression and alcohol use.

7. CLINICAL ENCOUNTER WITH A PATIENT PRESENTING WITH DIABETIC KETOACIDOSIS (DKA)

In this encounter, the trainee is meeting a young patient for the first time who was recently admitted to the hospital for treatment of DKA. The exchange is an example of an opportunistic intervention that utilizes motivational interviewing to engage and explore the patient's understanding of her chronic medical condition. The trainee works collaboratively with the patient to create a self-management plan that the patient is confident in and willing to follow.

8. CLINICAL ENCOUNTER WITH A PATIENT STRUGGLING WITH ADHERING TO MEDICATION

In this encounter, the trainee is meeting with an older man whom he has known for many years in outpatient treatment. He was recently diagnosed with atrial fibrillation, stabilized, and discharged home. During this outpatient encounter, the trainee uses the motivational interviewing spirit, strategies, techniques, and the elicit-provide-elicit framework to explore and address the patient's challenges related to medication adherence.

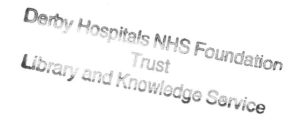

References, Videos, and Books

REFERENCES

CHAPTER 1

Bandura, A. (1977). *Social learning theory*. Englewood Cliffs, NJ: Prentice Hall.

Bem, D. M. (1967). Self-perception: An alternative interpretation of cognitive dissonance phenomena. *Psychology Review, 74*, 183–200.

Festinger, L. (1957). *A theory of cognitive dissonance*. Stanford, CA: Stanford University Press.

Greaves, C. J., Middlebrook, A., O'Laughlin, L., Holland, S., Piper, J., Steele, A., ... Daly, M. (2008). Motivational interviewing for modifying diabetes risk: A randomised controlled trial. *British Journal of General Practice, 58*(553), 535–540.

Markland, D., Ryan, R. M., Tobin, V. J., et al. (2005). Motivational interviewing and self-determination theory. *Journal of Social and Clinical Psychology, 24*, 811–831.

Miller, W. R. (1983). Motivational interviewing with problem drinkers. *Behavioural Psychotherapy, 11*(2), 147–172

Miller, W. R., & Rollnick, S. (1991). *Motivational interviewing: Preparing people to change addictive behavior*. New York, NY: Guilford Press.

Miller, W. R., & Rollnick, S. (2013). *Motivational interviewing: Helping people change* (3rd ed.). New York, NY: Guilford Press.

Miller, W. R., & Rose, G. S. (2009). Toward a theory of motivational interviewing. *American Psychologist, 64*(6), 527–537.

Resnicow, K., & McMaster, F. (2012). Motivational interviewing: Moving from why to how with autonomy support. *International Journal of Behavioral Nutrition and physical Activity, 9*, 19.

Rogers, C. R. (1957). The necessary and sufficient conditions of therapeutic personality change. *Journal of Consulting Psychology, 21*, 95–103.

Rogers, C. R. (1986). Carl Rogers on the development of the person-centered approach. *Person Centered Review, 1*, 257–259.

Rubak, S., Sandbaek, A., Lauritzen, T., & Christensen, B. (2005). Motivational interviewing: A systematic review and meta-analysis. *British Journal of General Practice, 55*(513), 305–312.

Rubak, S., Sandbaek, A., Lauritzen, T., Borch-Johnsen, K., & Christensen, B. (2009). General practitioners trained in motivational interviewing can positively affect the attitude t behaviour change in people with type 2 diabetes. *Scandinavian Journal of Primary Health Care, 27*(3), 172–179.

Sjoling, M., Lundberg, K., Englund, E., Westman, A., & Jong, M. C. (2011). Effectiveness of motivational interviewing and physical activity on prescription on leisure exercise in subjects suffering from mild to moderate hypertension. *BMC Research Notes, 4*, 352.

Swenson, S. L., Buell, S., Zettler, P., White, M., Ruston, D. C., & Lo, B. (2004). Patient-centered communication: Do patients really prefer it? *Journal of General Internal Medicine, 19*, 1069–1079.

Westra, H. A., Aviram, A., & Doell, F. K. (2011). Extending motivational interviewing to the treatment of major mental health problems: Current directions and evidence. *Canadian Journal of Psychiatry, 56*(11), 643–650.

CHAPTER 2

Armstrong, M. J., Mottershead, T. A., et al. (2011). Motivational interviewing to improve weight loss in overweight and/or obese patients: A systematic review and meta-analysis of randomized controlled trials. *Obesity Reviews, 12*(9), 709–723.

Harland, J., White, M., Drinkwater, C., Chinn, D., Farr, L., & Howel, D. (1999). The Newcastle exercise project: A randomised controlled trial of methods to promote physical activity in primary care. *British Medical Journal, 319*(7213), 828–832.

Lai, D. T., Cahill, K., Qin, Y., & Tang, J. L. (2010). Motivational interviewing for smoking cessation. *Cochrane Database of Systematic Reviews* (1), CD006936.

Miller, W. R. (1983). Motivational interviewing with problem drinkers. *Behavioural Psychotherapy, 11*(2), 147–172.

Miller, W. R., & Rollnick, S. (1991). *Motivational Interviewing, preparing people to change addictive behavior*. New York, NY: Guilford Press.

Miller, W. R., & Rollnick, S. (2002). *Motivational interviewing: Preparing people for change* (2nd ed.). New York, NY: Guilford Press.

Miller, W. R., & Rollnick, S. (2013). *Motivational interviewing: Helping people change* (3rd ed.). New York, NY: Guilford Press.

Miller, W. R., & Rose, G. S. (2009). Toward a theory of motivational interviewing. *American Psychologist, 64*(6), 527–537.

Rogers, C. (1965). *Client centered therapy*. Boston, MA: Houghton-Mifflin.

Rollnick, S., Miller, W. R., & Butler, C. C. (2008). *Motivational interviewing in health care: Helping people change behavior*. New York, NY: Guilford Press.

Rubak, S., Sandbaek, A., Lauritzen, T., Borch-Johnsen, K., & Christensen, B. (2009). General practitioners trained in motivational interviewing can positively affect the attitude to behaviour change in people with type 2 diabetes. One year follow-up of an RCT, ADDITION Denmark. *Scandinavian Journal of Primary Health Care, 27*(3), 172–179.

Rubak, S., Sandbaek, A., Lauritzen, T., & Christensen, B. (2005). Motivational interviewing: A systematic review and meta-analysis. *British Journal of General Practice, 55*(513), 305–312.

Rusch, N., & Corrigan, P. W. (2002). Motivational interviewing to improve insight and treatment adherence in schizophrenia. *Psychiatric Rehabilitation Journal, 26*(1), 23–32.

Sjoling, M., Lundberg, K., Englund, E., Westman, A., & Jong, M. C. (2011). Effectiveness of motivational interviewing and physical activity on prescription on leisure exercise time in subjects suffering from mild to moderate hypertension. *BMC Research Notes, 4*, 352.

Smedslund, G., Berg, R. C., Hammerstrøm, K. T., Steiro, A., Leiknes, K. A., Dahl, H. M., & Karlsen, K. (2011). Motivational interviewing for substance abuse. *Cochrane Database of Systematic Reviews*, (5), CD008063.

Westra, H. A., Aviram, A., & Doell, F. K. (2011). Extending motivational interviewing to the treatment of major mental health problems: Current directions and evidence. *Canadian Journal of Psychiatry/Revue Canadienne de Psychiatrie, 56*(11), 643–650.

CHAPTER 3

Arkowitz, H., & Westra, H. A. (2009). Introduction to the special series on motivational interviewing and psychotherapy. *Journal of Clinical Psychology, 65*(11), 1149–1155.

Barnes, A. J., & Gold, M. A. (2012). Promoting healthy behaviors in pediatrics: Motivational interviewing. *Pediatrics in Review, 33*(9), e57–68.

Chanut, F., Brown, T. G., & Dongier, M. (2005). Motivational interviewing and clinical psychiatry. *Journal of Clinical Psychiatry, 50*, 715–721.

Douaihy, A., Stowell, K. R., Kohnen, S., Salloum, I. M. (2008). Substance use disorders. In D. Kupfer, M. Horner, D. Brent, D. Lewis, C. Reynolds, M. Thase, M. Travis. (Eds.), *Oxford American handbook of psychiatry* (pp. 615–688). New York, NY: Oxford University Press.

Miller, W. R., & Rollnick, S. (2013). *Motivational interviewing: Helping people change* (3rd ed.). New York, NY: Guilford Press.

Sussman, C., Khatkhate, G., Tavares, A., Johnson, K., Rivera, M., Miller, M. D., Douaihy, A. (2008). Psychotherapy. In D. Kupfer, M. Horner, D, Brent, D. Lewis, C. Reynolds, M. Thase, M. Travis. (Eds.), *Oxford American handbook of psychiatry* (pp. 98–102). New York, NY: Oxford University Press.

CHAPTER 4

Mason, P., & Butler, C. (2010). *Health behavior change: A guide for practitioners* (2nd ed.). New York, NY: Churchill Livingstone.

Miller, W. R., & Rollnick, S. (2009). Ten things that motivational interviewing is not. *Behavioural and Cognitive Therapy, 37*, 129–140.

Miller, W. R., & Rollnick, S. (2013). *Motivational interviewing: Helping people change* (3rd ed.). New York, NY: Guilford Press.

Prochaska, J. O., & Diclemente, C. C. (1983). Stages and processes of self-change of smoking: Toward an integrative model of change. *Journal of Consulting and Clinical Psychology, 51*, 390–395.

Rosengren, D. B. (2009). *Building motivational interviewing skills: A practitioner workbook.* New York, NY: Guilford Press.

Velicer, W. F., Prochaska, J. O., Fava, J. L., Norman, G. J., Redding, C. A. (1998). Smoking cessation and stress management: Applications of the transtheoretical model of behavior change. *Homeostasis in Health and Disease, 38(5–6)*, 216–233.

CHAPTER 5

Arora, N. K., Weaver, K. E., Clayman, M. L., Oakley-Girvan, I., & Potosky, A. L. (2009). Physicians' decision-making style and psychosocial outcomes among cancer survivors. *Patient Education and Counseling, 77*(3), 404–412.

Buckman, R., Tulsky, J. A., & Rodin, G. (2011). Empathic responses in clinical practice: Intuition or tuition. *Canadian Medical Association Journal, 183*(5), 569–571.

Gerteis, M., Edgeman-Levitan, S., Daley, J., & Delbanco, T. M. (Eds.). (1993). *Through the patient's eyes: Understanding and promoting patient-centered care.* San Francisco, CA: Jossey-Bass.

Guyatt, G., Montori, V., Devereaux, P. J., Schünemann, H., & Bhandari, M. (2004). Patients at the center: In our practice, and in our use of language. *ACP Journal Club, 140*(1), A11–A12.

McWhinney, I. R. (1985). Patient-centred and doctor-centred models of clinical decision making. In M. Sheldon, J. Brook, & A. Rector (Eds.), *Decision making in general practice* (pp. 31–46). London, UK: Stockton.

Mercer, S. W., & Reynolds, W. J. (2002). Empathy and quality of care. *British Journal of General Practice, 52*(Suppl.), S9–12.

Miller, W. R., & Rollnick, S. (2013). *Motivational interviewing: Helping people change.* New York, NY: Guilford Press.

Neuman, M., Bensing, J., Mercer, S., Ernstmann, N., Ommen, O., & Pfaff, H. (2009). Analysing the "nature" and "specific effectiveness" of clinical empathy: A theoretical overview and contribution towards a theory-based research agenda. *Patient Education and Counseling, 74,* 339–346.

Peters, E., Hibbard, J., Slovic, C., & Dieckmann, N. (2007). Numeracy skill and the communication, comprehension, and use of risk-benefit information. *Health Affairs (Millwood), 26*(3), 741–748.

Pollak, K. I., Arnold, R. M., Jeffrey, A. S., Alexander, S. C., Olsen, M. K., Abernethy, A. P., . . . Tulsky, J. A. (2007). Oncologist communication about emotion during visits with patients with advanced cancer. *Journal of Clinical Oncology, 25,* 5748–5752.

Street, R. L., & Haidet, P. (2011). How well do doctors know their patients? Factors affecting physician understanding of patients' health beliefs. *Journal of General Internal Medicine, 26*(1), 21–27.

CHAPTER 6

Miller, W. R., & Rollnick, S. (1991). *Motivational interviewing: Preparing people to change addictive behavior.* New York, NY: Guilford Press.

Miller, W. R., & Rollnick, S. (2013). *Motivational interviewing: Helping people change.* (3rd ed.). New York, NY: Guilford Press.

CHAPTER 7

Dew, M. A., DiMartini, A. F., DeVito Dabbs, A. J., Zuckoff, A., Tan, H. P., McNulty, M. L., . . . Humar, A. (2013). Preventive intervention for living donor psychosocial outcomes: Feasibility and efficacy in a randomized controlled trial. *American Journal of Transplantation, 13,* 2672–2684.

Miller, W. R., & Rollnick, S. (2013). *Motivational interviewing: Helping people change.* (3rd ed.). New York, NY: Guilford Press.

CHAPTER 8

Adams, J., & Murray, R. (1998). The difficult diagnosis: The general approach to the difficult patient. *Emergency Medicine Clinics of North America, 16,* 689–700.

Boyle, G., Fr. (2010). *Tattoos on the heart: The power of boundless compassion.* New York, NY: Free Press.

Butler, C. C., & Evans, M. (1999). The "heartsink" patient revisited. The Welsh Philosophy and General Practice Discussion Group. *British Journal of General Practice, 49,* 230–233.

Epstein, R. M. (1999). Mindful practice. *Journal of the American Medical Association, 282,* 833–839.

Gaba, D. M., & Howard, S. K. (2002). Patient safety: Fatigue among clinicians and the safety of patients. *New England Journal of Medicine, 347*, 1249–1255.

Groves, J. E. (1978). Taking care of the hateful patient. *New England Journal of Medicine, 298*(16), 883–887.

Haas, L. J., Leiser, J. P., Magill, M. K., & Sanyer, O. N. (2005). Management of the difficult patient. *American Family Physician, 72*(10), 2063–2068.

Hull, S. K., & Broquet, K. (2007). How to manage difficult patient encounters. *Family Practice Management, 14*(6), 30–34.

Jackson, J. L., & Kroenke, K. (1999). Difficult patient encounters in the ambulatory clinic: Clinical predictors and outcomes. *Archives of Internal Medicine, 159*, 1069–1075.

Mathers, N., Jones, N., & Hannay, D. (1995). Heartsink patients: A study of their general practitioner, *British Journal of General Practice, 45*(395), 293–296.

Miller, W. R., & Rollnick, S. (2013). *Motivational interviewing: Helping people change* (3rd ed.). New York, NY: Guilford Press.

Robinson, G., Beasley, R., & Aldington, S. (2006). From medical student to junior doctor: The difficult patient *Student British Medical Journal, 14*, 265–308.

Shea, S. C. (1998). *Psychiatric interviewing: The art of understanding* (2nd ed.). Philadelphia, PA: Saunders.

Steinmetz, D., & Tabenkin, H. (2001). The difficult patient as perceived by family physicians. *Family Practice, 18*, 495–500.

Winnicott, D. W. (1949). Hate in the countertransference. *International Journal of Psychoanalysis, 30*, 69–74.

Wilson, H. (2005). Reflecting on the difficult patient. *Journal of the New Zealand Medical Association, 118*(1212), U1384.

CHAPTER 9

Academic ED SBIRT Research Collaborative. (2010). The impact of screening, brief intervention and referral for treatment in emergency department patients' alcohol use: A 3-, 6- and 12-month follow-up. *Alcohol Alcohol, 45*(6), 514–519.

Accreditation Council for Graduate Medical Education (ACGME). (2007). New program requirements. Effective July 1, 2007. ACGME, Chicago IL.

Aubrey, L. L. (1998). *Motivational interviewing with adolescents presenting for outpatient substance abuse treatment*. Unpublished Ph.D. dissertation. University of New Mexico, Albuquerque, NM.

Beauchamp, T. L., & Childress, J. F. (2009). *Principles of biomedical ethics*. New York, NY: Oxford University Press.

Bell, K. R., Temkin, N. R., Esselman, P. C., Doctor, J. N., Bombardier, C. H., Fraser, R. T., … Dikmen, S. (2005). The effect of a scheduled telephone intervention on outcome after moderate to severe traumatic brain injury: A randomized trial. *Archives of Physical Medicine and Rehabilitation, 86*(5), 851–856.

Bernstein, E., & Bernstein, J. (2008). Effectiveness of alcohol screening and brief motivational intervention in the emergency department setting. *Annals of Emergency Medicine, 51*(6), 751–754.

Bernstein, E., Bernstein, J., & Levenson, S. (1997). Project ASSERT: An ED-based intervention to increase access to primary care, preventive services, and the substance abuse treatment system. *Annals of Emergency Medicine, 30*(2), 181–189.

Bernstein, J., Bernstein, E., Tassiopoulos, K., Heeren, T., Levenson, S., & Hingson, R. (2005). Brief motivational intervention at a clinic visit reduces cocaine and heroin use. *Drug and Alcohol Dependence, 77*(1), 49–59.

Beutler, L. E., & Harwood, T. M. (2002). What is and can be attributed to the therapeutic relationship? *Journal of Contemporary Psychotherapy, 32*, 25–33.

Bien, T. H., Miller, W. R., & Tonigan, S. (1993). Brief interventions for alcohol problems: A review. *Addiction, 88*, 315–336.

Burke, B. L., Arkowitz, H., & Menchola, M. (2003). The efficacy of motivational interviewing: A meta-analysis of controlled clinical trials. *Journal of Consulting and Clinical Psychology, 71*, 843–861.

DiClemente, C. C. (2003). *Addiction and change: How addictions develop and addicted people recover.* New York, NY: Guilford Press.

Engle, D. E., & Arkowitz, H. (2006). *Ambivalence in psychotherapy: Facilitating readiness to change.* New York, NY: Guilford Press.

Erickson, S. J., Gerstle, M., & Feldstein, S. W. (2005). Brief interventions and motivational interviewing with children, adolescents, and their parents in pediatric health care settings: A review. *Archives of Pediatric and Adolescent Medicine, 159*(12), 1173–1180.

Gentilello, L. M., Ebel, B. E., Wickizer, T. M., Salkever, D. S., & Rivara, F. P. (2005). Alcohol interventions for trauma patients treated in emergency departments and hospitals: A cost benefit analysis. *Annals of Surgery, 241*(4), 541–550.

Gentilello, L. M., Rivara, F. P., Donovan, D. M., Jurkovich, G. J., Daranciang, E., Dunn, C. W., et al. (1999). Alcohol interventions in a trauma center as a means of reducing the risk of injury recurrence. *Annals of Surgery, 230*(40), 473–483.

Handmaker, N. S., Miller, W. R., & Manicke, M. (1999). Findings of a pilot study of motivational interviewing with pregnant drinkers. *Journal of Studies on Alcohol, 60*, 285–287.

Heather, N. (1996). The public health and brief interventions for alcohol consumption: The British experience. *Addictive Behaviors, 21*, 857–868.

Heather, N., Rollnick, S., Bell, A., & Richmond, R. (1996). Effects of brief counselling among male heavy drinkers identified on general hospital wards. *Drug and Alcohol Review, 15*(1), 29–38.

Hettema, J., Steele, J., & Miller, W. (2005). Motivational interviewing. *Annual Review of Clinical Psychology, 1*, 91–111.

Humeniuk, R., Henry-Edwards, S., Ali, R., Poznyak, V., & Monteiro, M. (2010). *Brief intervention. The ASSIST-linked brief intervention for hazardous and harmful substance use: Manual for use in primary care.* Geneva, Switzerland: WHO Press.

Institute of Medicine. (2001). *Crossing the quality chasm: A new health system for the 21st century.* Washington, DC: NIH.

Iyengar, S. S., & Lepper, M. R. (2000). When choice is demotivating: Can one desire too much of a good thing? *Journal of Personality and Social Psychology, 79*, 995–1006.

Kelly, T. M., Daley, D. C., & Douaihy, A. B. (2012). Treatment of substance abusing patients with comorbid psychiatric disorders. *Addictive Behaviors, 37*, 11–24.

Koerber, A., Crawford, J., & O'Connell, K. (2003). The effects of teaching dental students brief motivational interviewing for smoking-cessation counseling: A pilot study. *Journal of Dental Education, 67*(4), 439–447.

Kushner, R. F. (1995). Barriers to providing nutrition counseling by physicians: A survey of primary care practitioners. *Preventive Medicine, 24*(6), 546–552.

Longabaugh, R., Woolard, R. F., Nirenberg, T. D., Minugh, A. P., Becker, B., Clifford, P. R., … Gogineni, A. (2001). Evaluating the effects of a brief motivational intervention for injured drinkers in the emergency department. *Journal of Studies on Alcohol, 62*(6), 806–816.

Lundahl, B., & Burke, B. L. (2009). The effectiveness and applicability of motivational interviewing: A practice-friendly review of four meta-analyses. *Journal of Clinical Psychology, 65*(11), 1232–1245.

Lundahl, B. W., Kunz, C., Brownell, C., Tollefson, D., & Burke, B. (2010). Meta-analysis of motivational interviewing: Twenty five years of empirical studies. *Research on Social Work Practice, 20,* 137–160.

Medical Professionalism Project: ABIM Foundation. (2002). Medical professionalism in the new millennium: A physician charter. *Annals of Internal Medicine, 136*(3), 243–246.

Miller, W. R. (1983). Motivational interviewing with problem drinkers. *Behavioural Psychotherapy. 11,* 147–172.

Miller, W. R., Benefield, R. G., & Tonigan, J. S. (1993). Enhancing motivation for change in problem drinking: A controlled comparison of two therapist styles. *Journal of Consulting and Clinical Psychology, 61,* 455–461.

Miller, W. R., & Moyers, T. B. (2006). Eight stages in learning motivational interviewing. *Journal of Teaching in the Addictions, 5*(1), 3–17.

Miller, W. R., & Rollnick, S. (1995). What is motivational interviewing? *Behavioural and Cognitive Psychotherapy, 23,* 325–334.

Miller, W. R., & Rollnick, S. (2009). Ten things that motivational interviewing is not. *Behavioural and Cognitive Psychotherapy, 37,* 129–140.

Miller, W. R., & Rollnick, S. (2013). *Motivational interviewing: Helping people change* (3rd ed.). New York, NY: Guilford Press.

Miller, W. R., & Sanchez, V. C. (1994). Motivating young adults for treatment and life-style. In G. S. Howard & P. E. Nathan (Eds.), *Alcohol use and misuse by young adults* (pp. 55–81). Notre Dame, IN: University of Notre Dame Press.

Mokdad, A., Marks, K., Stroup, D., & Gerberding, J. (2004). Actual causes of death in the United States, 2000. *Journal of the American Medical Association, 291,* 1238–1245.

Monti, P. M., Barnett, N. P., Colby, S. M., Gwaltney, C. J., Spirito, A., Rohsenow, D. J., & Woolard, R. (2007). Motivational interviewing versus feedback only in emergency care for young adult problem drinking. *Addiction, 102*(8), 1234–1243.

Monti, P. M., Colby, S. M., Barnett, N. P., Spirito, A., Rohsenow, D. J., Myers, M., et al. (1999). Brief intervention for harm reduction with alcohol-positive older adolescents in a hospital emergency department. *Journal of Consulting and Clinical Psychology, 67*(6), 989–994.

Neighbors, C. J., Barnett, N. P., Rohsenow, D. J., Colby, S. M., & Monti, P. M. (2010). Cost-effectiveness of a motivational intervention for alcohol-involved youth in a hospital emergency department. *Journal of Studies on Alcohol and Drugs, 71*(3), 384–394.

Nock, M. K., & Kazdin, A. E. (2005). Randomized controlled trial of a brief intervention for increasing participation in parent management training. *Journal of Consulting and Clinical Psychology, 73*(5), 872–879.

Norcross, J. C. (2002). *Psychotherapy relationships that work: Therapist contributions and responsiveness to patients.* New York, NY:Oxford University Press.

Patterson, G. R., & Forgatch, M. S. (1985). Therapist behavior as a determinant for client noncompliance: A paradox for the behavior modifier. *Journal of Consulting and Clinical Psychology, 53,* 846–851.

Project MATCH Research Group. (1998). Matching alcoholism treatments to client heterogeneity: Project MATCH three-year drinking outcomes. *Alcoholism: Clinical and Experimental Research, 23,* 1300–1311.

Rollnick, S., Mason, P., & Butler, C. (1999). *Health behavior change: A guide for practitioners.* New York, NY: Churchill Livingstone.

Rollnick, S., Miller, W. R., & Butler, C. C. (2008). *Motivational interviewing in health care: Helping patients change behavior.* New York, NY:Guilford Press.

Rubak, S., Sandbaek, A., Lauritzen, T., & Christensen, B. (2005). Motivational interviewing: A systematic review and meta-analysis. *British Journal of General Practice, 55*(513), 305–312.

Schermer, C. R., Moyers, T. B., Miller, W. R., & Bloomfield, L. A. (2006). Trauma center brief interventions for alcohol disorders decrease subsequent driving under the influence arrests. *Journal of Trauma, 60*(1), 29–34.

Senft, R. A., Polen, M. R., Freeborn, D. K., & Hollis, J. F. (1997). Brief intervention in a primary care setting for hazardous drinkers. *American Journal of Preventive Medicine, 13*(6), 464–470.

Soria, R., Legido, A., Escolano, C., Lopez Yeste, A., & Montoya, J. (2006). A randomised controlled trial of motivational interviewing for smoking cessation. *British Journal of General Practice, 56*(531), 768–774.

Spirito, A., Monti, P. M., Barnett, N. P., Colby, S. M., Sindelar, H., Rohsenow, D. J., ... Myers, M. (2004). A randomized clinical trial of a brief motivational intervention for alcohol-positive adolescents treated in an emergency department. *Pediatrics, 145*(3), 396–402.

Stotts, A. L., Schmitz, J. M., Rhoades, H. M., & Grabowski, J. (2001). Motivational interviewing with cocaine-dependent patients: A pilot study. *Journal of Consulting and Clinical Psychology, 69*(5), 858–862.

The Academic ED SBIRT Collaborative. (2007). An evidence-based alcohol ccreening, brief intervention and referral to treatment (SBIRT) curriculum for emergency department (ED) providers improves skills and utilization. *Substance Abuse, 28*(4), 79–92.

Valanis, B., Lichtenstein, E., Mullooly, J. P., Labuhn, K., Brody, K., Severson, H. H., & Stevens, N. (2001). Maternal smoking cessation and relapse prevention during health care visits. *American Journal of Preventive Medicine, 20*(1), 1–8.

Valanis, B., Whitlock, E. E., Mullooly, J., Vogt, T., Smith, S., Chen, C., & Glasgow, R. E. (2003). Screening rarely screened women: Time-to-service and 24-month outcomes of tailored interventions. *Preventive Medicine, 37*(5), 442–450.

Vansteenkiste, M., Williams, G. C., & Resnicow, K. (2012). Toward systematic integration between self-determination theory and motvational interviewing as examples of top-down and bottom-up intervention development: Autonomy or volition as a fundamental theoretical principle. *International Journal of Behavioral Nutrition and Physical Activity, 9,* 23.

Vasilaki, E., Hosier, S., & Cox, W. (2006). The efficacy of motivational interviewing as a brief intervention for excessive drinkings: A meta-analytic review. *Alcohol and Alcoholism, 41*(3), 328–335.

Wutzke, S. E., Shiell, A., Gomel, M. K., & Conigrave, K. M. (2001). Cost effectiveness of brief interventions for reducing alcohol consumption. *Social Science and Medicine, 52*(6), 863–870.

Yach, D., Hawkes, C., Gould, C., & Hoffman, K. (2004). The global burden of chronic diseases. *Journal of the American Medical Association, 291,* 2616–2622.

CHAPTER 10

Antiss, T. (2009). Motivational interviewing in primary care. *Journal of Clinical Psychology in Medical Settings, 16*(1), 87–93.

Bem, D. (1967). Self-perception: An alternative interpretation of cognitive dissonance phenomena. *Psychological Review, 74*(3), 183–200.

Bodenheimer, T., Wagner, E., & Grumbach, K. (2002). Improving primary care for patients with chronic illness: The chronic care model, Part 2. *Journal of the American Medical Association, 288*(15), 1909–1914.

Brug, J., Spikmans, F., Aartsen, C., Breedveld, B., Bes, R., & Ferieria, L. (2007). Training dietitians in basic motivational interviewing skills results in changes in their counseling style and in lower saturated fat intakes in their patients. *Journal of Nutrition Education and Behavior, 39*(1), 8–12.

Duffey, K. J., & Popkin, B. M. (2007). Shifts in patterns and consumption of beverages between 1965 and 2002. *Obesity, 15*(11), 2739–2747.

Hettema, J., Steele, J., & Miller, W. (2005). Motivational interviewing. *Annual Review of Clinical Psychology, 1*, 91–111.

Iyengar, S. S., & Lepper, M. R. (2000). When choice is demotivating: Can one desire too much of a good thing? *Journal of Personality and Social Psychology, 79*, 995–1006.

Lundahl, B., & Burke, B. L. (2009). The effectiveness and applicability of motivational interviewing: A practice-friendly review of four meta-analyses. *Journal of Clinical Psychology, 65*(11), 1232–1245.

Lundahl, B. W., Kunz, C., Brownell, C., Tollefson, D., & Burke, B. (2010). Meta-analysis of motivational interviewing: Twenty five years of empirical studies. *Research on Social Work Practice, 20*, 137–160.

Miller, W. R. (1983). Motivational interviewing with problem drinkers. *Behavioura Psychotherapy, 11*, 147–172.

Miller, W. R., & Rollnick, S. (2009). Ten things that motivational interviewing is not. *Behavioural and Cognitive Psychotherapy, 37*, 129–140.

Miller, W. R., & Rollnick, S. (2013). *Motivational interviewing: Helping people change* (3rd ed.). New York, NY: Guilford Press.

Miller, W. R., & Rose, G. S. (2009). Toward a theory of motivational interviewing. *American Psychologist, 64*(6), 527–537.

Miller, W. R., Yahne, C. E., Moyers, T. B., Martinez, J., & Pirritano, M. (2004). A randomized trial of methods to help clinicians learn motivational interviewing. *Journal of Counseling and Clinical Psychology, 16*(6), 1050–1062.

Moller, A. C., Deci, E. L., & Ryan, R. M. (2006). Choice and ego-depletion: The moderating role of autonomy. *Personality and Social Psychology Bulletin, 32*(8), 1024–1036.

Vansteenkiste, M., Williams, G. C., & Resnicow, K. (2012). Toward systematic integratino between self-determination theory and motvational interviewing as examples of top-down and bottom-up intervention development: Autonomy or volition as a fundamental theoretical principle. *International Journal of Behavioral Nutrition and Physical Activity, 9*, 23.

Wagner, E., Davis, C., Schaefer, J., Von Korff, M., & Austin, B. (1999). A survey of leading chronic disease management programs: Are they consistent with the literature? *Managed Care Quarterly, 7*(3), 56–66.

Wang, Y. C., Bleich, S. N., & Gortmaker, S. L. (2008). Increasing caloric contribution from sugar-sweetened beverages and 100% fruit juices among US children and adolescents, 1988–2004. *Pediatrics, 121*(6), e1604–e1614.

CHAPTER 11

Barnes, A. J., & Gold, M. A. (2012). Promoting healthy behaviors in pediatrics: Motivational interviewing. *Pediatrics in Review, 33*(9), e57–68.

Brown, R. A., Ramsey, S. E., Strong, D. R., Myers, M. G., Kahler, C. W, … Abrams, D. B. (2003). Effects of motivational interviewing on smoking cessation in adolescents with psychiatric disorders. *Tobacco Control, 12*(Suppl 4), IV3–10.

Channon, S. J., Huws-Thomas, M. V., Rollnick, S., Hood, K., Cannings-John, R. L., Rogers, C., & Gregory, J. W. (2007). A multicenter randomized controlled trial of motivational interviewing in teenagers with diabetes. *Diabetes Care, 30*(6), 1390–1395.

Duff, A. J., & Latchford, G. J. (2010). Motivational interviewing for adherence problems in cystic fibrosis. *Pediatric Pulmonology, 45*(3), 211–220.

Erickson, S. J., Gerstle, M., & Feldstein, S. W. (2005). Brief interventions and motivational interviewing with children, adolescents, and their parents in pediatric care settings. *Archives of Pediatrics and Adolescent Medicine, 159,* 1173–1180.

Gold, M. A., & Delisi, K. (2008). Motivational interviewing and sexual and contraceptive behaviors. *Adolescent Medicine: State of the Art Reviews, 19,* 69–82.

Gold, M. A., & Kokotailo, P. K. (2007). Motivational interviewing. *Adolescent Health Update, American Academy of Pediatrics, 20*(1), 1–10.

Hagen, J. F., Shaw, J. S., & Duncan, P. M. (2008). *Bright futures: Guidelines for health supervision of infants, children, and adolescents* (3rd ed.). Elk Grove Village, IL: American Academy of Pediatrics.

Kelly, T. M., & Bukstein, O. G. (2004). Evaluation and treatment of substance use problems among adolescents in emergency departments. *Clinical Pediatric Emergency Medicine, 5*(3), 164–172.

Kokotailo, P. K., & Gold, M. A. (2008). Motivational interviewing with adolescents. *Adolescent Medicine: State of the Art Reviews, 19,* 54–68.

Miller, W. R., & Rollnick, S. (2013). *Motivational interviewing: Helping people change* (3rd ed.). New York, NY: Guilford Press.

Monti, P. M., Colby, S. M., Barnett, N. P., Spirito, A., Rohsenow, D. J., . . . Lewander, W. (1999). Brief intervention for harm reduction with alcohol-positive older adolescents in a hospital emergency department. *Journal of Consulting and Clinical Psychology, 67*(6), 989–994.

Naar-King, S., & Suarez, M. (2011). *Motivational interviewing with adolescents and young adults.* New York, NY: Guilford Press.

Olson, A. L., Gaffney, C. A., Lee, P. W., & Starr, P. (2008). Changing adolescent health behaviors: The healthy teens counseling approach. *American Journal of Preventive Medicine, 35*(5S), S359–S364.

Resnicow, K., Davis, R., & Rollick, S. (2006). Motivational interviewing for pediatric obesity: Conceptual issues and evidence review. *Journal of the American Dietetic Association, 106,* 2024–2033

Rollnick, S., Miller, W. R., & Butler, C. (2008). *Motivational interviewing in health care: helping patients change behavior.* New York, NY: Guilford Press.

Suarez, M., & Mullins, S. (2008). Motivational interviewing and pediatric health behavior interventions. *Journal of Developmental & Behavioral Pediatrics, 29*(5), 417–428.

Teixeira, P. J., Silva, M. N., Mata, J., Palmeira, A. L., & Markland, D. (2012). Motivation, self-determination, and long-term weight control. *International Journal of Behavioral Nutrition and Physical Activity, 9,* 22.

Walpole, B., Dettmer, E., Morrongiello, B., McCrindle, B., & Hamilton, J. (2011). Motivational interviewing as an intervention to increase adolescent self-efficacy and promote weight loss: Methodology and design. *BMC Public Health, 11,* 459.

CHAPTER 12

Heru, A. M. (2006). Family psychiatry: From research to practice. *American Journal of Psychiatry, 163*(6), 962–968.

Miller, W. R., & Rollnick, S. (2013). *Motivational interviewing: Helping people change.* (3rd ed.). New York, NY: Guilford Press.

Rey, J., & Birmaher, B. (2009). Using family therapy. In *Treating child and adolescent depression* (pp. xx–xx). Baltimore, MD: Lippincott Williams & Welkins.

Stanton, M. D. (1981). Strategic approaches to family therapy. In A. S. Gurman & D. P. Kniskern (Eds.), *Handbook of family therapy* (pp. xx–xx). New York, NY: Brunner/Mazel.

Sussman, C., Khatkhate, G., Tavares, A., Johnson, K., Rivera, M., Miller, M. D., Douaihy, A. (2008). Psychotherapy. In D. Kupfer, M. Horner, D, Brent, D. Lewis, C. Reynolds, M. Thase, M. Travis. (Eds.), *Oxford American handbook of psychiatry* (pp. 98–102). New York, NY: Oxford University Press.

Walsh, F. (2003). Family resilience: A framework for clinical practice. *Family Process, 42*, 1.

CHAPTER 13

Screening

Screening for Unhealthy Alcohol Use

Babor, T. F., & Kadden, R. M. (2005). Screening and interventions for alcohol and drug problems in medical settings: What works? *Journal of Trauma, 59*(3), S80–S87.

Ballesteros, J., Duffy, J. C., Querejeta, I., Ariño, J., & González-Pinto, A. (2004). Efficacy of brief interventions for hazardous drinkers in primary care: Systematic review and meta-analyses. *Alcoholism, Clinical and Experimental Research, 28*(4), 608–618.

Bien, T. H., Miller, W. R., & Tonigan, J. S. (1993). Brief interventions for alcohol problems: A review. *Addiction, 88*, 315–335.

Canagasaby, A., & Vinson, D. C. (2005). Screening for hazardous or harmful drinking using one or two quantity-frequency questions. *Alcohol and Alcoholism, 40*(3), 208–213.

Miller, W. R., & Sanchez, V. C. (1994). Motivating young adults for treatment and lifestyle change. In G. Howard (Ed.), *Issues in alcohol use and misuse by young adults* (pp. 55–82). Notre Dame, IN: University of Notre Dame Press.

Sexual Behaviors

Berg, R. C., Ross, M. W., & Tikkanen, R. (2011). The effectiveness of MI4MSM: How useful is motivational interviewing as an HIV risk prevention program for men who have sex with men? A systematic review. *AIDS Education and Prevention, 23*(6), 533–549.

Koblin, B., Chesney, M., Coates, T., EXPLORE Study Team. (2004). Effects of a behavioural intervention to reduce acquisition of HIV infection among men who have sex with men: The EXPLORE randomized controlled study. *Lancet, 364*, 41–50

Lundhal, B. W., Kunz, C., et al. (2010). A meta-analysis of motivational interviewing: Twenty five of empirical studies. *Research on Social Work Practice, 20*(2), 137–160.

Chronic Pain

Douaihy, A. B., Jensen, M. P., & Jou, R. J. (2005). Motivating behavior change in patients with chronic pain. In B. McCarberg, S. D. Passik (Eds.), *Expert guide to pain management* (pp. 217–229). Philadelphia, PA: American College of Physicians.

Fahey, K. F., Rao, S. M., Douglas, M. K., Thomas, M. L., Elliott, J. E., & Miaskowski, C. (2008). Nurse coaching to explore and modify patient attitudinal barriers interfering with effective cancer pain management. *Oncology Nursing Forum, 35*(2), 233–240.

Habib, S., Morrissey, S., & Helmes, E. (2005). Preparing for pain management: A pilot study to enhance engagement. *Journal of Pain, 6*, 48–54.

Jensen, M., Nielson, W., & Kerns, R. (2003). Toward the development of a motivational model of pain self-management. *Journal of Pain, 4*, 477–492.

Molton, I. R., Jensen, M. P., Nielson, W., Cardenas, D., & Ehde, D. M. (2008). A preliminary evaluation of the motivational model of pain self-management in persons with spinal cord injury-related pain. *Journal of Pain, 9*(7), 606–612.

Osborne, T. L., Raichle, A. K., & Jensen, M. P. (2006). Psychologic interventions for chronic pain. *Physical Medicine and Rehabilitation Clinics in North America, 17*, 415–433.

Eating Disorders

Armstrong, M. J., Mottershead, T. A., Ronksley, P. E., Sigal, R. J., Campbell, T. S., & Hemmelgarn, B. R. (2011). Motivational interviewing to improve weight loss in overweight and or obese patients: A systematic review and meta-analysis of randomized controlled trials. *Obesity Reviews, 12*(9), 709–723.

Brewell-Weiss, C., & Mills, J. (2009). *Motivational interviewing as a prelude to intensive eating disorder treatment.* Paper presented at the Annual Meeting of the Eating Disorder Research Society, Brooklyn, NY, Sept. 24–26, 2009.

MacDonald, P., Hibbs, R., Corfield, F., & Treasure, J. (2012). The use of motivational interviewing in eating disorders: A systematic review. *Psychiatric Research, 200*, 1–11.

Hardcastle, S. J., Taylor, A. H., Bailey, M. P., Harley, R. A., & Hagger, M. S. (2013). Effectiveness of a motivational interviewing intervention on weight loss, physical activity, and cardiovascular disease risk factors: A randomized controlled trail with a 12-month post intervention follow-up. *International Journal of Behavioral Nutrition and Physical Activity, 10*(40), 1–16.

Substance Use in Pregnancy

American College of Obstetricians and Gynecologists. (2006). *Drinking and reproductive health: A fetal alcohol spectrum disorders prevention tool kit.* Retrieved February 2014, from http://mail.ny.acog.org/website/FASDToolKit.pdf.

Floyd, R. L., Sobell, M., Velasquez, M. M., Ingersoll, K., Nettleman, M., Sobell, L., ... Project CHOICES Efficacy Study Group. (2007). Preventing alcohol-exposed pregnancies: A randomized controlled trial. Project CHOICES Efficacy Study Group. *American Journal of Preventive Medicine, 32*, 1–10.

Hettema, J. E., & Hendricks, P. S. (2010). Motivational interviewing for smoking cessation: A meta-analytic review. *Journal of Consulting and Clinical Psychology, 78*(6), 868–884.

Palliative Care

deHaes, H., & Teunissen, S. (2005). Communication in palliative care: A review of recent literature. *Current Opinions in Oncology, 17*(4), 345–350.

Miller, W. R., & Rollnick, S. (2013). *Motivational Interviewing: Helping people change* (3rd ed.). New York, NY: Guilford Press.

Pollak, K. I., Childers, J. W. & Arnold, R. M. (2011). Applying motivational interviewing techniques to palliative care communication. *Journal of Palliative Medicine, 14*(5), 587–592.

Psychiatric Disorders

Arkowitz, H., & Burke, B. L. (2008). Motivational interviewing as an integrative framework for the treatment of depression. In H. Arkowitz, H. A. Westra, W. R. Miller, & S. Rollnick (Eds.), *Motivational interviewing in the treatment of psychological problems* (pp.145–172). New York, NY: Guilford Press.

Britton, P. C., Patrick, H., Wenzel, A. Williams, G. C. (2011). Integrating motivational interviewing and self-determination theory with cognitive behavioral therapy to prevent suicide. *Cognitive and Behavioral Practice, 18*(1), 16–27.

Burke, B. L. (2011). What can motivational interviewing do for you? *Cognitive and Behavioral Practice, 18*, 74–81.

Flynn, H. A. (2011). Setting the stage for the integration of motivational interviewing and cognitive behavioral therapy in the treatment of depression. *Cognitive and Behavioral Practice, 18*, 46–54.

Simpson, H. B., & Zuckoff, A. (2011). Using motivational interviewing to enhance treatment outcome in people with obsessive compulsive disorder. *Cognitive and Behavioral Practice, 18*, 28–37.

Westra, H. A., Aviram, A., & Doell, F. K. (2011). Extending motivational interviewing to the treatment of major mental health problems: Current directions and evidence. *Canadian Journal of Psychiatry, 56*(11), 643–650.

Substance Use Disorders

Daley, D. C., & Zuckoff, A. (1999). *Improving treatment compliance: Counseling and systems strategies for substance abuse and dual disorders.* Center City, MN: Hazelden.

Daeppen, J. B., Bertholet, N., & Gaume, J. (2010). What process research tells us about brief intervention efficacy. *Drug and Alcohol Review, 29*, 612–616.

Hettema, J., Steele, J., & Miller, W. R. (2005). Motivational interviewing. *Annual Review of Clinical Psychology, 1*, 91–111.

Landhal, B. W., & Burke, B. L. (2009). The effectiveness and applicability of motivational interviewing: A practice-friendly review of four meta-analyses. *Journal of Clinical Psychology, 65*, 1232–1245.

Smedslund, G., Berg, R. C., Hammerstrøm, K. T., Steiro, A., Leiknes, K. A., Dahl, H. M., & Karlsen, K. (2011). Motivational interviewing for substance abuse. *Cochrane Database of Systematic Reviews* (5): CD008063.

Chapter 14

Institute of Medicine. (1991). *The computer-based patient record: An essential technology for health care.* (R. S. Dick & E. B. Steen, Eds.). Washington, DC: National Academy Press.

Institute of Medicine. (1997). *The computer-based patient record: An essential technology for health care* (Rev. ed., R. S. Dick, E. B. Steen, & D. E. Detmer, Eds.). Washington, DC: National Academy Press.

Makoul, G. (2001). The SEGUE framework for teaching and assessing communications skills. *Patient Education and Counseling, 45*, 23–34.

Makoul, G. (2003). The interplay between education and research about patient-provider communication. *Patient Education and Counseling, 50*, 79–84.

McGrath, J. M., Arar, N. H., & Pugh, J. A. (2007). The influence of electronic medical record usage on nonverbal communication in the medical interview. *Health Informatics, 13*(2), 105–118.

Brendtsen, P., Johansson, K., & Akerlind, I. (2006). Feasibility of an email-based electronic screening and brief intervention (e-SBI) to college students in Sweden. *Addiction Behavior, 31*(5), 777–787.

Walker, J., Ahern, D., Le, L. X., & Deblanco, T. (2009). Insights for internists: "I want the computer to know who I am". *Journal of General Internal Medicine, 24*, 727–732.

Amrhein, P. C., Miller, W. R., Yahne, C. E., Palmer, M., & Fulcher, L. (2003). Patient commitment language during motivational interviewing predicts drug use outcomes. *Journal of Consulting and Clinical Psychology, 71,* 862–878.

Aspegren, K. (1999). BEME Guide No 2. Teaching and learning communication skills in medicine- a review with quality grading of articles. *Medical Teacher, 21,* 563–570.

Dunn, C., DeRoo, L., & Rivera, F. P. (2001). The use of brief interventions adapted from motivational interviewing across behavioural domains: A systematic review. *Addiction, 96,* 1725–1742.

Dweck, C. (2012). *Mindset: How you can fulfill your potential.* London, U.K.: Constable and Robinson.

Falender, C. A., & Shafranske, E. P. (2007). Competence in competency-based supervision: Construct and application. *Professional Psychology: Research and Practice, 38,* 232–240.

Forsberg, L., Berman, A. H., Kallmen, H., Hermansson, U., & Helgason, A. R. (2008). A test of the validity of motivational interviewing integrity code. *Cognitive Behavioral Therapy, 37,* 183–191.

Kurtz, S., Silverman, J., & Draper, J. (1998). *Teaching and learning communication skills in medicine.* Abingdon, UK: Radcliffe Medical.

Lane, C., Huws-Thomas, M., Hood, K., Rollnick, S., Edwards, K., & Robling, K. (2005). Measuring adaptations of motivational interviewing: The development and validation of the behavior change counseling index (BECCI). *Patient Education and Counseling, 56,* 166–173.

Lane, C., Hood, K., & Rollnick, S. (2008). Teaching motivational interviewing: Using role play is as effective as simulated patients. *Medical Education, 42,* 637–644.

Madison, M. D., Loignon, A. C., & Lane, C. (2009). Training in motivational interviewing: A systematic review. *Journal of Substance Abuse Treatment, 36,* 101–109.

Martino, S., Haeseler, F., Belitsky, R., Pantalon, M., & Fortin, A. H. (2007). Teaching brief motivational interviewing to year three medical students. *Medical Education, 41,* 160–167.

Miller, W. R. (2004). Motivational interviewing in service to health promotion. *American Journal of Health Promotion, 18*(3), A1–A10.

Miller, W. R., Hendrick, K. E., & Orlofsky, D. R. (1991). The Helpful Responses Questionnaire: A procedure for measuring therapeutic empathy. *Journal of Clinical Psychology, 47*(3), 444–448.

Miller, W. R., & Mount, K. A. (2001). A small study of training in motivational interviewing: Does one workshop change clinician and patient behavior? *Behavioural and Cognitive Psychotherapy, 29,* 457–471.

Miller, W. R., & Moyers, T. B. (2006). Eight stages in learning motivational interviewing. *Journal of Teaching in the Addictions, 5*(1), 3–17.

Miller, W. R., & Rollnick, S. (2002). *Motivational interviewing: Preparing people for change* (2nd ed.). New York, NY: Guilford Press.

Miller, W. R., & Rollnick, S. (2013). *Motivational interviewing: Helping people change* (3rd ed.). New York, NY: Guildford Press.

Miller, W. R., Yahne, C. E., Moyers, T. B., Martinez, J., & Pirritano, M. (2004). A randomized trial of methods to help clinicians learn motivational interviewing. *Journal of Counseling and Clinical Psychology, 72,* 1050–1062.

Motivational Interviewing Network of Trainers (MINT). (2012). About MINT. Retrieved February 2014, from http://www.motivationalinterviewing.org/about_mint.

Mounsey, A. L., Bovbjerg, V., White, L., & Gazewood, J. (2006). Do students develop better motivational interviewing skills through role-play with standardized patients or with student colleagues? *Medical Education, 40,* 775–780.

Moyers, T. B., Martin, T., Manuel, J. K., Miller, W. R., & Ernst, D. (2009). *The motivational interviewing treatment integrity (MITI) code: Version 3.1.1.* Albuquerque, NM: University of New Mexico.

Moyers, T. B., Miller, W. R., & Hendrickson, S. M. L. (2005). What makes motivational interviewing work? Therapist interpersonal skills as a predictor of patient involvement within motivational interviewing sessions. *Journal of Consulting and Clinical Psychology, 73*(4), 590–598.

Papadakis, M. A., Croughan-Minihane, M., Fromm, L. J., Wilkie, H. A., & Ernester, V. L. (1997). A comparison of two methods to teach smoking-cessation techniques to medical students. *Academic Medicine, 72,* 725–727.

Poirier, M. K., Clark, M. M., Cerhan, J. H., Pruthi, S., Geda, Y. E., & Dale, L. C. (2004). Teaching motivational interviewing to first year medical students to improve counseling skills in health behaviour change. *Mayo Clin Proceedings, 79,* 327–331.

Rubak, S., Sandbaek, A., Lauritzen, T., Borch-Johnsen, K., & Christensen, B. (2009). General practitioners trained in motivational interviewing can positively affect the attitude to behavior change in people with type 2 diabetes. *Scandinavian Journal of Primary Health Care, 29,* 213–218.

Soderlung, L. L., Madson, M. B., Rubak, S., & Nilsen, P. (2011). A systematic review of motivational interviewing training for general healthcare practitioners. *Patient Education and Counseling, 84,* 16–26.

Thomson O'Brien, M., Freemantle, N., Oxman, A., Wolf, F., Davis, D., & Herrin, J. (2001). Continuing education meetings and workshops: Effects on professional practice and health care outcomes. *Cochrane Database of Systematic Reviews* (1): 1–31.

CHAPTER 16

Miller, W. R., & Rollnick, S. (2013). *Motivational interviewing: Helping people change* (3rd ed.). New York, NY: Guilford Press.

VIDEOS

Can Listening Save Time? A Story from Dr Dr Ng Min Yin. 8-minute video with Dr. Ng and Stephen Rollnick. Video link: http://vimeo.com/67088727

Alaina: 13-year-old with Nail-biting. Video of 10-minute primary care office visit, illustrating MI principles discussed in the journal article: Barnes, A. J., & Gold, M. A. (2012). Promoting healthy behaviors in pediatrics: Motivational interviewing. *Pediatrics in Review, 33*(9), e57-68). Video link: http://link.brightcove.com/services/player/bcpid15 55958052001?bckey=AQ~~,AAABNTGpvPE~,4qE3VldHW5YmHnFjijevknrzxpJlgs3 F&bctid=1802805262001 Transcript available at: http://pedsinreview.aappublications. org/content/33/9/e57/suppl/DC1

Motivational interviewing: Helping people change. (W. R. Miller, T. B. Moyers, & S. Rollnick). This two-part DVD set, or streaming video package, offers a detailed illustration of Motivational Interviewing, based on the revised and updated *Motivational Interviewing, 3rd edition* (2013). This material introduces the new four-process method of Motivational Interviewing. The DVD includes over 6 hours of video material, including a discussion between Drs. William R. Miller, Theresa B. Moyers and Stephen Rollnick, as well as 14 example interviews using MI to illustrate real-world applications. Video link: http://www.changecompanies.net/motivational_interviewing.php

Motivational Interviewing—An MI learning Resource: The first 15 minutes. This resource includes interviews with accomplished trainers, knowledgeable researchers and skilled practitioners covering a wide range of topics. Along with learning about MI, the DVDs include demonstrations of MI sessions in the areas of addiction, mental health, corrections and health care. Based on the research, practice and wisdom of William Miller & Stephen Rollnick. Video link: http://www.youtube.com/watch?v=cPd1aLOfwF4

The Effective Physician: MI Demonstration. Demonstration of the motivational interviewing approach in a brief medical encounter. Produced by University of Florida Department of Psychiatry. Video link: http://www.youtube.com/watch?v=URiKA7CKtfc&feature=watch_response*The Effective Pharmacist: MI Demonstration.* Demonstration of the motivational interviewing approach to the practice of pharmacy. Produced by University of Florida Department of Psychiatry. Video link: http://www.youtube.com/watch?v=5UU63mfNnD4

The Effective Dentist: MI Demonstration. Demonstration of the motivational interviewing approach in the practice of dentistry. Produced by University of Florida Department of Psychiatry. Video link: http://www.youtube.com/watch?v=f8QSA_5PEFM

The Ineffective Physician: Non-Motivational Approach. Demonstration of confrontational patient counseling (to contrast with motivational interviewing approach). Produced by University of Florida Department of Psychiatry. Video link: http://www.youtube.com/watch?v=80XyNE89eCs

Motivational Interviewing—Evoking Commitment to Change. In this weight-loss video clip, the physician works together with the patient to develop a specific focus. The provider does this by asking open-ended questions, providing affirmation, using reflective listening and summarizing for the patients (OARS). He also helps the patient to scale the importance of the issue and the patient's confidence level for change behavior. Video Link: http://www.youtube.com/watch?v=dm-rJJPCuTE

Motivational Interviewing about STD Testing. Video of counselor and young woman. Video link: http://www.youtube.com/watch?v=c9x7w0kWApY

Motivational Interviewing (MI) for Addictions Video. Video with MI expert and trainer Cathy Cole. Video link: http://www.youtube.com/watch?v=EvLquWI8aqc&feature=c4-overview&playnext=1&list=TLu77M2bUv5M4

Motivational Interviewing: Facilitating Change across Boundaries. Dr. William R. Miller, one-hour lecture at Columbia University, 2009. Video Link: http://www.youtube.com/watch?v=6EeCirPyq2w

Culture and Change: Stage of Change Tasks and Cultural Competence. Dr. Carlo Clemente, one-hour lecture at Columbia University, 2009. Video Link: http://www.youtube.com/watch?v=Z79h0M8xW-o

Dr. Joel Porter presents at the 3rd International Symposium on Motivational Interviewing, Melbourne, Australia, 2013. Video Link: http://vimeo.com/69405688

Ken McMaster Interviews Daryl about Going Straight. In this demonstration of motivational interviewing, Ken McMaster interviews Daryl about change after release from prison. Video Link: http://vimeo.com/68899209

MI in Practice: The Chicago Interviews. Prof. William R. Miller demonstrates motivational interviewing. An international group of clinicians provide commentary. Video Link: http://vimeo.com/67456556

ICCS: How MI Helps. In this presentation, Rik Bes talks about the use of MI in improving communication skills between HCPs and their patients. Video Link: http://vimeo.com/65628987

Bill Miller on M-3. Prof. Miller speaks about the key changes, which make the third edition of the standard text on Motivational Interviewing such a unique and rich resource for anyone who is interested in MI. Video Link: http://vimeo.com/65379303

Motivational Interviewing Webinar (May 6, 2010). Presented by Chris Dunn, PhD and Kari Stephens, PhD. Video Link: http://vimeo.com/60488916

Introduction to Motivational Interviewing (MI) for Non-Clinicians—Session 1. (Hosted by Mid-America ATTC). This webinar will review the basics of MI and will provide an overview of the primary concepts. Video Link: http://vimeo.com/58551783

Introduction to Motivational Interviewing (MI) for Non-Clinicians—Session 2. (Hosted by Mid-America ATTC). Continuation of Session 1, reviewing the basics of MI and providing and overview of the primary concepts. Video Link: http://vimeo.com/59697208

MI Part I: Introduction to Motivational Interviewing (E. Stellon). Part 1 of 4-part series on Motivational Interviewing. Video Link: http://vimeo.com/52569942

MI Part II: Key Concepts of Motivational Interviewing (E. Stellon). Part 2 of 4-part series on Motivational Interviewing. Video Link: http://vimeo.com/52569940

MI Part III: Tools and Techniques for Motivational Interviewing (E. Stellon). Part 3 of 4-part series on Motivational Interviewing. Video Link: http://vimeo.com/52569941

MI Part IV: Motivational Interviewing Role Plays (E. Stellon). Part 4 of 4-part series on Motivational Interviewing. Video Link: http://vimeo.com/52695126

The Motivational Interviewing (MI) Journey: A New Nursing Practice Model. (Health Sciences Institute) Video Link: http://vimeo.com/44960683

Five Essential Strategies in Motivating Clients to Change. Dr. Marilyn Herie shares her "top 5" motivational strategies with an emphasis on practical tips and tools. Video Link: http://vimeo.com/37325847

Motivational Interviewing Role Play. In this unscripted role play, Dr. Stan Steindl demonstrates how MI can be used in time-limited settings to effect behavior change. Video Link: http://vimeo.com/37220976

Motivational Interviewing: An Introduction. (B. Matulich). The basic concepts of motivational interviewing. Video Link: http://www.youtube.com/watch?v=s3MCJZ7OGRk

Motivational Interviewing: Setting the Scene. (B. Matulich). Develop an understanding of empathic counseling skills, central to using this technique. Video Link: http://www.youtube.com/watch?v=aTe4LpGz_E

Motivational Interviewing: The Spirit and Principles. (B. Matulich). Learn when and how to use advice and other more directive elements of motivational interviewing. Video Link: http://www.youtube.com/watch?v=nim6211oaN4

Motivational Interviewing: Clients Arguing for Change—Introducing DARN-C—Desire, Ability, Reason, Need-Commitment. (B. Matulich). Learn when and how to use advice and other more directive elements of motivational interviewing. Video Link: http://www.youtube.com/watch?v=Pwu99NIGiXU

Motivational Interviewing: Core Clinician Skills—Introducing OARS—Open questions, Affirmations, Reflections, Summaries. (B. Matulich). Using MI to roll with resistance, resolve ambivalence, encourage change and commitment talk, and help people carry through changes in health behaviours. Video Link: http://www.youtube.com/watch?v=-zEpwxJlRQI

Motivational Interviewing: Recommendations and Conclusion (B. Matulich). Encourage change and commitment talk, and help people carry through changes in health behaviours. Video Link: http://www.youtube.com/watch?v=se7gJCjNo2Q

BOOKS

Arkowitz, H., Westra, H. A., Miller, W. R., & Rollnick, S. (Eds.). (2008). *Motivational interviewing in the treatment of psychological problems. Applications of motivational interviewing.* New York, NY: Guilford Press.

Berger, B. A., & Villaume, W. A. (2013). *Motivational Interviewing for Health Care Professionals*. Washington, DC: American Pharmacists Association.

Dart, M. A. (2011). *Motivational interviewing in nursing practice: Empowering the patient*. Sudbury, MA: Jones and Bartlett.

Fields, A. E. (2004). *Curriculum-based motivation group: A five session motivational interviewing group intervention*. Vancouver, WA: Hollifield Associates.

Fields, A. E. (2006). *Resolving patient ambivalence: A five-session motivational interviewing intervention*. Vancouver, WA: Hollifield Associates.

Fuller, C., & Taylor, P. (2008). *A toolkit of motivational skills: Encouraging and supporting change in individuals* (2nd ed.). Hoboken, NJ: Wiley.

Hohman, M. (2012). *Motivational interviewing in social work practice. Applications of motivational interviewing*. New York, NY: Guilford Press.

Matulich, B. (2013). *How to do motivational interviewing: A guidebook* (2nd ed.). San Diego, CA: Publisher Bill Matulich.

Miller, W. R., & Rollnick, S. (1991). *Motivational interviewing: Preparing people to change addictive behaviors*. New York, NY: Guilford Press.

Miller, W. R., & Rollnick, S. (2002). *Motivational interviewing: Preparing People for Change* (2nd ed.). New York, NY: Guilford Press.

Miller, W. R., & Rollnick, S. (2013). *Motivational interviewing: Helping People Change Applications of Motivational Interviewing*. (3rd ed.). New York, NY: Guilford Press.

Murphy, C. M., & Maiuro, R. D. (2009). *Motivational interviewing and stages of change of intimate partner violence*. New York, NY: Springer.

Naar-King, S., & Suarez, M. (2011). *Motivational interviewing with adolescents and young adults. Applications of motivational interviewing*. New York, NY: Guilford Press.

Rollnick, S., Mason, P., & Butler, C. (1999). *Health behavior change: A guide for practitioners*. New York, NY: Churchill Livingston.

Rollnick, S., Miller, W. R., & Butler, C. (2008). *Motivational interviewing in health care: Helping patients change behavior*. New York, NY: Guilford Press.

Rosengren, D. B. (2009). *Building motivational interviewing skills. Applications of motivational interviewing*. New York, NY: Guilford Press.

Sobell, L. C., & Sobell, M. A. (2011). *Group therapy for substance use disorders. A motivational cognitive-behavioral approach*. New York, NY: Guilford Press.

Wagner, C. C., & Ingersoll, K. S. (2012). *Motivational interviewing in groups. Applications of motivational interviewing*. New York, NY: Guilford Press.

Westra, H. A. (2012). *Motivational interviewing in the treatment of anxiety. Applications of motivational interviewing*. New York, NY: Guilford Press.

Index